19

Commissioning Editor: Timothy Horne
Development Editor: Lulu Stader
Project Manager: Janaki Srinivasan Kumar
Designer/Design Direction: Charles Gray

SYSTEMS OF THE BODY

The Digestive System

BASIC SCIENCE AND CLINICAL CONDITIONS

SECOND EDITION

Margaret E. Smith PhD DSc

Professor of Experimental Neurology
School of Clinical and Experimental Medicine
College of Medical and Dental Sciences
University of Birmingham
Birmingham, UK

Dion G. Morton MD DSc

Professor of Surgery
Academic Department of Surgery
University Hospital Birmingham
Birmingham, UK

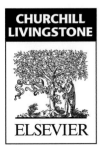

CHURCHILL
LIVINGSTONE

ELSEVIER

EDINBURGH LONDON NEW YORK OXFORD PHILADELPHIA ST LOUIS SYDNEY TORONTO 2010

CHURCHILL
LIVINGSTONE
ELSEVIER

First Edition © 2010 Elsevier Limited.
Second Edition © 2010 Elsevier Limited. All rights reserved.

ISBN 978-0-7020-3367-4

British Library Cataloguing in Publication Data
A catalogue record for this book is available from the British Library

Library of Congress Cataloging in Publication Data
A catalog record for this book is available from the Library of Congress

1006268284

Notices
Knowledge and best practice in this field are constantly changing. As new research and experience broaden our understanding, changes in research methods, professional practices, or medical treatment may become necessary.

Practitioners and researchers must always rely on their own experience and knowledge in evaluating and using any information, methods, compounds, or experiments described herein. In using such information or methods they should be mindful of their own safety and the safety of others, including parties for whom they have a professional responsibility.

With respect to any drug or pharmaceutical products identified, readers are advised to check the most current information provided (i) on procedures featured or (ii) by the manufacturer of each product to be administered, to verify the recommended dose or formula, the method and duration of administration, and contraindications. It is the responsibility of practitioners, relying on their own experience and knowledge of their patients, to make diagnoses, to determine dosages and the best treatment for each individual patient, and to take all appropriate safety precautions.

To the fullest extent of the law, neither the Publisher nor the authors, contributors, or editors, assume any liability for any injury and/or damage to persons or property as a matter of products liability, negligence or otherwise, or from any use or operation of any methods, products, instructions, or ideas contained in the material herein.

The Publisher

ELSEVIER your source for books, journals and multimedia in the health sciences
www.elsevierhealth.com

Printed in China

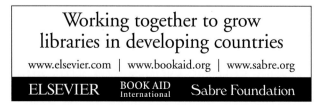

Working together to grow
libraries in developing countries

www.elsevier.com | www.bookaid.org | www.sabre.org

ELSEVIER   BOOK AID International   Sabre Foundation

The Publisher's policy is to use **paper manufactured from sustainable forests**

Many medical schools in the UK and other countries are using systems-based courses. In addition, many are taking a problem-based learning approach to the systems. This textbook provides the basic science needed by the medical students following such courses, and places it in a clinical context. The first edition of *The Digestive System* is a basic text that has been used on many university courses over the past 8 years, including those taught by the authors at the University of Birmingham. During that time, it has been highly commended by the Royal Society of Medicine and the Society of Authors, and has been translated into Portuguese and Chinese.

Over the past few years, the approach taken in this textbook to emphasize the importance of a knowledge of basic science for the understanding of medicine was found to stimulate the students to think, rather than just learn didactically. It has helped to motivate them at a very early stage in their courses. In the second edition of *The Digestive System*, much of the material has been updated.

The subject matter of each chapter is illustrated by the problems encountered in carefully selected clinical situations. Additional case studies have been included in this second edition. The clinical cases chosen are those that demonstrate the relevance of many aspects of basic science to the understanding of each specific clinical problem and by inference, to the understanding of medicine as a whole. The clinical problems chosen are ones that illustrate a number of different aspects of each area of the digestive system, and not all of them are common diseases. Indeed, some of them are uncommon, or even rare. However, common, relevant diseases are described (mostly in boxes), where relevant, in the text. This aspect has been expanded in this second edition. The last chapter draws together information on the common diseases of the digestive system. It has been found that this case-based approach stimulates the student to learn more about the system and its diseases and helps to motivate them to study basic science.

The book has a further purpose; to demonstrate the importance of integration of knowledge of the digestive system with that of the other systems of the body. In medicine, no physiological system can be successfully studied in isolation from the others. Various systems and many organs can be involved in a disease state, either as the primary foci of the lesion or the result of secondary complications. Furthermore, the treatment of disease by drug therapy or surgical intervention can have untoward side-effects that affect systems other than manifesting the primary defect. With these considerations in mind, many of the cases and problems given in *The Digestive System* address relevant aspects of other physiological systems. The approach taken by this book will therefore ensure not only a better understanding of the functioning of body as a whole but also the causes and treatment of disease.

We are grateful for the help given by various people in the preparation of both editions of this book. Mr John Hamburger of Birmingham University Dental School read The Mouth chapter, and he and Dr Linda Shaw made some useful general suggestions. Mr Hamburger and Dr John Rippin kindly provided the photographs for The Mouth chapter. The late Professor Roger Coleman and Dr Rosemary Waring of the School of Bioscience at Birmingham University provided some useful information for The Liver chapter. Dr Peter Guest, consultant radiologist at the University Hospital, Birmingham provided many of the X-rays and clinical photographs. Professor Cliff Bailey of the Department of Biological Sciences at the University of Aston made useful comments on the Absorptive and Post-absorptive States chapter. Professor Barry Hirst of the Department of Physiological Sciences at the University of Newcastle upon Tyne suggested some important revisions concerning ion transport in Chapters 2 and 3 of this second edition. Dr Chris Tselepis of the School of Cancer Studies in the University of Birmingham made useful suggestions for revision of the section on iron absorption in Chapter 8. The encouragement of Dexter Smith and the drawing skills of Dr Imogen Smith (for two of the figures) were much appreciated.

CONTENTS

OVERVIEW OF THE DIGESTIVE SYSTEM

1

Chapter objectives

After studying this chapter you should be able to:

1. Understand the key mechanisms of secretion, absorption and motility in the gastrointestinal system.

2. Understand the coordinated and integrated functioning of the digestive system.

3. Understand how function of the digestive system depends on other systems, such as the cardiovascular system.

Introduction: overall function of the digestive system

The cells of the body require adequate amounts of raw materials for their energy requiring and synthetic processes. The raw materials are obtained from the external environment through the ingestion of food. The overall function of the digestive system is to transfer the nutrients in food from the external environment to the internal environment, where they can be distributed to the cells of the body via the circulation. In this chapter, the general principles and basic mechanisms involved in the functioning of the digestive system will be discussed in the context of the system as a whole. The importance of the integration of the digestive system with the other body systems is well illustrated by the problems encountered in non-occlusive ischaemic disease of the gut: a condition in which the defect originates in the vascular system, but serious consequences result from abnormal absorption in the small intestine (see Case 1.1: 1 and Case 1.1: 2).

Components of the digestive system

Figure 1.1 illustrates the component organs of the gastrointestinal tract, and the associated organs that are essential for the functioning of the digestive system. The gastrointestinal tract consists of the mouth, oesophagus, stomach, small intestine and large intestine. The food is taken into the mouth and moved into the pharynx by the activity of skeletal muscle, then along the rest of the tract by the activity of smooth muscle. The food material is brought to an appropriate semi-fluid consistency, and the nutrients in it are dissolved and degraded by secretions that enter the tract at different locations. These processes are aided by the contractions of the muscles that serve to mix the secretions with the food.

The associated organs situated outside the gastrointestinal tract that are essential for the digestive process are exocrine glands that secrete important digestive juices. These are as follows:

- The three pairs of salivary glands which produce saliva which has a range of functions, but most importantly it provides lubrication of the upper gastrointestinal tract to allow the food to be moved along

- The exocrine pancreas which secretes pancreatic juice which contains most of the important digestive enzymes required to degrade the food into molecules which can be absorbed

- The exocrine liver which produces bile, a secretion which is important for fat digestion and absorption. The bile is also a medium for the excretion of waste metabolites and drugs.

Saliva is released into the mouth. Pancreatic juice and bile enter the duodenum in the upper small intestine (Fig. 1.1). The release of these juices is stimulated when a meal is present in the gastrointestinal tract.

Case 1.1 Non-occlusive ischaemic disease of the gut: 1

An elderly patient, who was being treated with digitalis for congestive heart failure, suddenly developed severe, constant, abdominal pain. The consultant physician examined him and found that he was in circulatory shock, with a low arterial blood pressure, a thready pulse and a sinus tachycardia (rapid heart rate). His abdomen was exquisitely tender to palpitation, with diffuse peritonism (tenderness). The physician suspected from the clinical findings that the patient was suffering from non-occlusive ischaemic disease of the gut. In this condition, the decreased cardiac output results in decreased intestinal perfusion and this, together with other mechanisms, results in the flow of blood to the gastrointestinal tissues being cut off. This disease is often fatal.

Upon consideration of the details of this case, we can ask the following questions:

- What are the main causes of the sudden development of this condition in patients with cardiac failure?
- What are the physiological consequences of reduced flow of blood for the functioning of the small intestine?
- What is the origin of the patient's pain?
- How are the normal homeostatic mechanisms which control the flow of blood to the gastrointestinal tract perturbed in this condition?
- How can this patient be treated?

Physiological processes of the digestive system

The physiological processes that are important for the functioning of the digestive system are:

- Digestion
- Absorption
- Motility
- Secretion (and excretion).

Digestion

Digestion is the process whereby large molecules are broken down to smaller ones. Food is ingested as large pieces of matter, containing high molecular weight substances such as protein and starch that are unable to cross the cell membranes of the gut epithelium. Before these complex molecules can be utilized they are degraded to smaller molecules, such as glucose and amino acids.

Absorption

The mixture of ingested material and secretions in the gastrointestinal tract contains water, minerals and vitamins

Defect, diagnosis and treatment

Decreased cardiac output results in decreased intestinal perfusion with blood. As the velocity of flow decreases, the viscosity of the blood increases and the blood tends to stagnate in the small vessels. Then microthrombi develop and disseminate in the blood vessels of the mesenteric circulation. There is also a generalized vasoconstriction of the blood vessels that diverts the arterial flow to essential organs. This causes small vessels to collapse. The consequent increase in resistance to flow in the splanchnic circulation, together with the decreased cardiac output and reduced arterial blood pressure results in severely reduced blood flow to the intestines, which eventually become ischaemic.

Reduced blood flow to the gastrointestinal tract results in lack of oxygen and reduced energy substrate supply to the tissues (hypoxia). The result is widespread necrosis of the gastrointestinal mucosa which is most sensitive to hypoxia. This quickly leads to disruption of its functions. The necrosis starts at the tips of the villi that become hypoxic first. It seems probable also that disruption of the brush border of the enterocytes exposes the underlying tissue to the effects of the digestive proteolytic enzymes in the lumen. The intestines become permeable to toxic substances from the contents of the gut lumen, such as bacteria and bacterial toxins, and toxic substances from the necrotic cells. These substances enter the portal circulation. In summary, the barrier function of the gut is lost. There is a profound toxaemia and impairment of the normal body defences, resulting in septic shock. Loss of fluid, electrolytes and blood from the gut will also occur. (This effect mirrors loss in the skin in burns). The loss of the external barrier allows penetration of bacteria into the body as well as fluid loss from it.

The abdominal pain is due to the inflammatory response to ischaemia that accompanies the necrosis. The abdominal tenderness (peritonism) is due to transmural ischaemia of the intestinal wall, which in turn results in secondary inflammation of the parietal peritoneum. Differentiation of this condition from occlusive arterial disease is difficult. Selective angiography, a technique involving the introduction of a radio-opaque substance into the blood, followed by X-radiography, may show narrowed and irregular branches of the superior mesenteric artery, and impaired filling of intramural vessels. In contrast, occlusive disease (such as an embolus) would more often be associated with loss of blood flow to major branches of the mesenteric arteries.

Management of this condition requires measures to maintain the cardiac output, blood pressure, and tissue oxygenation, treatment of infection, and replacement of fluid and electrolytes lost from the gastrointestinal tract. Surgery for heart failure is not safe in the presence of gut infarction. If peritonitis is present, abdominal surgery is required to remove the necrotic intestinal tissue.

---

as well as complex nutrients. The products of digestion and other small molecules and ions and water are transported across the epithelial cell membranes, mainly in the small intestine. This is the process of absorption. The transported molecules enter the blood or lymph for circulation to the tissues. This process is central to the digestive system, and the other physiological processes of the gastrointestinal tract subserve it.

Motility

The gastrointestinal tract is a tube of variable diameter, approximately 15 feet long in living human adults. It extends through the body from the mouth to the anus. The food must be moved along it to reach the appropriate sites for mixing, digestion and absorption. Two layers of smooth muscle line the gastrointestinal tract, and contractions of this muscle mix the contents of the lumen and move them through the tract. The process of motility is under the control of nerves and hormones.

Secretion

Exocrine glands secrete enzymes, ions, water, mucins and other substances into the digestive tract. The glands are situated within the gastrointestinal tract, in the walls of the stomach and intestines, or outside it (salivary glands, pancreas, liver, see above). Secretion is under the control of nerves and hormones.

Some substances are excreted, by the liver, into the gastrointestinal tract as components of bile. The gut lumen is continuous with the external environment and its contents are therefore technically outside the body. The faeces eliminated by the intestinal tract are composed mainly of bacteria that have proliferated in the tract, and undigested material such as cellulose, a component of plant cell membranes that cannot be absorbed. Undigested residues are largely material which was never actually inside the body, and is therefore not excreted but eliminated from the body. However, a small portion of the faecal material consists of excreted substances such as the pigments (breakdown products of haemoglobin) that impart the characteristic colour to the faeces.

Quantities of material processed by the gastrointestinal tract

During the course of the day, an adult usually consumes about 800 g of food and upto 2 litres of water. However, the ingested material is a small part of the material that enters

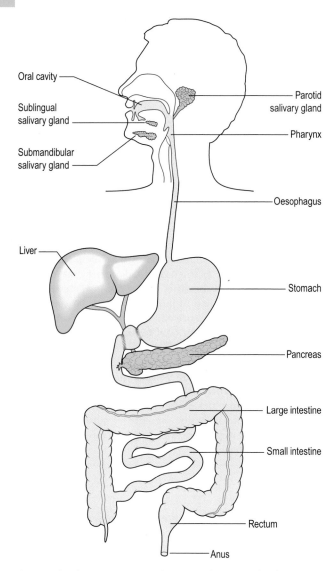

Fig. 1.1 The digestive system and associated exocrine glands.

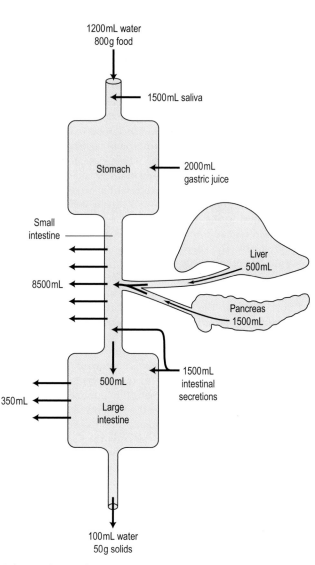

Fig. 1.2 Volumes of material handled by the gastrointestinal tract. The food and fluid ingested, may amount to 2 L per day. In addition to the material ingested, large volumes of secretions enter the tract. Most of the nutrients and water are normally absorbed in the small intestine but a small proportion is absorbed in the colon.

the gastrointestinal tract because secretion into the tract may amount to 7–8 L of fluid, the exact amount depending on the frequency and composition of the meals eaten. Figure 1.2 indicates the approximate volumes of fluid entering or leaving the gastrointestinal tract during the average day, and the locations where the processes occur.

Thus 9–10 L of fluid may enter the tract per day. Most of this has been processed when the chyme reaches the large intestine and only 5–10% of it is left to pass on into the colon. Most of this is absorbed in the colon and only approximately 150 g is eliminated from the body as faeces. The latter contain about 30–40% solids that are undigested residues and a few excreted substances (see above).

Regulation of ingestion

Intake of food should be adequate to meet the metabolic needs of the individual, but it should not be so much that it causes obesity. Food ingestion is determined by the sensation of hunger. Hunger induces an individual to search for an adequate supply of food. A desire for specific foods is known as appetite. Satiety is the opposite of hunger. It is a sensation that usually results from the ingestion of a meal in a normal individual. The control of hunger can be considered in relation to two categories of sensation:

1. Sensations from the stomach known as hunger contractions or hunger pangs, i.e. 'alimentary' regulation concerned with the immediate effects of feeding, on the gastrointestinal tract
2. Subjective sensations associated with low levels of nutrients in the blood, i.e. 'nutritional' regulation, concerned with the maintenance of normal stores of fat and glycogen in the body.

The regulation of food intake is coordinated by neurones in two areas of the brain, known as the feeding (or hunger) centre and the satiety centre. Figure 1.3 indicates some of the factors involved in the regulation of food intake, and the areas of the brain upon which they act. The feeding centre is located in the lateral hypothalamus. Stimulation of neurones in this area causes an animal to eat voraciously (hyperphagia). On the other hand, lesions of this area can cause a lack of desire for food and progressive inanition (loss of weight). In summary, this area excites the emotional drive to search for food. It controls the amount of food eaten and also excites the various centres in the brainstem that control chewing, salivation and swallowing.

The satiety centre is situated in the ventromedial nuclei of the hypothalamus. Stimulation of neurones in this area results in complete satiety, and the animal refuses to eat (aphagia), whereas lesions in this area can cause voracious eating and obesity. The satiety centre operates primarily by inhibiting the feeding centre.

The control of appetite appears to be via higher centres than the hypothalamus, including areas in the amygdala, where sensations of smell have an important role in this control, and cortical areas of the limbic system. These areas are closely coupled to the feeding and satiety centres in the hypothalamus.

Alimentary regulation of feeding

The regulation of feeding by sensation from the alimentary tract is short-term regulation. The feeling of hunger when the stomach is empty is due to stimulation of nerve fibres in the vagus nerve that causes the stomach to contract. These contractions are known as hunger contractions, or hunger 'pains'. They are triggered by low blood sugar, which stimulates the vagus nerve fibres. However, feelings of hunger or satiety at different times of the day depend to a large extent on habit. Individuals who are in the habit of eating three meals a day at regular times, but miss a meal on an occasion are likely to feel hungry, even if adequate nutritional stores are present in the tissues. The mechanisms responsible for this are not understood.

Other factors are also important in the alimentary control of hunger, such as distension of the stomach or duodenum. This causes inhibition of the feeding centre and reduces the desire for food. It depends mainly on the activation of mechanoreceptors in these areas of the tract, which results in signals being transmitted in sensory fibres in the vagus nerves. The chemical composition of the food in the duodenum is also important. Thus fat in the duodenum stimulates satiety via release of the hormone cholecystokinin (CCK) into the blood, from the walls of the duodenum (see Ch. 5).

Functional activity of the oral cavity, such as taste, salivation, chewing and swallowing is also important in monitoring the amount of food that passes through the mouth. Thus, the degree of hunger is reduced after a certain amount of food has passed through the mouth. However, the inhibition of hunger by this mechanism is

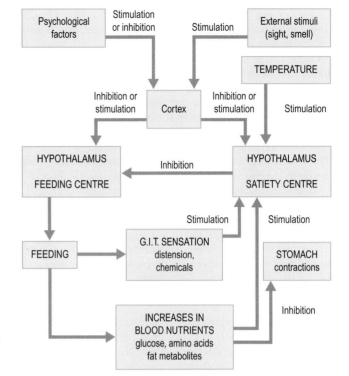

Fig. 1.3 Schematic representation of the role of some factors involved in the regulation of food intake.

short-lived, lasting only 30 min or so. The functional significance of this is probably that the individual is stimulated to eat only when the gastrointestinal tract can cope efficiently with food, so that digestion, absorption and metabolism can work at an appropriate pace.

Nutritional regulation of feeding

The regulation of feeding via nutrient levels in the blood serves to help maintain body energy stores. An individual who has been fasting for some time tends to eat more when presented with food, than one who has been eating regular meals. Conversely if an animal is force-fed for some time, it eats very little when the force-feeding ceases but food is made available. The activity of the feeding centre is therefore geared to the nutritional status of the body. The factors that reflect this and control the feeding and satiety centres are the levels of glucose, amino acids and fat metabolites available to them. Glucose is very important in this respect. When blood glucose levels fall, an animal increases its feeding. This returns its blood glucose concentration to normal. Furthermore, an increase in blood glucose concentration increases the electrical activity in neurones in the satiety centre. Neurones in the satiety centre, but not other areas of the hypothalamus, concentrate glucose, and this may be related to its role in the control of hunger. The control of feeding by blood glucose levels is known as the 'glucostatic' theory of hunger. To a lesser extent, an increase in the concentration of amino acids in the blood can also reduce feeding, and a decrease enhances feeding.

The extent of feeding in an animal depends on the amount of adipose tissue in the body, indicating a role for fat metabolites in the control of feeding behaviour. If adipose tissue mass is low, feeding is increased. It seems likely that lipid metabolites exert a negative feedback control of feeding. This is known as the 'lipostatic' theory of hunger. The nature of the metabolites responsible for this effect is unknown. However, the average concentration of unesterified fatty acid in the blood is approximately proportional to the quantity of adipose tissue fat in the body. Thus, free fatty acids or their metabolites probably also regulate long-term feeding habits, and so enable the individual's nutritional stores to remain constant.

Obesity can be due to an abnormality of the feeding mechanism, resulting from either psychogenic factors or from an abnormality of the hypothalamic feeding centres. These can be genetic or environmental factors; overeating in childhood is probably one environmental determinant of obesity. Excessive feeding results in increased energy input over energy output. However, this may occur only during the phase when obesity is developing. Once the fat has been deposited the obesity will be maintained by normal food intake. It can only be reduced if energy input is lower than energy output. This can be achieved only by reducing food intake, or by increasing energy output via exercise.

Various drugs have been used in the treatment of obesity. These include amphetamines that increase activity levels and inhibit the feeding centre in the hypothalamus. More recently developed drugs include endocannabinoids that are involved in metabolic homeostasis. These also act by (among other mechanisms) modulation of central nervous system pathways, to suppress hunger via the feeding centre. A promising new drug, orlistat (tetrahydrolipstatin), acts by inhibiting pancreatic lipase, the enzyme that breaks down neutral fat (triacylglycerol) in the small intestine (see Ch. 8). Undegraded triacylglycerol is not absorbed in the digestive tract. Although this drug provides an effective treatment for obesity, the absorption of fat-soluble vitamins may also be reduced and the diet should be supplemented with these vitamins to increase the amount absorbed.

Modern treatment of obesity can include surgery to restrict the ability of the stomach to distend, hence providing the sensation of satiety (through suppression of the feeding centre in the hypothalamus), or even, in severe cases, wiring of the jaw to restrict food intake.

Inanition is the opposite of obesity. It can be caused by food deprivation, hypothalamic abnormalities, psychogenic abnormalities or a catabolic state such as that present in advanced cancer. Anorexia nervosa is an abnormal state, believed to be of psychogenic origin, in which the desire for food is lost.

Body temperature is also important in the regulation of feeding. Exposure of an animal to cold causes it to eat more than usual. This has physiological significance because increased food intake increases the metabolic rate, and therefore heat production. It also increases fat deposition for insulation. Exposure to heat in an animal causes it to eat less than normal. These effects involve interaction between centres in the hypothalamus that regulate temperature and the centres that regulate food intake.

Thirst

The sensation of thirst occurs when there is an increase in plasma osmolality, a decrease in blood volume, or a decrease in arterial blood pressure. However, thirst can be satisfied by drinking water before sufficient is absorbed to correct these changes. Receptors located in the mouth, pharynx and upper oesophagus are involved in this rapid response. However, the relief of thirst by this mechanism is short-lived. Complete satisfaction of thirst occurs only when the plasma osmolality, blood volume, and arterial blood pressure are returned to normal. Body fluid hyperosmolality is the most potent of these stimuli. An increase of only 2% can cause thirst. Water intake is regulated by neurones in the hypothalamus in the 'thirst centre'. Some of these cells are osmoreceptors that are stimulated by an increase in osmolality. The neural pathways involved in the response are not clear, but they may be the same pathways that regulate the release of antidiuretic hormone (ADH, vasopressin), which controls water reabsorption in the kidney tubules. ADH is released from the posterior pituitary in response to changes in osmolality, blood volume and arterial blood pressure (see the companion volume *The Endocrine System*). Thirst and vasopressin work in concert to maintain the water balance of the body. This axis is disrupted in the hyperglycaemia associated with diabetes mellitus. The raised serum glucose concentration increases the osmolality thereby stimulating thirst. In addition the increase in plasma glucose (which results in excretion of glucose in the urine, causes an osmotic diuresis (excessive production of urine). For this reason patients with new onset diabetes often present with polydipsia and polyuria (see Ch. 9). The resulting hypovolaemia (low blood volume) exacerbates the situation by stimulating thirst even more.

Distribution of blood to the digestive organs

The proper functioning of the digestive system depends on the gastrointestinal tract and associated organs receiving an adequate supply of oxygen and nutrients to meet their metabolic needs. These substances are carried to the tissues by the blood circulation. The blood vessels that supply the digestive organs located in the abdomen (and the spleen) comprise the splanchnic circulation. Over 25% of the output from the left ventricle of the heart can flow through the splanchnic circulation. It is the largest of the regional circulations arising from the aorta. A major function of the splanchnic circulation is to provide fuel to enable the processes of secretion, motility, digestion, absorption, and excretion, to take place. It also functions as a storage site for a large volume of blood that can be mobilized when the need arises. Thus, during exercise, for example, the blood is diverted away from the digestive organs to the skeletal and heart musculature.

The distribution of the blood in the splanchnic circulation to the various abdominal organs is indicated in Figures 1.4 and 1.5. Three major arteries in the splanchnic circulation, the coeliac artery, the inferior mesenteric artery and the superior mesenteric artery, supply the abdominal organs. The coeliac artery supplies the liver, stomach, spleen and pancreas. Approximately 20% of the liver's blood supply arises from the hepatic branch of the coeliac artery. The rest is supplied by blood in the portal vein (see Ch. 6), which is returning from the stomach, spleen, pancreas, and small and large intestines that are supplied by other branches of the coeliac artery and branches of the superior and inferior mesenteric arteries. The blood vessels of the splanchnic circulation are therefore arranged both in series and parallel (Fig. 1.4), and most of its blood flows through the liver, either directly, or after passing through other abdominal organs. It leaves the liver via the hepatic veins to drain back to the inferior vena cava. The branches of the major arteries give rise to smaller branches that penetrate the organs of the gastrointestinal tract and their muscular coats. These smaller branches divide to give rise to an extensive network of small arteries in the submucosa. These in turn give rise to the mucosal arterioles that carry the blood to the capillaries. This arrangement of blood vessels leads to considerable overlap in the distribution of blood by adjacent arteries, and helps to prevent loss of blood flow to a specific region if a major arterial branch is occluded by a thrombus or embolus. It is not uncommon to find the inferior mesenteric artery to be occluded in elderly patients, but this rarely gives rise to symptoms because the blood supply is sustained from the superior mesenteric bowel.

The problems seen in a more serious condition where generalized ischaemia of the gut is present are described in described in Case 1.1: 3 and Case 1.1: 4.

Membrane transport

The processes of absorption and secretion both depend on the transport of molecules or ions across the plasma membrane of the cell. The mechanisms involved in these two processes share many common characteristics.

Net transport of a substance by passive diffusion is down its concentration or electrical gradient and it is proportional to the surface area of the membrane across which it is taking place. However, molecules are usually moving across a cell membrane in both directions. Absorption involves net transport from the intestinal lumen to the blood or lymph. Secretion involves transport into the lumen of a glandular duct or the lumen of the gastrointestinal tract.

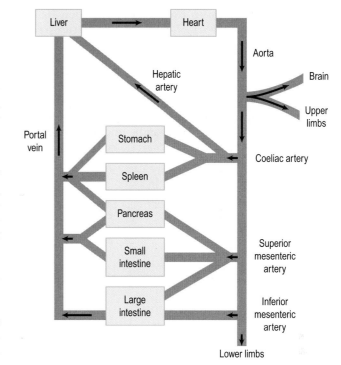

Fig. 1.4 Arrangement of the blood supply to the abdominal organs. The coeliac artery directly provides only approximately 20% of the blood supply of the liver. This provides it with oxygenated arterial blood. The rest of the output of the coeliac artery supplies the stomach and spleen with oxygenated blood. The superior mesenteric artery supplies the pancreas and small intestines and provides part of the oxygenated blood supply of the large intestine. The inferior mesenteric artery also supplies the large intestine with oxygenated blood. The venous blood arising from the abdominal organs contains the absorbed nutrients that have been absorbed from the intestines. This constitutes the portal blood that transports the nutrients in the portal vein to the liver.

Transport of an unionized substance across a membrane can be described by the Fick equation:

$$\frac{ds}{dt} = P(C_i - C_o)A$$

(ds/dt, rate of transport, P, permeability constant, C_i concentration inside, C_o concentration outside, A, surface area). It is worth noting that the huge surface area of the small intestine makes this organ ideal for the processes of absorption and secretion. In addition the high blood flow through the splanchnic circulation ensures $(C_i - C_o)$ is maximized. The problems experienced when there is a reduced surface area for absorption are described in Case 1.1: 3.

Potential difference

In the case of a charged ion the transport is proportional to the sum of the concentration gradient and the potential difference across the membrane. The potential difference across the membranes of secretory cells and absorptive cells (enterocytes) varies from region to region in the digestive system (see Ch. 7). An ion that diffuses passively across a membrane will distribute itself on the two sides of the membrane until electrochemical equilibrium is reached. At this point the forces caused by the electrical potential gradient and the concentration difference are equal and opposite, and there are no net forces on the ion, and no net movement occurs. The electrical potential difference across a membrane can be calculated from the Nernst equation:

$$E_i - E_o = \frac{RT}{zF} \ln \frac{[X^+]_o}{[X^+]_i}$$

where $E_i - E_o$ is the electrical potential difference across the membrane, z is the number of charges on the ion, F is the Faraday number, R is the gas constant, T is the absolute temperature, $[X^+]_o$ and $[X^+]_i$ are the concentrations of the ion (in this case a cation) on the two sides of the membrane.

Mechanisms of transport

Some substances are transported solely by passive diffusion. Others are transported slowly by passive diffusion and more rapidly by special mechanisms. The special mechanisms include active transport and facilitated diffusion.

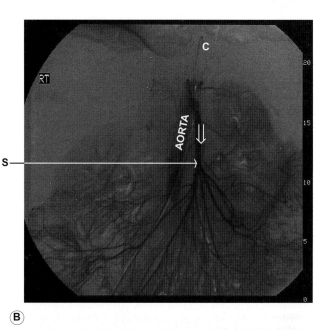

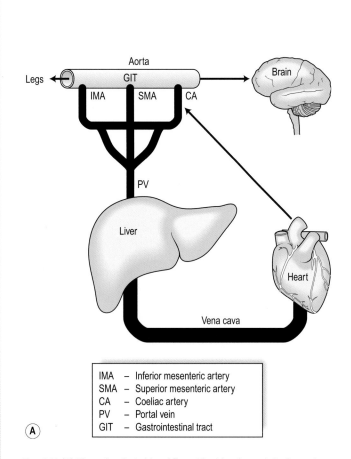

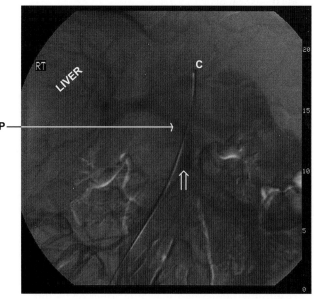

Fig. 1.5 (A) The splanchnic blood flow. The blood supply is dependent on three arteries, and drains via the portal system to the liver, before returning to the systemic circulation. The blood flow is demonstrated in the accompanying arteriograms (B and C). The contrast material has been injected through a catheter (C) into the superior mesenteric artery (S), and flows through the capillary beds in the wall of the small bowel, before collecting in the portal vein (P) and draining into the liver.

Active transport

Table 1.1 shows the criteria used to distinguish active and passive transport processes. A source of energy is required for active transport to take place. Passive transport requires no measurable amount of energy. If an active transport mechanism exists for the absorption of a substance it can be transported against a concentration gradient or, in the case of an ion, against an electrical gradient. In the small intestine the serosal surface of the membrane is positive with respect to the luminal surface. Thus net absorption of cations into the blood must be accomplished by means of active transport. Active transport of an ion may involve exchange for another ion of the same charge, or it may be accompanied by transport of an ion of the opposite charge. These arrangements preserve the electrical status of the cell. Furthermore, in secretory tissues the rate of transport for an actively transported fluid (for example saliva, bile) can be constant until a pressure above the systolic arterial pressure of the blood serving the secreting tissue is reached.

Passive diffusion is transport down a concentration gradient and the rate of transport is proportional to the concentration difference of the substance across the membrane, over a wide range of concentration differences. However, for active transport the rate is only proportional to the concentration gradient at low concentration differences. This is because at high concentrations the process becomes saturated and a transport maximum (Tm) is reached (Fig. 1.6). Active transport of a substance is much faster than passive transport of that substance.

A 10°C rise in temperature can result in a 3–5-fold increase in the rate of an active transport process. Finally, an active transport process is unidirectional. Thus glucose, for example, is actively transported from the lumen of the small intestine into the blood but it is not actively transported in the opposite direction.

Facilitated diffusion

Transport via facilitated diffusion does not occur against a concentration gradient. However, for a given substance, it is a more rapid than passive diffusion. Like active transport, it is proportional to the concentration difference across the membrane only at low favourable concentration gradients. At high concentration differences the mechanism becomes saturated, usually because it depends on the binding of the substance to a carrier

---

Case 1.1 Non-occlusive ischaemic disease of the gut: 3

Effects on membrane transport

Under hypoxic conditions, cellular metabolism becomes anaerobic. Adenosine, a metabolite of ATP is degraded to hypoxanthine. The enzyme hypoxanthine oxidase then catalyses the conversion of hypoxanthine to superoxide and hydroxyl free radicals, which are cytotoxic. These compounds oxidize cell membrane lipids, and this in turn causes irreversible changes in the permeability of cell membranes and disruption of active transport systems in the cell plasma membranes. As a consequence, the cells can no longer maintain their normal intracellular composition and they die. Because of its high metabolic activity the mucosa has the highest requirement for oxygen of all layers of the gastrointestinal tract, and consequently it is the most sensitive to anoxia. Necrosis of the absorptive cells reduces the surface area for absorption and disrupts the specialized transport mechanisms for the absorption of nutrients. In addition, because the normal barrier to diffusion has been removed as the mucosal cells die, toxic metabolites and other substances diffuse into the blood. Under normal conditions mucosal cell loss would result in rapid cell proliferation and replacement. As this process requires oxygen, it will not take place unless the blood supply is restored. Thus, aggressive treatment of the heart failure is central to the survival of these patients.

Table 1.1 Comparison between active and passive transport

Criterion	Passive	Active
1. Effect of opposing concentration or electrical gradient	No net transport against a gradient	Transport against a gradient
2. Variation with concentration difference	Transport proportional to concentration difference over a wide range	Transport proportional only at low concentrations, saturation at high concentrations
3. Energy supply	Not required	Required, glucose, O_2, ATP, etc.
4. Inhibitors	Not inhibited by metabolic or competitive inhibitors	Inhibited by metabolic inhibitors (F^-, DNP, etc.)
5. Temperature change	No appreciable effect	Sensitive to temperature change (Q_{10} is high)
6. Direction	Bidirectional	Unidirectional

DNP, dinitrophenol; Q_{10}, effect of a 10°C increase in temperature.

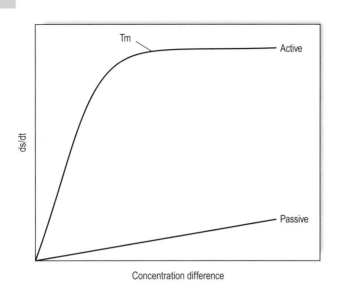

ds/dt

Tm

Active

Passive

Concentration difference

Fig. 1.6 The effect of concentration gradient on active and passive transport processes. Tm, transport maximum, ds/dt, rate of transport.

protein in the membrane. Facilitated diffusion can be inhibited competitively, by substances that bind to the same site as the natural substrate.

Pinocytosis

Some large macromolecules or particles may be absorbed in the small intestine via pinocytosis (endocytosis). This process involves the molecule becoming surrounded by the cell membrane and engulfed into the cell. It resembles phagocytosis but pinocytotic vesicles are small (usually 100–200 nM in diameter) while phagocytosed particles are larger (e.g. bacteria). The macromolecules usually attach to specific receptors that are concentrated in small, coated pits in the membrane. The cytoplasmic surface of the pit is coated with a dense material containing contractile filaments. After the protein molecule has attached to its receptors, the entire pit invaginates into the cell and its borders close over the attached macromolecules together with a small amount of fluid. The invaginated portion of the membrane breaks away from the rest of the membrane. Thus, the endocytosed particle is surrounded by the plasma membrane of the cell and engulfed. It is then a membrane-bound particle within the cytoplasm of the cell. The process is active, requiring energy in the form of ATP within the cell, and Ca^{2+} ions in the extracellular fluid. Inside the cell Ca^{2+} may activate the contractile microfilaments to pinch the vesicles off the cell membrane.

Motility

Smooth muscle in the gastrointestinal tract

The muscle of the gastrointestinal tract is arranged mainly in two layers, an outer longitudinal coat, and an inner circular coat (Fig. 1.7A). In most regions of the gastrointestinal tract, the muscular coat is composed entirely of smooth muscle. However, skeletal muscle is present in the pharynx and the upper third of the oesophagus, and the external anal sphincter.

The smooth muscle of the gastrointestinal tract is of two types, phasic and tonic. Phasic muscle contracts and relaxes in a matter of seconds (i.e. phasically). This type of smooth muscle is present in the main body of the oesophagus, the gastric antrum and the small intestine. Tonic muscle contracts in a slow and sustained manner (i.e. tonically). The duration of tonic muscle contractions can be minutes or hours. This type of smooth muscle is present in the lower oesophageal sphincter, the ileocaecal sphincter and the internal anal sphincter. The differences between phasic and tonic muscle reflect the different functions they perform. Thus, phasic contraction of the antrum muscle empties food rapidly into the intestines, whereas the tonic contractions of the muscle of the ileocaecal sphincter keep the junction between the ileum and the colon closed for long periods of time and enables the entry of chyme into the colon to be carefully controlled. Whether the muscle is phasic or tonic depends on properties intrinsic to the muscle cells. Neurotransmitters and hormones alter the amplitude of phasic contractions, and the tone of tonic muscle. These differences relate to the electrical properties of the cells but the basic mechanisms underlying the contractile activity are similar in all smooth muscle cells.

The smooth muscle is composed of small spindle-shaped cells. Unlike those in skeletal muscle, these cells are not arranged in orderly sarcomeres. There are no striations, although thick and thin myofilaments are present. Actin and tropomyosin are the contractile proteins that constitute the thin filaments and myosin is the contractile protein of the thick filaments. Troponin is present only in negligible amounts, if at all. There are many more actin than myosin filaments. The ratio of thin to thick filaments is between 12:1 and 18:1. This can be contrasted with skeletal muscle, where the ratio is 2:1. The thin filaments are anchored either to the plasma membrane or to structures known as dense bodies that are attached to a network of another type of filament of intermediate thickness between the thick and thin filaments. These intermediate filaments form an internal skeleton on which the contractile filaments are anchored. Figure 1.7B shows the organization of the structures in smooth muscle. The dense bodies correspond to the Z lines in skeletal muscle. Contractions of smooth muscle occur by a sliding filament mechanism similar to that in skeletal and cardiac muscle, with cross-bridge formation occurring between the overlapping thick and thin filaments. The muscle cells are organized as sheets that behave as effector units because the individual cells are functionally coupled to one another. Opposing membranes of the cells are fused to form gap junctions or nexuses. These are low-resistance junctions that allow the spread of excitation from one cell to another. Contractions of the bundles of cells are therefore synchronous.

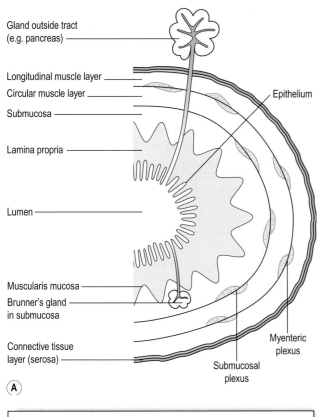

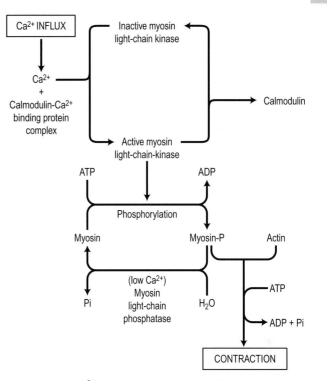

Fig. 1.8 Role of Ca^{2+} in the contraction of smooth muscle.

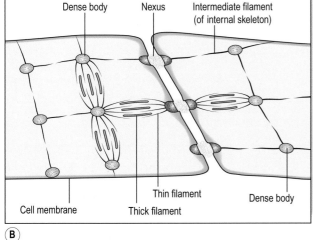

Fig. 1.7 (A) Layers of the gastrointestinal tract showing the locations of glands, the smooth muscle coats, and the enteric nerve plexi. (B) Structural features of visceral smooth muscle.

Initiation of smooth muscle contraction

Contraction of smooth muscle cells is triggered by Ca^{2+} influx. Neurotransmitters, hormones and other factors can promote Ca^{2+} influx. In resting muscle, the intracellular Ca^{2+} concentration is low (approximately $10^{-7}M$) and there is no interaction between actin and myosin. The extracellular Ca^{2+} concentration is approximately 2 mM. In phasic muscle cells Ca^{2+} enters via voltage-determined

Ca^{2+} channels (VDCCs). When the cell membrane is depolarized to threshold an action potential is generated and the VDCCs open. Ca^{2+} enters down its concentration gradient causing the cell to contract. The resulting influx of Ca^{2+} initiates the contractile response of the (non-pacemaker) cells. The intracellular events that trigger muscle contraction are outlined in Figure 1.8. Inside the cell, the Ca^{2+} binds to calmodulin, a Ca^{2+} binding protein. This complex activates a kinase enzyme on the light chain of the myosin molecules in the thick filaments. The activated myosin light chain kinase catalyses the phosphorylation of myosin, utilizing ATP that is dephosphorylated to form ADP. The phosphorylated myosin can then interact with actin, to split ATP, causing the movement of the cross bridges. The myofilaments slide past each other and the muscle contracts. The myosin is inactivated by dephosphorylation and the ADP formed is converted back to ATP. The process of contraction requires energy, so an ischaemic bowel can quickly become atonic, and passively dilate, resulting in abdominal distension (Fig. 1.9).

Control of smooth muscle

Action potentials are triggered in only a few cells by nervous and hormonal influences. These are known as pacemaker cells. The action potentials set up in these cells are transmitted throughout the muscle sheet. The pacemaker cells are most numerous in the longitudinal muscle layer. In these cells, the resting membrane potential (RMP) is continuously oscillating. This activity is known as the

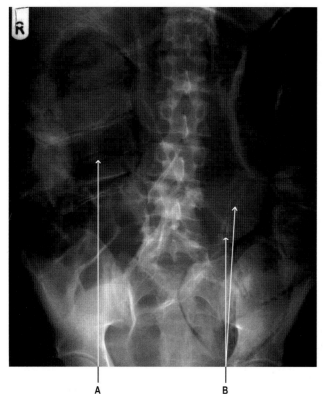

Fig. 1.9 A plain X-ray of large bowel ischaemia, showing dilated large bowel (A), with gas in the oedematous bowel wall, underneath the ischaemic mucosa (B).

basal electrical rhythm. The control of tension development in smooth muscle is exerted via changing the offset of this basal electrical rhythm (Fig. 1.10). If the amplitude of the depolarization phase of the oscillation reaches the threshold level, an action potential is triggered. The action potential is conducted via nexuses from cell to cell, causing Ca^{2+} influx, and contraction of the smooth muscle cells. With increased frequency of action potentials there is summation of the contractile response and the muscle contracts with increased force. The force generated is related to the intracellular Ca^{2+} concentration.

Action potentials occur spontaneously in pacemaker cells as the amplitude of the oscillations occasionally reaches the threshold potential in the absence of external stimulation. The muscle is therefore under a certain amount of tension even in the resting state. This property of spontaneous contraction is known as tone.

Increased Ca^{2+} influx leads to increased force of contraction. Conversely, because there is normally always a degree of tone present, a reduction in Ca^{2+} influx leads to a decrease in the force of contraction, i.e. relative relaxation. Control is exerted largely by shifts in the mean RMP (Fig. 1.10). If the membrane potential is shifted closer to threshold (depolarization), more oscillations reach threshold and more action potentials are generated and the force of contraction will be increased. If the membrane potential is shifted further from the threshold (hyperpolarization) fewer of the oscillations reach threshold, the frequency of action potentials decreases, and the force of contraction decreases.

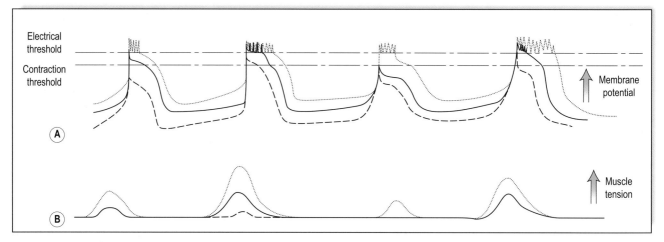

Fig. 1.10 Control of pacemaker cells in gastrointestinal smooth muscle. The generation of action potentials by the cell and their frequency depend on the amplitude of the oscillations in the membrane potential. (A) Oscillating membrane potential. The solid line represents a recording from a cell that is not under the influence of hormones or transmitters. Stimulation shifts the resting membrane potential towards the threshold for electrical excitation (depolarization), resulting in the generation of action potentials (dotted line). When the membrane potential exceeds the threshold level muscle tension is developed. Inhibition shifts the resting membrane potential further away from the threshold (hyperpolarization, dashed line). (B) Development of muscle tension. An increased frequency of action potentials causes the development of increased muscle tension via summation of the contractile response. The contraction threshold of the membrane potential may be slightly lower than the action potential threshold (see A). Solid line, tension developed in the absence of external stimulation. Dotted line, tension developed in response to stimulation.

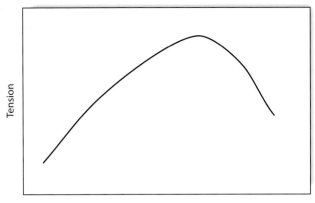

Fig. 1.11 Effect of stretch on tension development in smooth muscle. Tension is proportional to stretch at low or moderate levels of stretch, but excessive stretch results in reduced tension.

Smooth muscle contracts in response to stretch. This is known as the myogenic reflex. It is an intrinsic property of smooth muscle and does not occur in skeletal muscle. Figure 1.11 shows the relationship between the degree of stretch and the force of contraction in visceral smooth muscle. Stretching the membrane opens Ca^{2+} channels in it and Ca^{2+} flows into the cell. However, whereas moderate stretch results in depolarization of the membrane and muscle contraction, excessive stretch inhibits the force of contraction.

The membrane potential of the pacemaker cells can be controlled by neurotransmitters and hormones. These act on receptors to cause either depolarization or hyperpolarization of the cells. The nerve axons that enter smooth muscle release neurotransmitters from swellings, known as varicosities, along their length. No discrete neuromuscular junctions exist between the muscle cells and the nerve release sites. Indeed the varicosities are usually some distance from the muscle cells.

Control of secretion and motility

The control of secretion and motility in the gastrointestinal tract is by neural, hormonal and paracrine mechanisms. The neural control is via both extrinsic nerves of the autonomic nervous system and nerves in the intrinsic enteric nerve plexi of the gastrointestinal tract. In many instances the mediators of neural or hormonal control are peptides. In some cases a given peptide acts as both a neurotransmitter and a hormone. Table 1.2 shows some of the neuropeptides involved in control of the gastrointestinal tract.

Neural control

The gastrointestinal tract is innervated by both autonomic nerves and by nerves in the enteric plexi in the walls of the tract (Fig. 1.7A). The enteric nervous system

Table 1.2 Some biologically active peptides of the digestive system, their cellular sites of origin in the gastrointestinal tract, and their sites of action

Peptide	Main site of origin	Site of action
Gastrin	APUD cells (stomach antrum)	Secretory cells of stomach, pancreas
		Smooth muscle of gallbladder, small intestine
GRP	Intrinsic neurones (stomach)	Secretory and smooth muscle cells of stomach
Somatostatin	APUD cells (stomach)	Secretory cells of stomach
Secretin	APUD cells (duodenum)	Secretory cells of stomach, pancreas, liver, small intestine
Cholecystokinin	APUD cells (duodenum)	Secretory cells of stomach, pancreas
		Smooth muscle of gallbladder, blood vessels
Motilin	APUD cells (duodenum, jejunum)	Smooth muscle of small intestine
GIP	APUD cells (duodenum, jejunum)	Secretory cells of stomach
Enteroglucagon	APUD cells (ileum and colon)	Secretory cells of stomach
		Smooth muscle cells of stomach, intestines
VIP	Intrinsic neurones (throughout the GIT)	Secretory cells of salivary glands, small intestines, pancreas
		Smooth muscle of stomach and large intestine, sphincters, blood vessels

GRP, gastrin releasing peptide; GIP, gastric inhibitory peptide; VIP, vasoactive intestinal peptide. APUD cells are the endocrine cells of the gastrointestinal tract.

controls motility, secretion and blood flow. However, signals from the central nervous system, travelling in both sympathetic and parasympathetic nerves can alter the activity of the nerves in the intrinsic plexi.

Enteric nervous system

The enteric nervous system may be regarded as a third division of the autonomic nervous system, after the sympathetic and parasympathetic divisions. However, in contrast to the sympathetic and parasympathetic nerves, the enteric nerves can perform many functions independently of the central nervous system. The importance of this becomes apparent following surgical resection of segments of the bowel, which may result in disruption of the autonomic nerve supply, particularly the parasympathetic vagal nerves (see later, Fig. 1.13). Activity in the intrinsic enteric nerves ensures that effective peristalsis and food propulsion along the intestine is maintained after such operations.

Anatomy of the enteric nervous system

The enteric nervous system consists of two major plexi, together with lesser plexi, in the wall of the gastrointestinal tract. Figure 1.12 shows the anatomical arrangement of the enteric nervous system in the tract. The major plexi are the myenteric plexus (Auerbach's plexus), which is situated between the layers of longitudinal and circular smooth muscle, and the submucous plexus (Meissner's plexus), which lies in the mucosa. The myenteric plexus is involved mainly in the control of gastrointestinal motility. This is exemplified in Hirschsprung's disease where ganglion cells are missing from a region of the myenteric plexus (see Ch. 10), resulting in severe constipation, which in the neonate can be life threatening. The submucous plexus is more important in the control of secretion and blood flow. It is also important in receiving sensory

information from the gut epithelium and from stretch receptors in the wall of the tract. Smaller plexi reside within the smooth muscle layers and within the mucosa.

Within each plexus the neuronal cell bodies are arranged in ganglia. Intrinsic nerves of the enteric nervous system connect the plexi together, synapsing on to the ganglion cells. They also innervate smooth muscle, secretory glands and blood vessels of the tract. In addition many of them synapse with postganglionic sympathetic and parasympathetic nerves, or sensory nerves. These arrangements are shown schematically in Figure 1.12. The enteric nervous system is therefore composed of four categories of nerves, extrinsic fibres, intrinsic motor fibres, intrinsic interneurones, and sensory neurones. If the extrinsic nerves are sectioned there is little impairment of gastrointestinal function, except in the mouth, oesophagus and anal regions, where control by extrinsic nerves is more important than in the rest of the gastrointestinal tract. Such extrinsic control is clearly required in these regions for the ingestion of food and the expulsion of faeces.

Both excitatory and inhibitory nerves innervate the smooth muscle, blood vessels and glands of the gastrointestinal tract. In addition there are both excitatory and inhibitory interneurones in the plexi. Furthermore, enteric neurones (as well as gastrointestinal smooth muscle cells) exhibit spontaneous rhythmic activity (see below).

In general, stimulation of the myenteric plexus increases the motor activity of the gut, by increasing tonic contractions (tone), the intensity and rate of rhythmic contractions of the smooth muscle, and the velocity of waves of contraction (peristalsis) along the tract. However, some fibres in the myenteric plexus are inhibitory. Many different excitatory and inhibitory neurotransmitters are involved.

Intrinsic motoneurones

Intrinsic motor nerves are predominantly excitatory. Some of the excitatory neurones are cholinergic and their effects can be blocked by atropine, indicating that the receptors involved are muscarinic. However, other excitatory neurones release other transmitters such as substance P. Stimulation of excitatory motor nerves can cause contraction of both circular and longitudinal smooth muscle, relaxation of sphincter muscle, or glandular secretion. Stimulation of inhibitory motor fibres in the enteric nervous system causes smooth muscle relaxation. The inhibitory transmitters involved may be ATP or vasoactive intestinal peptide (VIP).

Intrinsic interneurones

Intrinsic interneurones can also be excitatory or inhibitory. The transmitter released by excitatory neurones is probably acetylcholine that acts on nicotinic receptors on postsynaptic neurones. The transmitters released by the inhibitory interneurones are largely unknown.

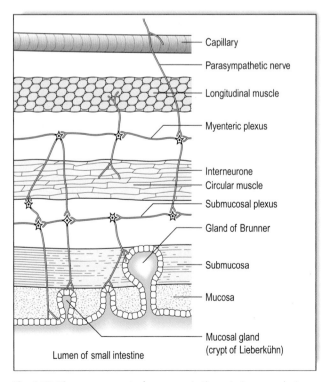

Capillary

Parasympathetic nerve

Longitudinal muscle

Myenteric plexus

Interneurone
Circular muscle

Submucosal plexus

Gland of Brunner

Submucosa

Mucosa

Mucosal gland
(crypt of Lieberkühn)

Lumen of small intestine

Fig. 1.12 The arrangement of neurones in the enteric nerve plexi.

Sensory neurones

Many afferent sensory neurones are present in the gastrointestinal tract. Some of these have their cell bodies in the enteric nervous system. They are stimulated by distension or irritation of the gut wall that activates mechanoreceptors and by substances in the food, which activate chemoreceptors. They form part of reflex pathways, which may or may not be influenced by control via extrinsic nerves. Some of these sensory fibres also terminate on interneurones that in turn can activate excitatory or inhibitory motor neurones.

Some afferent sensory fibres that have their cell bodies in the enteric nerve plexi, terminate in the sympathetic ganglia. Other sensory fibres from the gastrointestinal tract have their cell bodies in the dorsal root ganglia of the spinal cord or in the cranial nerve ganglia. These nerve fibres travel in the same nerve trunks as the autonomic nerves. They transmit information to the medulla, which in turn transmits efferent signals back to the gastrointestinal tract to influence its functions. Specific reflexes are described in the appropriate chapters in this book.

Control by autonomic nerves

At any one time, activity in autonomic nerves can alter the activity of the entire gastrointestinal tract, or of a discrete part of it, via its influences on the enteric nervous system. In addition, autonomic nerves may synapse directly on smooth muscle and secretory cells to influence their activity directly, although they synapse principally with enteric interneurones to influence function indirectly.

Parasympathetic nerves

Preganglionic nerves from both the cranial and sacral divisions of the parasympathetic nervous system supply the gastrointestinal tract. The cranial parasympathetic preganglionic nerve fibres travel in the vagus nerve, except for a few which innervate the mouth and pharyngeal regions. The vagal fibres innervate the oesophagus, stomach, pancreas, liver, small intestine and the ascending and transverse colon (Fig. 1.13). The preganglionic nerves of the sacral division of the parasympathetic nervous system, which innervate the tract, originate in the second, third and fourth segments of the sacral spinal cord and travel in the pelvic nerves to the distal part of the large intestine. The parasympathetic innervation of the tract is more extensive in the upper (orad) region and the distal (rectal and anal) regions than elsewhere. The preganglionic parasympathetic nerve fibres form excitatory synapses with postganglionic neurones in both the myenteric and submucosal plexi. These are mainly excitatory interneurones of the enteric nerve plexi. Stimulation of the parasympathetic nerves can have a diffuse, far-reaching effect to activate the entire enteric nervous system via these interneurones. In general, the effects of activity in the parasympathetic nerves is to stimulate secretion and motility in the gastrointestinal tract. The transmitter released by the preganglionic parasympathetic nerves is acetylcholine and it acts on nicotinic receptors on interneurones in the enteric nerve plexi.

Sympathetic nerves

The preganglionic sympathetic nerves that supply the gastrointestinal tract arise from segments T8–L2 in the thoracic spinal cord (Fig. 1.13). This is why pain from the gastrointestinal tract is referred to these somatic dermatomes (areas of the skin innervated by neurones which enter the spinal cord at the same level). The intestine is a midline embryological structure, so this 'autonomic' pain is referred to the midline. Thus, for example, appendicitis initially produces pain felt around the umbilicus (i.e. via segment T10 nerves). The fibres pass through the sympathetic chains and synapse with postganglionic neurones in the coeliac ganglion and various mesenteric ganglia. The postganglionic fibres travel together with blood vessels to innervate all regions of the tract. They terminate mainly on neurones in the enteric nerve plexi, although a few terminate directly on smooth muscle cells or secretory cells. In general, activity in the sympathetic nerves inhibits activity in the gastrointestinal tract, having opposite effects to stimulation of the parasympathetic nerves. Stimulation of postganglionic sympathetic nerve fibres can inhibit the release of acetylcholine from excitatory motoneurones, to cause relaxation of the smooth muscle indirectly. They can also cause constriction of sphincter

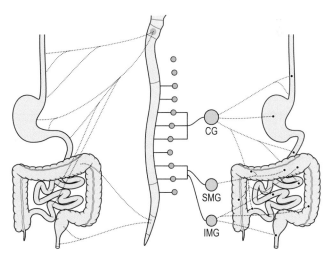

Fig. 1.13 The autonomic innervation of the gastrointestinal tract. LHS, dotted lines indicate the preganglionic parasympathetic innervation by the vagus nerve (cranial nerve 10) from the brainstem, and nerves of the sacral outflow of the spinal cord. RHS, the dotted lines indicate the postganglionic sympathetic innervation arising from the cervical ganglion (CG), the superior mesenteric ganglion (SMG) and the inferior mesenteric ganglion (IMG). The preganglionic sympathetic nerves arise in the thoracic and upper lumbar regions of the spinal cord, and pass through the paravertebral chains to ganglia.

muscle, or inhibit glandular secretion, and importantly, cause vasoconstriction of arterioles of the gastrointestinal tract, redirecting blood flow away from the splanchnic bed. Most effects of activation of sympathetic nerves are exerted indirectly via their connections in the enteric nervous system. Movement of food through the gastrointestinal tract can be completely blocked by strong activation of the sympathetic nervous system. The transmitter released by postganglionic nerve fibres is noradrenaline.

Endocrine control

The gastrointestinal tract is the largest endocrine organ in the body, but the hormone-secreting cells are diffusely distributed in the mucosa, scattered among numerous other types of cell, in contrast to other endocrine organs such as the pituitary, thyroid and adrenals, where the cells are organized 'en masse'. The endocrine cells of the gastrointestinal tract are APUD cells. This acronym stands for amine precursor uptake and decarboxylation, after the classical function of the cells, which may relate to their role in hormone synthesis. The APUD cells in different regions of the tract secrete different hormones. Table 1.2 indicates some of the peptides secreted, and the locations in the gastrointestinal tract where they are secreted.

The APUD cells that contain peptide hormones can be stained with silver. They contain dense core vesicles in which the peptide hormones are packaged. These cells are of two types: 'open' and 'closed' (Fig. 1.14).

The open cells in the gastrointestinal mucosa extend to the lumen of the tract and their luminal surface is covered with microvilli. In some cases only a thin neck of cytoplasm exists between the luminal margin and the basilar side of the cell. The secretory vesicles are at the

base of the cell. The open APUD cell is the most common type of endocrine cell in the gastrointestinal tract. It is found in areas extending from the pyloric antrum to the rectum. These cells sense chemical substances in the food. Thus they behave as chemoreceptors or 'taste' cells. In addition they may respond to mechanical stimulation.

The closed APUD cells are numerous in the oxyntic area of the stomach mucosa. They sometimes have horizontal processes. They usually make synaptic contacts with intrinsic nerve cells as well as with other APUD cells. Cells of both types release hormones into the interstitial spaces from where they are transported by diffusion or vesicular transport (cytopempsis) into the blood capillaries.

Upon stimulation both the open and the closed types of APUD cells release hormones. The hormones circulate in the blood to act at sites that may be distant from the location where they are secreted. Gastrin, for example, is a hormone secreted by the stomach antrum, but it acts on the liver and pancreas as well as the stomach. However, the hormones are secreted first into the interstitial spaces where they can regulate cells that are in close proximity to the hormone release sites. They can therefore have local and distant influences. The local influences are known as paracrine control.

Control of blood flow

The blood flow to the digestive organs is relatively low in the fasting state but it increases several-fold when a meal is present in the tract and the tissues are actively secreting digestive juices, or absorbing nutrients. Blood flow to the gut is controlled by many factors including haemodynamic factors such as cardiac output, systemic arterial pressure, blood viscosity and blood volume, which regulate the flow to all tissues in the body. Other factors include increased activity in sympathetic nerves that causes vasoconstriction and reduced blood flow, via release of noradrenaline that activates α-adrenergic receptors. However this effect is short-lived for several reasons, one of these being changes in local factors. Thus there is a reduction in oxygen tension (hypoxia), when the blood flow is reduced, and this induces vasodilatation. In addition sympathetic nerve stimulation relaxes gut smooth muscle which results in reduced mechanical resistance to blood flow to the gastrointestinal tract. Other substances which constrict the splanchnic blood vessels are circulating adrenaline, angiotensin II and vasopressin.

Stimulation of the parasympathetic nerves to the gastrointestinal tract causes an increase in blood flow by various indirect mechanisms. These are a result of the increased secretory activity of the tissues induced by parasympathetic nerve stimulation. Secretion requires an increased metabolism of the actively secreting tissues, which results in an increased production of metabolites such as K^+, amines and polypeptides, and CO_2, and reduced O_2 tension, all of which may cause localized

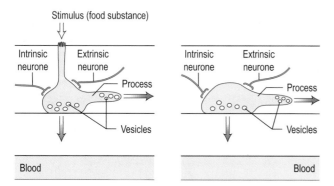

Fig. 1.14 Schematic representation of open and closed APUD cells. (A) open cell, (B) closed cell. The peptide hormones are stored in secretory vesicles, and released by exocytosis into the blood. They may also be secreted from extensions, or processes. They can also act in a paracrine manner on other cells, including other APUD cells, in the mucosa. Open cells can be stimulated by substances within the lumen of the gastrointestinal tract. Both open and closed cells can be stimulated by peptides released from other APUD cells, or by transmitters released from intrinsic or extrinsic nerves.

vasodilatation, with a consequent increase in blood flow. The transmitter released from these parasympathetic nerves may be VIP.

Stimulation of tissues to secrete can also result in the release of proteolytic enzymes, known as kallikreins, which activate precursors of the vasodilator bradykinin, in the intercellular spaces, to form the active vasodilator (see Ch. 2). These local responses are feedback mechanisms whereby the consumption of energy metabolites results in a greater supply of metabolites via increased blood flow. Other substances that dilate the blood vessels of the gastrointestinal tract are the hormones gastrin and cholecystokinin (CCK) that are released into the blood when food is present in the stomach and duodenum, respectively. These have a more localized effect, with gastrin increasing the blood flow to the stomach and CCK increasing blood flow to the pancreas and intestines.

During a meal, the different organs of the digestive system are activated in sequence to secrete, absorb or contract, and their demand for energy substrates and oxygen increases accordingly. These requirements are met by an increased blood supply to the individual component organs as they require them. Neural activity in efferent nerves from the higher centres in the brain, autonomic nerves, and enteric nerves, and hormones and local metabolites all interact to mediate the increased regional blood flow (hyperaemia) as each region requires it. During a meal there is also a generalized increase in blood flow due to an increased cardiac output. Thus when food enters the stomach, the release of gastrin and local metabolites in the stomach stimulates its blood flow. When the food enters the small intestine, the release of CCK and local metabolites results in increased blood flow to the small intestine.

The splanchnic circulation can be compromised in a number of pathological conditions that may arise in other organs of the body, such as haemorrhage and congestive heart failure, or by diseases of the digestive organs. Such diseases include nonocclusive ischaemic disease of the intestines, or cirrhosis of the liver. The effects of generalized abnormal activation of the sympathetic nervous system due to hypotension in congestive heart failure, on the blood vessels of the gastrointestinal tract, are described in Case 1.1: 4.

Control of gastrointestinal functions during a meal

In general, the presence of food in the gastrointestinal tract stimulates smooth muscle in the main body of the tract and the gall bladder, relaxes the smooth muscle of the sphincters, and stimulates secretion and blood flow in salivary glands, pancreas and liver. The control can be considered in three phases, depending on the location of the food:

1. The cephalic phase is due to the approach of food and the presence of food in the mouth.

Case 1.1 Non-occlusive ischaemic disease of the gut: 4

Involvement of control mechanisms

Arterial hypotension causes generalized activation of the sympathetic nervous system through baroreceptor and chemoreceptor mechanisms. This results in the release of noradrenaline from sympathetic nerves, which causes generalized vasoconstriction of the small blood vessels in the gastrointestinal circulation. Reflex responses involving the brain and kidneys result in the release of vasopressin and angiotensin II, respectively, both of which also cause vasoconstriction. The vasoconstriction of the small vessels exacerbates the effect on the mesenteric blood circulation of reduced perfusion pressure, increased blood viscosity, and microthrombi formation, and resistance to blood flow through the gut increases. Eventually the critical closing pressure of the small blood vessels is reached and they collapse, and the flow of blood through the intestines effectively ceases. The patient was being treated with digitalis, a cardiac glycoside, for his heart condition. Such drugs may exacerbate the ischaemia as they are known to cause vasoconstriction in the mesenteric circulation. Patients with hypotension can be treated with α-adrenergic vasoconstrictor drugs to elevate the arterial blood pressure. However, in patients with non-occlusive disease of the gut, this would also compound the problem of reduced perfusion of the gut, by their effect on the sympathetic receptors in the gastrointestinal tract.

2. The gastric phase is due to the presence of food in the stomach.
3. The intestinal phase is when the food is present in the small intestines.

The sequential effects of food or chyme in these various locations enables synchronization and coordination of activity of smooth muscle, secretory tissues and the vascular system of the different regions and organs.

Food in the mouth stimulates pressure receptors and chemo- (taste) receptors and this results in increased blood flow to the salivary glands and secretion of saliva that starts the digestion of starch. It also initiates the secretions of the stomach, pancreas and liver to prepare the gastrointestinal tract to perform its digestive and absorptive functions. At this time the motility of the stomach is transiently inhibited.

Food in the stomach causes increased blood flow to the stomach and secretion of gastric juice, and stimulates the smooth muscle of the stomach. This enables the stomach to churn the food present within it and start the digestion of the food. However, food in the stomach also stimulates the secretion of pancreatic juice, bile and intestinal juices in preparation for the chyme when it arrives in the small intestine where most digestion and absorption occurs.

In addition, it stimulates motility in the ileum and colon. This moves the chyme present in those regions into the next region to make way for the arrival of more chyme.

Chyme in the duodenum exerts the major control over gastrointestinal function. It inhibits gastric secretion and motility that transiently prevents further emptying of the stomach, allowing the processing of the food material already present in the small intestine. Food in the small intestine also stimulates secretion of intestinal juice, pancreatic juice and alkaline bile and the blood flow to the intestines, pancreas and liver. It also stimulates contraction of the gall bladder and relaxation of the sphincter of Oddi to allow the pancreatic juice and bile to enter the duodenum. These digestive juices can then perform the digestion of the complex nutrients, enabling absorption to take place in the small intestine.

THE MOUTH, SALIVARY GLANDS AND OESOPHAGUS

2

Chapter objectives

After studying this chapter you should be able to:

1. Describe the structures of the mouth and oesophagus.

2. Understand the mechanisms of taste, mastication, salivary secretion and swallowing.

Introduction

The functions of the mouth and oesophagus include:

- Mastication
- Taste
- Swallowing
- Lubrication
- Digestion
- Speech
- Signalling of thirst
- Protection of the body from harmful ingested substances.

The performance of all of these functions depends on the presence of saliva. In this chapter, the functional importance of saliva is illustrated by the problems encountered in individuals with xerostomia (dry mouth), a condition characterized by pathological changes in the salivary and mucous glands that result in impaired secretion (see Boxes 1 and 2). A second problem, involving denervation of structures following oral surgery is used to highlight the importance of nerves in control of functions in the mouth (see Boxes 3 and 5).

The mouth

Anatomical features of the mouth

The oral cavity (mouth) is closed by the apposition of the lips. The lips and the cheeks are composed mainly of skeletal muscle embedded in elastic fibro-connective tissue. Figure 2.4 shows the anatomical features of the oral cavity and the structures within it, including the tongue and the teeth. It also shows associated structures, such as the olfactory mucosa, which are important for the functioning of the digestive system.

Case 2.1 Xerostomia: 1

A 60-year-old woman visited her general practitioner and complained of a persistent dry mouth, difficulties in chewing and swallowing, and sore gritty, eyes. She also said that her food seemed tasteless. The doctor examined the patient's mouth. Her gums and teeth appeared inflamed and infected, and her tongue appeared lobulated. The patient was sent for investigation of salivary function.

The most frequent cause of dry mouth (xerostomia) is hypofunction of the salivary glands (which is often accompanied by hypofunction of the lacrimal glands). Figure 2.1 shows the appearance of the tongue in a patient with xerostomia.

The following questions will be addressed:

- What are the major causes of dry mouth? Which oral conditions are associated with xerostomia? Which systemic conditions are associated with xerostomia?
- How can salivary function be assessed?
- Why is saliva important for oral and dental health?
- Which functions of the mouth would be impaired in xerostomia?
- Why is saliva important for the functioning of the oesophagus?
- Which drugs or other treatments can be used to alleviate xerostomia and what side-effects might be expected from these treatments?

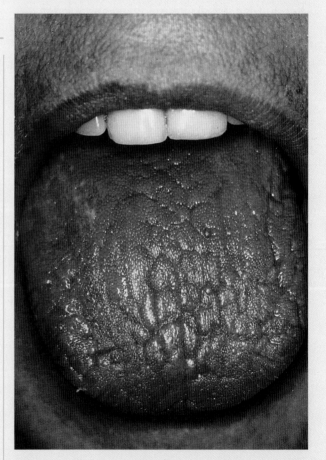

Fig. 2.1 The tongue of a patient with xerostomia, showing a characteristic grooved appearance. (Courtesy of Mr J. Hamburger, Dental School, University of Birmingham.)

Causes and diagnosis

Causes

Xerostomia is a fairly common condition. Its prevalence is approximately 2% of the general population. It affects more women than men. The incidence increases with age. It is associated with conditions that are commoner in middle and old age, possibly partly because of the higher incidence of people on medication in these age groups. The symptoms are dry eyes and dry mouth. The major causes are:

- Medication, especially tricyclic antidepressants and sympathomimetic drugs
- Head and neck irradiation
- Autoimmune inflammatory diseases such as Sjögren's syndrome, which targets exocrine glands in general.

Sjögren's syndrome

In some patients with Sjögren's syndrome the ducts of the submandibular glands are obstructed and the glands become swollen (Fig. 2.2). In such patients the submandibular glands in the neck are clearly located. Characteristically in Sjögren's syndrome, there is atrophy of acinar tissue. It should be noted however, that there is normally an average loss of approximately 40% of acinar tissue between the ages of 40 and 65 years. Ductal hyperplasia and focal periductal infiltrates of lymphocytes (largely helper T cells) are also seen in Sjögren's syndrome.

Figure 2.3 shows a histological section of a minor salivary gland in a patient with Sjögren's syndrome, in which focal aggregates of lymphocytes can be clearly seen. In non-autoimmune inflammatory disease, the infiltration with lymphocytes is more diffuse. Atrophy of the mucous glands in the buccal mucosa may also be present. Primary Sjögren's syndrome is characterized by dry mouth and eyes, but a secondary form exists in which these symptoms are accompanied by connective tissue disease, usually rheumatoid arthritis or lupus erythematosus, primary biliary cirrhosis, polymyositis, and a number of other conditions. In some patients with HIV disease the condition resembles Sjögren's syndrome. Diabetes mellitus and diabetes insipidus can also cause symptoms of xerostomia as these conditions are accompanied by dehydration resulting from copious urine flow.

Symptomatic xerostomia

The 'perception' of oral dryness, in the absence of actual oral dryness, termed 'symptomatic xerostomia', can be the result of sensory or cognitive disorder. In addition, altered perception of oral sensation (oral dysaesthesia) is a feature of anxiety, although acute anxiety can actually cause clinical symptoms and signs of xerostomia.

Diagnosis

A simple test for xerostomia that can be carried out in the surgery involves swabbing the tongue with 5% citric acid, and measuring the volume of saliva that can be spat out into a graduated tube. Alternatively, a Curby cup can be placed over the opening of Stensen's duct. This creates a vacuum and saliva can be collected. Saliva can also be collected with a pre-weighed sponge. Swallowing difficulty can also be assessed, i.e. whether water has to be taken with dry food for swallowing to be accomplished (e.g. the 'cream cracker' test). All of these tests have to be interpreted with care, but on the basis of such tests patients are initially categorized into 'responders' who have functional salivary gland tissue and 'non-responders' who do not. Scintigraphy (scintiscanning) is a technique involving intravenous administration of a radioisotope, usually technetium pertechnetate, a gamma emitter with a short half-life. This is taken up into the salivary acinar cells. Uptake with time can be

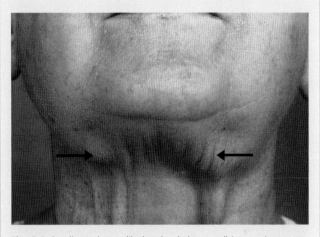

Fig. 2.2 Swollen submandibular glands (arrowed) in a patient with Sjögren's syndrome. The inflammatory process can cause the ducts to become blocked with mucoid saliva. The ducts may also be narrowed (stenosis). As a consequence, the glands swell. (Courtesy of Mr J. Hamburger, Dental School, University of Birmingham.)

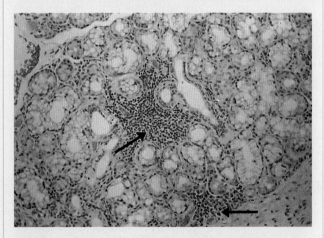

Fig. 2.3 Histological section of a minor salivary gland of the lip in a patient with Sjögren's syndrome. Focal infiltrates of lymphocytes are indicated by the arrows. (Courtesy of Mr J. Hamburger, Dental School, University of Birmingham.)

measured using a Geiger counter. Responders by definition have functioning Na⁺/K⁺/Cl⁻ co-transporters that can carry Cl⁻ ions or technetium pertechnetate across the acinar cell membrane. Water moves passively across the membrane as a consequence.

Non-responders have no functional epithelium and therefore cannot handle pertechnetate correctly. In Sjögren's syndrome, there is a slow uptake of the isotope, a low peak value and a prolonged excretory phase.

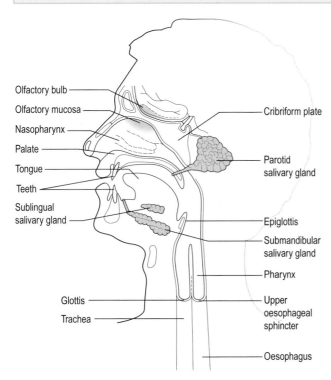

Fig. 2.4 Structures in the mouth, and associated structures.

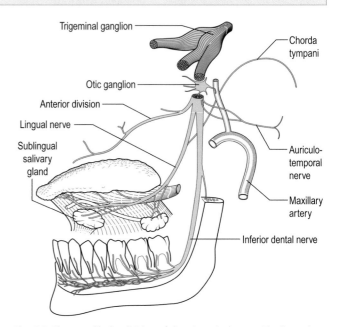

Fig. 2.5 The mandibular division of the trigeminal nerve. The lingual nerve innervates the anterior two-thirds of the tongue and the sublingual and submandibular salivary glands. The inferior dental nerve innervates the tooth pulp, periodontal ligaments and gums. The anterior division innervates the muscles of mastication (not shown). The auriculotemporal nerve innervates structures of the ear (not shown).

Innervation

The innervation of many structures of the mouth is via the four branches of the mandibular division of the trigeminal nerve (Fig. 2.5). These are:

1. The anterior division, which innervates the lateral pterygoid, temporal, and masseter muscles which are involved in mastication (see below)

2. The auriculotemporal nerve, which innervates structures of the ear

3. The inferior dental nerve, which innervates the lower lip and the tooth pulp, periodontal ligaments and gums

4. The lingual nerve, which innervates the anterior two-thirds of the tongue, the floor of the mouth, and the gum on the lingual side of the lower teeth.

The lingual nerve is joined by the chorda tympani that run through the lateral pterygoid muscle. The chorda tympani carries sensory taste fibres from the lingual nerve to the facial nerve, and secretomotor (parasympathetic) fibres from the facial nerve to the lingual nerve. These fibres innervate the submandibular and sublingual salivary glands. Nerve damage is not uncommon following dental procedures, and this is described for a patient who had undergone a wisdom tooth extraction (see Box 3).

Anatomy and histology of the tongue

The tongue has a freely moveable portion known as the body, and a basal or root portion that is attached to the floor of the oral cavity, and forms part of the anterior wall of the pharynx. It is divided into anterior and posterior regions by the sulcus terminalis, a V-shaped groove with the apex of the V directed posteriorly. It is composed largely of skeletal muscle fibres and glands, and is covered by a mucous membrane. Some of the muscle fibres are intrinsic, and are confined to the tongue. These are arranged vertically, transversely and longitudinally. There are also extrinsic fibres, which originate outside the tongue, mainly on the mandible and hyoid bone, and pass into the tongue (Fig. 2.7A). The glands are located

Case 2.2 Denervation following wisdom tooth extraction: 1

An 18-year-old man was admitted to hospital to have an impacted wisdom tooth extracted. The operation involved reflection of a flap of tissue to allow extraction of the tooth. In this patient the inferior dental nerve ran unusually close to the apical part of the tooth root and the nerve was accidentally damaged. (Figure 2.6 shows an X-radiograph from a subject in whom the dental nerve is abnormally close to the root of a wisdom tooth). Unfortunately, in the patient the lingual nerve was also damaged during the surgical procedure because it also ran unusually close to the tooth. As a result, after the anaesthetic had worn off, the side of the patient's tongue and the lower lip on the operated side of his mouth were numb.

Perusal of this case history may provoke the following questions:

- Would the damage to the inferior dental nerve and the lingual nerve affect the patient's ability to chew, swallow, or his speech?
- Would the nerve damage affect the patient's sense of taste?
- Would the patient have defective salivary secretion and defective sense of taste?
- Would loss of pain sensation be a problem for this patient? Why was the patient's lower lip numb?

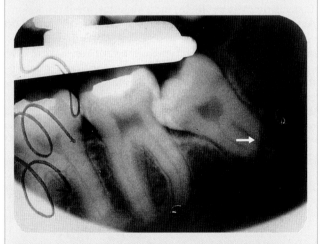

Fig. 2.6 An X-ray in a patient in which the inferior dental nerve (arrow) runs close to a wisdom tooth. In this individual, the root of the tooth has become grooved as it developed around the abnormally close nerve.

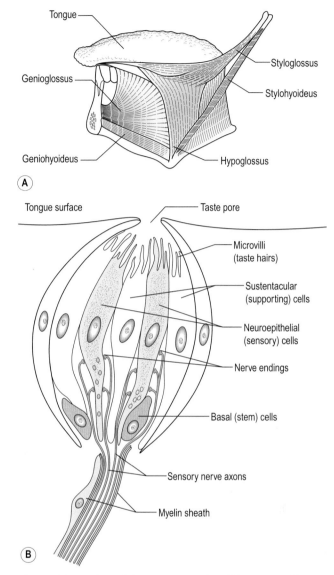

Fig. 2.7 (A) Locations of the extrinsic muscles of the tongue. (B) Structure of a taste bud.

between the muscle fibres. The glands in the base of the tongue are mainly mucous and their ducts open behind the sulcus terminalis. In the body of the tongue, the glands are mainly serous and their ducts open anterior to the sulcus. Near the tip, the glands are mixed and their ducts open onto the inferior surface of the tongue.

On the upper surface of the tongue are numerous small protuberances, or papillae, which give the tongue its roughened appearance. Different types of papillae are present and these have different distributions on the tongue; fungiform and foliate papillae are present on the anterior and lateral surface and circumvallate papillae are on the base of the tongue. Papillae contain numerous nerve endings that sense touch. Most papillae have associated taste buds (see below). Lymphatic nodules (the lingual tonsil) protrude from the surface of the posterior one third of the tongue and give it a nodular, irregular appearance. Between the nodules are crypts where the epithelium is infiltrated with numerous lymphocytes. The inferior surface of the tongue is smooth and is underlain by a submucosa.

Taste

Taste buds

There are several thousand taste buds on the human tongue. Each circumvallate papilla contains several hundred taste buds. The taste buds contain the gustatory (taste) receptor cells. Figure 2.7B shows the structure of a taste bud. They are located in the oral (stratified squamous) epithelium, mainly in association with the papillae, but can be situated elsewhere in the oral cavity such as the palate and the epiglottis. They lie within the epithelium. They have a pale, barrel-shaped appearance with a depression, the taste pore, in the surface. This is an aperture that provides communication with the exterior. It contains three types of cell: supporting (sustentacular) cells, neuroepithelial taste cells, and basal cells. The supporting cells lie at the periphery, and are arranged like the staves of a barrel. The neuroepithelial cells, 10–14 in each taste bud, lie more centrally. Two types of neuroepithelial sensory cell can be distinguished under the electron microscope; one type contains clear vesicles within its cytoplasm and the other contains dense core vesicles. The presence of different vesicles is consistent with the presence of different transmitter substances. These are stored in the vesicles prior to being released from the cell. Both the sensory cells and the support cells have long apical microvilli, or taste hairs, which project into the taste pore. The taste hairs lie in amorphous polysaccharide material that is secreted by the supporting cells. The basal cell is located peripherally near the basal lamina. These are the stem cells for the other cell types. There are club-shaped endings of sensory nerves lying between the cells. Chemical (taste) stimuli are received by the neuroepithelial cells and transmitted via the release of neurotransmitters from the cells to the nerve endings. The secretions of the serous glands of the papillae wash away food material and permit new taste stimuli to be received by the receptors.

Taste sensation

The solubilization of food constituents by saliva enables the sense of taste to be experienced. Thus, taste depends on the detection of chemicals that are dissolved in the saliva and for this reason, taste is compromised in xerostomia (see Box 4). There are four submodalities: salt, sour (acid), sweet and bitter. Dissolved substances with these properties stimulate the receptors (the taste buds) on the tongue. Acid is the most potent stimulus; in humans, sucking a lemon can lead to the maximum rate of secretion, which can be 7–8 mL of saliva per minute. A taste bud responds to several or all of these submodalities, but each taste bud is most sensitive to one particular taste. However, all taste buds respond to all four stimuli, given high enough concentrations of the appropriate chemicals. The taste buds that respond primarily to each submodality are situated as follows:

- Sour: the posterior sides of the tongue
- Salt: the anterior sides
- Sweet: the front of the tongue
- Bitter: the rear of the tongue.

There are however, no obvious structural differences in taste buds in the different regions. The differences in sensitivity are partly due to precise projections of the afferent nerves to the central nervous system and partly to the patterns of impulses from a population of chemoreceptors. The nerves from the taste buds in the anterior of the tongue pass in the chorda tympani (a branch of the facial nerve) and those from the taste buds in the posterior third travel in the glossopharyngeal nerve. These nerves project to the tractus solitarius (Fig. 2.8). The sensory nerves from the taste buds in the palate and epiglottis ascend in the vagus nerve. The possible pathological sequelae following damage to some of the nerves during oral surgery are discussed in Box 5.

The dissolved chemicals in the saliva diffuse into the taste pore from the fluid layer on the tongue. Appropriate chemicals, such as NaCl, are detected by receptor molecules on the taste hairs, and this results in a depolarization of the cell membrane (receptor potential) of the taste bud cell which causes the release of an excitatory transmitter that evokes a generator potential in the sensory nerve endings (see the companion volume *The Nervous System*). The mechanism of the response to salt (NaCl) has been well studied (Fig. 2.9).

Smell

Taste as defined by the layman includes smell (olfaction). Activation of olfactory receptors, in conjunction with central nervous system processing of their responses, enables many different types of odour, or flavours, to be distinguished. Smell has more primary qualities than taste. These include floral, ethereal, musky, camphor, putrid and pungent submodalities. Blockage of the nose by the common cold, or olfactory nerve lesions, renders taste discrimination crude as it then relies only

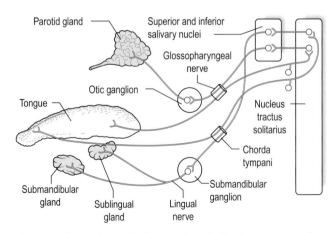

Fig. 2.8 Reflex pathway for the secretion of saliva in response to the stimulation of taste bud receptors.

Case 2.1 Xerostomia: 3

Consequences for the functioning of the mouth and oesophagus

Lubrication

Saliva is necessary to aid chewing, swallowing and speech because of the lubricant properties conferred on it by its mucin content. Therefore these functions are all compromised in xerostomia. Saliva is necessary for mastication because it coats the food and lubricates it, making it more easily moved about in the mouth. During swallowing it is more easily moved back into the pharynx where it stimulates the pressure receptors that initiate the process, enabling it to pass smoothly into the oesophagus. Individuals with xerostomia therefore require fluid intake with food to enable chewing and swallowing to take place. The lubricant properties of saliva also assist the passage of the food bolus down the oesophagus and prevent abrasion of the walls by hard material in the swallowed food.

Digestion

Lack of salivary α-amylase does not result in malabsorption of starch if pancreatic α-amylase secretion is adequate, as the amylases from the two sources have similar catalytic actions in starch digestion, and adequate amounts of α-amylase are secreted by the pancreas.

Solution

Saliva is important for taste as it depends on substances dissolved in saliva. It is also important for the solution of substances that are absorbed by mouth.

Moistness

Lack of saliva signals thirst. Thirst is therefore a constant sensation in xerostomia.

Protection

Saliva is also important for oral and dental health: it washes the mouth, buffers acids in the food, and contains antimicrobial substances. Infections of the mouth are rare following dental surgery even though it is difficult to maintain aseptic conditions in the mouth. However, infections of the mouth and associated structures are common in xerostomia without the protective properties of saliva. In addition the constant rinsing of the oesophagus by saliva and its buffering and antimicrobial properties, help to protect the oesophagus from damage by acids, and to prevent infections.

Dental and oral health

Dental health depends on saliva for many reasons including its continuous rinsing of the oral and buccal cavities to wash away particles in which microorganisms grow, its ability to buffer acids (saliva is more alkaline at high rates of flow), its specific and non-specific immune functions due to the presence of immunoglobulins, the antimicrobial constituents sialoperoxidase, thiocyanate and lysozyme, and the presence of calcium phosphate, which prevents demineralization of the teeth. As a consequence of the decreased production of saliva various oral diseases are associated with xerostomia. These are dental caries, gum disease, mucosal ulceration and atrophy, infections of the mouth (e.g. candida), and ascending infection of the salivary glands.

In addition, in the absence of saliva, retention of dentures is more difficult. Patients who have a dry mouth because they are being treated with tricyclic antidepressants, ganglion-blocking drugs, or parasympathomimetic drugs (for hypertension), may experience difficulty in oral function if they wear dentures.

Case 2.2 Denervation following wisdom tooth extraction: 2

Consequences for the functioning of the mouth

Chewing, swallowing and speech

Chewing depends on activation of periodontal receptors that results in impulses in sensory nerve fibres in the inferior dental nerve being transmitted to the chewing centre. However, in practice, chewing is not usually much impaired following such nerve damage. The tongue, which is innervated by the lingual nerve, moves the food around in the mouth to aid chewing. Therefore if the tongue is partially denervated the process of mastication could be impaired, but this is not usually a serious problem.

The swallowing reflex is initiated when the tongue moves the food bolus to the back of the mouth where it activates pressure receptors in the pharynx. However, swallowing is usually not seriously affected after such nerve damage, because only a small part of the musculature is likely to be affected.

Articulation of many sounds depends on fine control of the movements of the muscles of the tongue. These reflexes partly depend on tactile information from the tongue, but in practice, unilateral damage to these nerves, accompanying wisdom tooth extraction, does not affect speech to any significant extent.

Taste

Some nerve fibres in the lingual nerve carry sensory information from the taste buds on the tongue (via the chorda tympani). Loss of some taste sensation on one side of the tongue could occur in the patient but it is not usually a serious problem.

Salivary secretion

The patient is unlikely to suffer from a dry mouth because between meals the mouth is kept moist by saliva from the smaller glands in the oral and buccal mucosa. When food is eaten or at the approach of food over half of the increased flow comes from the parotid glands. The lingual nerve innervates the submandibular and sublingual salivary glands but not the parotids (Fig. 2.5). The latter are innervated by fibres in the glossopharyngeal nerve. Thus interference with the flow of saliva is not a serious problem after unilateral lingual nerve damage accompanying a wisdom tooth extraction.

Loss of pain sensation

The numbness experienced by this patient due to the damaged lingual nerve could be a serious problem because the patient could injure his tongue by biting it without realizing it. He may also burn the tongue and other tissues in his mouth by drinking liquid that is too hot. The patient's lower lip was also numb, because of this structure is innervated by the inferior dental nerve. Thus injury could also occur due to accidental biting or scalding of the lip. Fortunately for this patient, sensation in the affected areas would probably return over the subsequent few weeks.

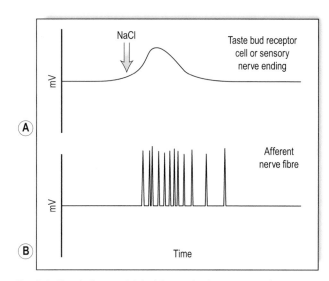

Fig. 2.9 Electrical potentials in (A) taste bud receptors and (B) primary afferent nerves from the taste receptors.

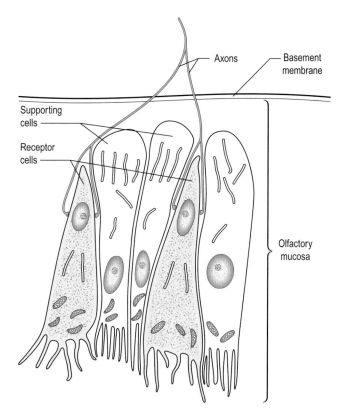

Fig. 2.10 Structure of the olfactory mucosa.

upper nasopharynx (Fig. 2.4). The odorant molecules are borne to the olfactory mucosa via the inspired air, or air in the oral cavity during feeding. The chemical odours are detected by receptors in bipolar cells present in the mucosa (Fig. 2.10). There are about 10 million chemoreceptor cells in the human olfactory mucosa. Immobile cilia on the surface of the cells detect odorants dissolved in the mucous layer that overlies the mucosa. The chemical odorants depolarize the receptor cell and this triggers a discharge in the sensory nerve. Coding for a particular smell, like coding for taste, depends on the response of a population of receptors. The information is integrated in cortical structures.

Teeth

The teeth are embedded in the bone of the upper and lower jaws. They are arranged in two arcs. The upper arc is larger

erupt between the ages of approximately 6 months and 2 years of age. These teeth are shed between 6 and 13 years of age and are gradually replaced by permanent adult teeth. The latter number eight in each half jaw (i.e. 32 in total). The anterior five adult teeth replace the milk teeth.

The sharp incisor teeth are specialized for biting, while the larger, more flattened molars are specialized for grinding. Figure 2.11 shows the basic structure of a tooth. Each tooth has a basic similar structure with a visible crown projecting above the gingiva (gum) and a root that is buried in the alveolus of the maxilla or the mandible.

At the junction between the crown and the root is the neck. In the centre of each tooth is the pulp cavity that is filled by connective tissue. The latter communicates via small pores (apical foramina) with the surrounding connective tissue or periodontal membrane, which holds the tooth in its socket (alveolus). This arrangement forms a peg and socket type of joint that permits slight movement. The hard tissues of the pulp are:

- Dentine: a calcified tissue similar to bone, which surrounds the pulp cavity and forms the bulk of the tooth
- Enamel: the hardest material which is mainly composed of apatite crystals and covers the dentine of the crown
- Cementin: which, like dentine, is similar to bone, and covers the dentine of the root.

Saliva is important for oral and dental health. The problems encountered by individuals with xerostomia are described in Box 4.

Mastication (chewing)

The sight, smell and thought of food elicit the secretion of saliva before food enters the mouth. However, the palatability of food also depends on orally sensed properties after food has been taken into the mouth, such as taste, texture and temperature. Once present in the mouth, the food is chewed, a process known as mastication. This involves movements of the jaw and the tongue. It is controlled by sensations from touch and pressure receptors located in the oral mucosa and the periodontium (area around the teeth), as well as from stretch and other receptors in the masticatory muscles, temporomandibular joints and periosteum.

Mastication process

The vertical (up and down) movements of the mandibles result in biting by the incisor teeth. After a piece of food has been taken into the mouth, both vertical movements and horizontal (side to side) movements enable the molars to crush and break the food into fragments of a size suitable for swallowing. These movements also mix the food with the saliva. This serves several functions including taste and digestion (see below). Chewing depends on the presence of saliva in the mouth. Saliva contains mucins that give it its lubricant property (see below). It coats the food and makes it slippery and more easily moved about in the mouth. Consequently, patients with xerostomia experience difficulty in chewing (see Box 4).

The muscles of mastication are capable of exerting considerable force. The biting forces exerted by the incisors and molars are 110–250 N and 390–900 N, respectively. The potential biting force is much greater than the force needed in ordinary chewing. The occlusal contact area between the molars and between the premolars is much more decisive than the biting force in determining the efficiency of mastication in a person with normal dentition. The efficiency of mastication is reduced in those who wear dentures, and they often tend to eat foods that are not difficult to chew; the toughness of the foods chosen seems to be related to the biting force that can be exerted on the dentures. The narrow selection of food, for example the omission of meat in the diet, can lead to nutritional deficiency.

Control of mastication

The muscles of mastication are the lateral pterygoids that are responsible for jaw opening, and the masseters, the temporalis, and the medial pterygoid muscles that are responsible for jaw closing (Fig. 2.12A). The muscles of closing are more powerful than those involved in opening. There is a reciprocal arrangement between the opening

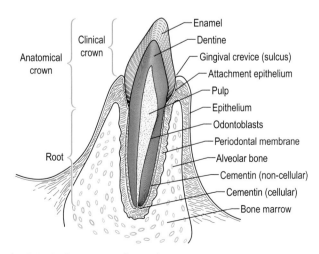

Fig. 2.11 Basic structure of a tooth.

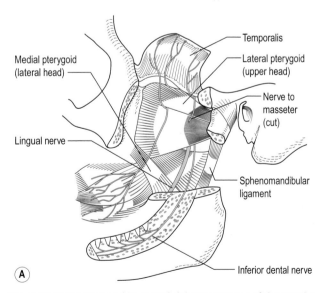

Fig. 2.12 Mastication and its control. (A) Arrangement of the muscles of mastication. The lateral pterygoid is responsible for jaw opening, and the medial pterygoid, the masseters and the temporalis are responsible for jaw closing.

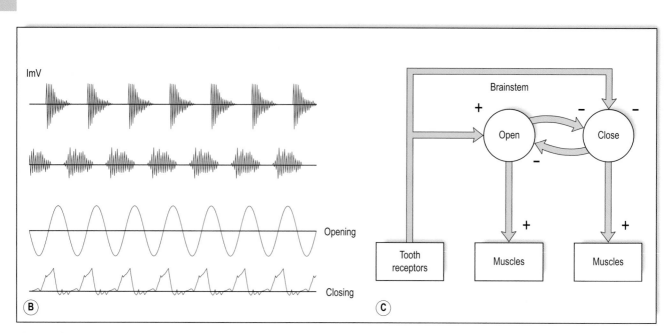

Fig. 2.12 (Cont'd) (B) The Pattern of electrical activity (EMG) in the muscles of opening and closing. (C) Simplified representation of a pattern generator that could control the opening and closing of jaws.

and closing muscles. The control is exerted by neural mechanisms. Two important aspects of the control are:

1. The generation of the movements
2. The regulation of the bite.

Generation of movements

A single bite is a voluntary process involving the cerebral cortex, as are other movements involving skeletal muscles. However, chewing is not a reflex. It is probably a programmed pattern of movements organized in the central nervous system. It involves neurones in the nucleus of the fifth cranial nerve. The 'chewing centre' is built into the organization of this group of neurones. Electrical stimulation of the cortical masticatory area in an anaesthetized animal induces rhythmic jaw movements similar to those observed during chewing. When the electrical changes in the membranes of the neurones are recorded they are seen to exhibit a bursting activity, the bursts being associated with jaw opening and jaw closing (Fig. 2.12B). This pattern is involuntary and is present even if the sensory input is absent. Chewing therefore probably depends on a pattern generator (similar to the pattern generator seen in the respiratory centre, see the companion volume *The Respiratory System*). Such generators are rather primitive basic activities. Figure 2.12 shows the arrangements of the pathways involved in the generation of this chewing activity and its modulation.

Regulation of the bite

As the jaws close, the teeth come into contact with food, or the opposing set of teeth. Two questions arise:

1. How is the bite terminated?
2. How is the force applied regulated?

Stimulation of mechanoreceptors associated with the teeth is important. Many sensory receptors are present in the tooth pulp and the periodontal ligaments. Stimulation of these receptors sends impulses in fibres in the lingual nerve (Fig. 2.5). Activation of the receptors causes information to be transmitted to the brainstem, to inhibit jaw closing when the biting force rises, and therefore to regulate the force applied. This is sometimes described as the jaw-opening reflex because if a tooth is tapped, for example an upper incisor, the jaw opens. The lingual nerve afferents ascend via the trigeminal nerve to the brainstem. When these receptors are stimulated, the amplitude of the jaw movement bursting responses changes and activity in the masseter jaw closing muscles increases. These inputs therefore modify the activity of the pattern generator, and contribute to the control of the chewing force. The texture of food is perceived during chewing by excitation of mechanoreceptors in the periodontal ligaments. Slight displacement of a tooth during chewing, causes the periodontal ligaments to be stretched and this deforms and excites the receptors. Each afferent responds maximally to one particular direction of applied force. The pressure stimulus threshold for perception of a stimulus applied to a tooth is >10mN and is higher for the molars than for the incisors or canines. The threshold level depends on the velocity of application of the force. Nevertheless, people who have lost their teeth can control masticatory force, indicating that tactile sensation in the periodontal ligaments is not the only input controlling the biting force. In fact muscle spindles in the masticatory muscles, temporomandibular joints and periosteum may also contribute.

Role of tongue movements in mastication

The density of mechanoreceptors is high in the front of the oral cavity and low in the posterior part. The tip of the tongue has the highest density. Two-point discrimination on the tip of the tongue can be less than 1 mm. Tactile information from the oral cavity and the tongue is transmitted to the brain via the trigeminal nerve. The tongue is a sophisticated motor organ that moves rhythmically in concert with the lower jaw (usually without being bitten) during chewing. The tongue can perform these movements because of the arrangement of its musculature (Fig. 2.7). The extrinsic muscles enable it to change its overall position. These, together with the intrinsic muscles that terminate on the mucosa or on other muscles of the tongue, enable it to both alter its shape and perform rapid movements. The nerve endings in the papillae transmit the senses of touch, pressure, temperature and pain. There are also proprioreceptors within the muscles, and abundant muscle spindles, in the human tongue, and these are also important for the intricate movements involved in chewing. The tongue mixes saliva with the crushed food by alternations from one side to the other, coating it with mucus.

Saliva

Saliva is secreted by three major pairs of salivary glands:

1. The parotid glands
2. The submandibular glands (submaxillary glands in animals)
3. The sublingual glands.

There are also numerous other, small glands scattered throughout the oral and buccal mucosa.

The parotids are the largest of the glands. Each parotid is located below and anterior to the ear, between the ramus of the mandible and the mastoid process, with an extension onto the face. Its main duct (Stensen's duct) passes forward to penetrate the cheek and opens into the mouth opposite the second molar tooth.

The submandibular gland lies in the floor of the mouth beneath the body of the mandible, extending below its lower border into the side of the neck. It has a duct (Wharton's duct) that opens beneath the tip of the tongue. In some patients with Sjögren's syndrome (see Box 2) the ducts of the submandibular glands are obstructed, and the glands become swollen (Fig. 2.2). In such patients, the location of the submandibular glands in the neck are clearly indicated.

The sublingual gland is actually a collection of glands that lie near to the duct of the submandibular gland beneath the mucous membrane of the floor of the mouth. Each of these sublingual glands has a separate duct that opens beneath the tongue.

The three pairs of glands differ with respect to the type of acini present, and they secrete saliva that differs in composition with respect to the mucus content. The parotids have acini that contain only serous cells. They produce a watery secretion that has a high content of α-amylase but very little mucus. Most acini of the submandibular glands are serous, but some are mucous, and

some are mixed and contain mucous cells with serous crescents or demilunes (Fig. 2.13). The saliva secreted by these glands has a weak α-amylase activity but contains lysozyme that is secreted by the serous demilunes. The sublingual glands contain mainly mucous acini but some of these have serous demilunes. Very few pure serous acini are present in the sublingual gland. Consequently, they produce a particularly thick mucous secretion.

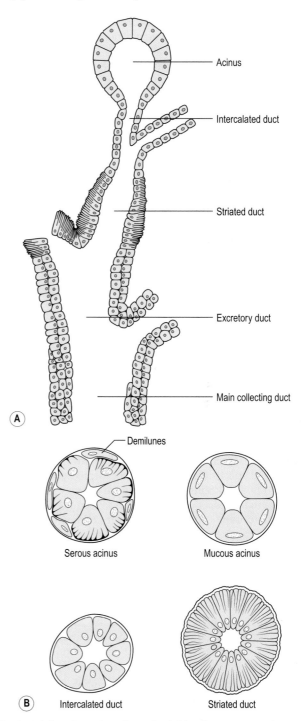

Fig. 2.13 (A) Regions of a salivary gland. (B) Cell types present in different regions.

Composition of saliva

Saliva in the mouth is a mixture of secretions from all the glands present. Human saliva contains less than 1% total solids. The ions present include Na^+, K^+, Ca^{2+}, Mg^{2+}, PO_4^{3-} and HCO_3^-. Saliva is supersaturated with calcium phosphates that help to prevent demineralization of the teeth. Specific phosphoproteins (proline-rich proteins and statherin) that inhibit the precipitation of calcium phosphate crystals from the supersaturated saliva onto the teeth, are also present. The alkalinity or acidity of saliva depends on the rate of flow (see below) but the pH is usually within the range 6.2 to 8.0. There are probably around 50 different proteins in saliva, the major ones being the enzyme α-amylase, and mucins, which are glycoproteins. Those present in smaller amounts include the enzymes lysozyme and sialoperoxidase (see below), as well as lactoferrin, histatins and various immunoglobulins, all of which have protective functions in the mouth. R proteins that bind cobalamins (collectively known as vitamin B_{12}, see Ch. 8) and keep the cobalamins in an absorbable form, are also present.

Salivary glands

Structure and histology

Figure 2.13A shows the structure of part of a mixed salivary gland. The glands are branched structures. The acini where the primary salivary secretion originates are located at the termini of these branches. In many respects the structure of a salivary gland resembles that of an exocrine gland of the pancreas. Figure 2.14 shows these features in a histological section of a human salivary gland. The cells which surround the acini are either serous and secrete α-amylase but no mucins, or mucous and secrete the glycoprotein mucins. The acinar cells also secrete substances across the basal membrane into the interstitial spaces. These include the proteolytic enzymes known as kallikreins, which have a role in controlling the regional blood flow to the glands (see Fig. 2.17). The basal membrane of the serous acinar cell has thin finger-like projections that increase the surface area for secretion (Fig. 2.13B). The secretions of the acinar cells drain into intercalated ducts (Fig. 2.13A) that are lined with columnar epithelium. These cells probably add constituents to the secretion as it passes down the ducts. The small, intercalated ducts from a number of acini merge to form larger striated ducts that are lined by taller cells. The basal membranes of these cells have numerous infoldings. Between the infoldings are rows of mitochondria that impart a striated appearance to the cells, under the microscope. These striated ducts drain into larger, excretory ducts, which in turn drain into a large collecting duct that opens into the mouth. The cells lining the striated ducts and the excretory ducts modify the secretion as it flows past them.

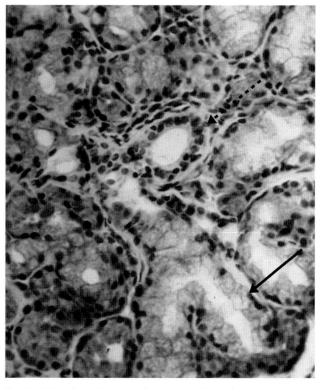

Fig. 2.14 Histological section of a normal salivary gland, showing duct cells (solid arrows) and acinar cells (dashed arrows). (Courtesy of Dr J. Rippin, Dental School, University of Birmingham.)

Somewhat sparsely distributed myoepithelial cells are present around the ducts and the acini of a salivary gland. These cells support the glandular elements and contract when the glands are stimulated, to assist the extrusion of the saliva from the ducts.

Functions of saliva

The secretion of saliva in response to food has been studied experimentally in animals by surgically making a permanent fistula at the throat, or by inserting a cannula in the appropriate duct under anaesthesia. In humans a variety of methods are used to assess salivary function. Some of these are discussed in Box 2.

Lubrication

The lubricant property of saliva depends on its content of mucins. These glycoproteins form a gel that coats the food and makes it more easily moved about in the mouth. This lubricant property of saliva enables chewing and swallowing to be performed.

Digestion

α-Amylase is the major digestive enzyme in saliva. It hydrolyses α-1,4 glycosidic linkages in starch (see Ch. 8).

The efficiency of mastication is important for salivary amylase to penetrate the food bolus. Despite the short exposure of saliva in the mouth, the salivary digestion of starch is important because it continues after the food has reached the stomach. Gastric acid in the stomach inactivates α-amylase but as the bolus of food takes time to disintegrate in the stomach, salivary digestion can continue within it for as long as half an hour. When the acid has completely penetrated the food the enzyme is inactivated. α-Amylase works best at a slightly alkaline pH. The starch in potatoes or bread may be digested to the extent of up to 75% by salivary α-amylase before the enzyme is inactivated by acid in the stomach.

Small amounts of other enzymes are also present in saliva, including lysozyme, sialoperoxidase, lingual lipase, ribonuclease, deoxyribonuclease and kallikreins. These salivary components are not important for the digestive process, although lysozyme and sialoperoxidase provide important protective functions (see below).

Protective functions of saliva

Saliva has many properties that enable it to promote oral and dental health:

- The large volume of the fluid produced enables the buccal cavity to be continually rinsed, thereby removing ingested substances and particles from it.

- It contains mucins that impart a slippery character to the secretion. It coats the mouth, thereby protecting it against abrasion by sharp pieces of food.

- The alkaline pH of the saliva produced when a meal is being eaten buffers acids present in the food. The copious secretion of saliva prior to vomiting protects the mouth from gastric acid in the vomit by virtue of its mucus content and its pH. Buffering of the acids in food prevents the erosion of tooth enamel.

- It is bacteriostatic because it contains an antimicrobial substance, thiocyanate, and an enzyme, sialoperoxidase which catalyses the reaction of metabolic products of bacteria, such as that of hydrogen peroxide with salivary thiocyanate:

$$H_2O_2 + CNS^- \xrightarrow{\text{Sialoperoxidase}} \text{oxidation products,}$$

$H_2O_2 +$	CNS^-	oxidation products,
Hydrogen	thiocyanate	e.g. $OSCN^-$
peroxide	(saliva)	hypothiocyanate
(bacterial		(toxic to bacteria)
activity)		

The oxidized derivatives produced in this reaction are highly toxic to bacterial systems. The oxidation products oxidize −SH groups on many enzymes including some of those involved in energy metabolism. Saliva also contains the enzyme lysozyme that acts on the cell walls of certain bacteria, including some streptococci, causing lysis and death. However, most organisms that colonize the mouth resist lysozyme attack by developing protective cell capsules. Nevertheless, infections in the mouth are rare, even after oral or dental surgery when aseptic precautions are difficult to maintain, because of the bacteriostatic properties of saliva.

Control of water intake

Thirst is the desire for increased water intake and it is perceived as a dry mouth. The sensation is signalled by receptors in the oropharynx and upper gastrointestinal tract but the mechanisms involved in the response of the receptors are still poorly understood. However, the relief of thirst sensation via these receptors is short-lived. The desire for increased water intake accompanies an increase in plasma hypertonicity or a reduction in blood volume or pressure (see Ch. 1). The sensation of thirst is initially satisfied by the act of drinking, but this occurs before sufficient water is absorbed from the gastrointestinal tract to correct these disturbances. The desire to drink is completely satisfied only when the plasma osmolarity, volume and pressure are adjusted to within the normal range.

Speech

Speech depends on the movements and positioning of the tongue, lips and cheeks, during controlled expiration. As movements of the tongue are facilitated by the lubricant effect of saliva, speech can be difficult in xerostomia. Speech is a function that is not directly related to the digestive process and will not be considered further here.

Absorption in the mouth

Absorption of low molecular weight molecules can occur, to some extent, directly from the oral cavity. This route of absorption can be useful for absorption of certain drugs, especially when a rapid treatment response is required. Such drugs are usually placed under the tongue. One example is glyceryl trinitrate that is used to treat an angina attack. It can also be a useful route for drugs which are unstable at the pH of the stomach, or which are rapidly metabolized by the liver. Drugs that are absorbed from the oral cavity enter the systemic circulation directly and therefore escape the 'first-pass' metabolism that occurs in the liver, unlike substances that are absorbed into the portal system (see Ch. 6). An example of a drug that is rapidly inactivated in the liver is isoprenaline that is sometimes used to treat heart block. This drug can be effective if given sublingually. Unfortunately, high molecular weight substances are not well absorbed from the mouth.

Mechanisms of secretion

The basal rate of secretion of saliva is very low during sleep; approximately 0.05 mL/min. In the resting, awake state it increases to about 0.5 mL/min that is just enough to keep the mouth moist. During the course of the day 1–2 L of saliva are secreted. Most of it is swallowed. The proteins in saliva are broken down in the gastrointestinal tract by digestive enzymes. The amino acids and peptides produced, together with the water and ions, are re-absorbed across the walls of the intestines.

Figure 2.15 is a simplified representation of a salivary secretory unit (a salivon) that consists of an acinus and a duct. The blood flows first past the duct and then past the acinus. The blood supply constitutes a portal system, because substances reabsorbed from the duct cells into the blood capillaries surrounding the duct are transported to the capillaries surrounding the acinus via an efferent arteriole, prior to being returned to the heart via the veins. The acinar cells secrete the primary saliva that passes down the ducts. The primary secretion consists of an ultrafiltrate of plasma to which some components synthesized by the acinar cells (such as α-amylase and mucins) have been added. It is therefore almost isotonic with plasma. The rates of secretion of the primary juice and the α-amylase concentration vary with the type of stimulation, but the ionic composition of the primary juice is fairly constant. The main ionic constituents of primary saliva are Na^+, K^+, Cl^- and HCO_3^-.

As the primary juice flows past the duct cells it undergoes secondary modification via transport systems in the membranes of the secretory and striated duct cells. Certain substances are produced by the duct cells and secreted into the saliva and others are extracted from the saliva by the cells. Na^+ and Cl^- are extracted from the saliva and K^+ is added to it. In fact Na^+ and K^+ are exchanged by an active mechanism in the duct cells. However, more Na^+ is extracted than K^+ is added by this mechanism, and the duct epithelium has a very low permeability to water. Consequently secondary saliva becomes more hypotonic as it flows down the ducts and in the human, saliva is always hypotonic compared to plasma. The tonicity is higher at high flow rates.

The HCO_3^- in saliva is produced from CO_2 and water in the duct cells via the reactions:

$$\text{carbonic anhydrase}$$
$$CO_2 + H_2O \rightleftharpoons H_2CO_3 \rightleftharpoons H^+ + HCO_3^-$$

The duct cells are rich in carbonic anhydrase, an enzyme which catalyses the formation of carbonic acid from CO_2 and water. HCO_3^- is secreted across the membranes into the ducts in exchange for Cl^- (Fig. 2.15).

The composition of saliva changes with rate of flow because at fast flow rates there is less time for the exchange processes occurring in the ducts to modify the composition. Thus at high flow rates the composition approaches that of the primary juice. Figure 2.16 shows the changes in the concentration of some ions in the saliva flowing from the ducts, with the rate of flow, and compares them with the concentration of those ions in the plasma. The concentrations of Na^+ ions and HCO_3^-

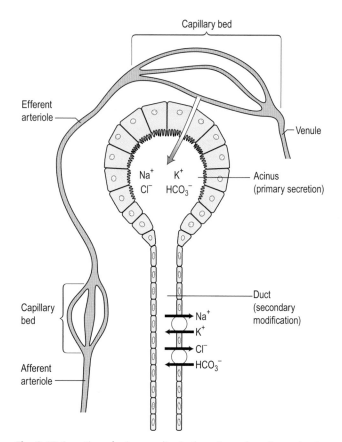

Fig. 2.15 Secretion of primary saliva in the acinus of a salivary gland, and secondary modification in the duct.

ions increase with rate of flow until a plateau is reached, whilst the concentration of K^+ ions decreases to reach a plateau at low flow rates. Na^+ is exchanged for K^+, but the Na^+: K^+ exchange ratio is 3:1. It is only at low flow rates that the active transport processes for these ions in the ducts makes a measurable difference to their concentrations in the saliva. At maximum rates of flow the tonicity of human saliva is approximately 70% of that of plasma. The ducts extract more ions than they deliver to the saliva, and the osmotic gradient is therefore in the direction of the plasma, but the ducts are relatively impermeable to water and so the saliva is always hypotonic to plasma. Table 2.1 compares the ionic composition of primary saliva produced in the acinus, secondary saliva produced at a low flow rate (unstimulated), and secondary saliva produced at a high flow rate (stimulated).

The pH of resting human saliva is only slightly alkaline, and its HCO_3^- concentration is lower than that of the primary juice. The reasons are unclear. However, it becomes more alkaline with increasing rate of flow as the concentration of HCO_3^- ions increases. At maximum rates of flow the pH may reach a value of 8.0 and the HCO_3^- concentration is higher than that of the primary juice (Table 2.1). At high rates of flow the secretion of HCO_3^- is stimulated. As it is removed from the cell more is produced by the intracellular mechanism.

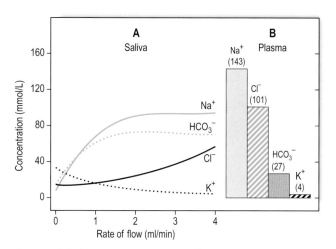

Fig. 2.16 (A) Changes in concentration of some ions in saliva with rate of flow. (B) Concentrations of the same ions in blood plasma.

Table 2.1 Concentrations of some important constituents in primary and secondary saliva

Ions (mmol/L)	Primary saliva	Secondary saliva	
		Unstimulated	*Stimulated*
Na$^+$	145	2	85
K$^+$	4	25	18
Cl$^-$	100	23	55
HCO$_3^-$	24	4	40
α-amylase (g/L)		<0.1	1.0
Flow rate (mL/min)		0.5	3.5

The ionic composition of the primary juice is similar to that of blood plasma. The differences in ionic compositions of the primary and secondary salivas are due to the modifications that take place as the saliva flows down the ducts. Thus Na$^+$ is extracted and K$^+$ is added in the ducts. HCO$_3^-$ secretion is stimulated at high rates of flow. The fate of Cl$^-$ is complex; it is exchanged for HCO$_3^-$, and is transported down the electrical gradient created by the transport of Na$^+$. In stimulated saliva there is less time for such modifications to take place, as the flow rate is faster. The composition of the stimulated secondary juice is therefore intermediate between that of the primary juice and the unstimulated secondary juice. The concentration of α-amylase is higher at high flow rates as its secretion from the acinar cells is stimulated.

Control of secretion

In the human, the secretion of saliva is mainly in response to nerve stimulation. The efferent control is via autonomic nerves. The glands are innervated by both parasympathetic and sympathetic nerves. The postganglionic sympathetic nerve fibres have their cell bodies in the superior cervical ganglion. The preganglionic parasympathetic nerve fibres travel in branches of the facial (cranial nerve VII) and the glossopharyngeal (cranial nerve XI) nerves. These synapse with postganglionic fibres in or near the glands. There is a parasympathetic innervation of all acini and most usually also have a sympathetic innervation. Several nerve fibres supply each acinus but not every cell is innervated. However, the acinar cells are electrically coupled so that the membrane depolarization brought about by nerve impulses in the innervated cells is transmitted to the neighbouring cells. Myoepithelial cells in the vicinity of the acini are innervated by the same nerve fibres. The duct cells and the myoepithelial cells and the arterioles of the gland, are also innervated by both parasympathetic and sympathetic nerves.

Nerve stimulation increases changes in both the composition and the volume of the secretion. Simulation of either the parasympathetic nerves or the sympathetic nerves increases the rate of secretion. However, the parasympathetic nerves provide a stronger and longer lasting stimulus. If the parasympathetic supply is interrupted the glands atrophy, but interruption of the sympathetic nervous supply causes no major defect in salivary secretion. The parasympathetic nerves release acetylcholine, substance P and vasoactive intestinal peptide (VIP), while the sympathetic nerves release noradrenaline.

The processes which are stimulated by parasympathetic nerve activity include the flow of saliva, the release of α-amylase and mucins from the acinar cells, transport events in the duct cells, the extrusion of the saliva from the ducts, the blood flow, and the metabolism and growth of the acinar and duct cells. Stimulation of the sympathetic nerves is a transient effect causing the release of saliva rich in α-amylase, mucins, HCO$_3^-$ and K$^+$, and contraction of the myoepithelial cells. It also causes vasoconstriction that reduces the blood flow to the glands. This effect may be exaggerated when an individual is frightened and may explain why some people experience a dry mouth when they are afraid. Circulating catecholamines reinforce the effect of sympathetic nerve stimulation. Acinar cell membranes have both α- and β-adrenergic receptors. Other hormones are not a major influence in the control of secretion of saliva, although both vasopressin and aldosterone can stimulate Na$^+$/K$^+$ exchange in the duct dells.

Cellular mechanisms of control

The acinar cells of the resting glands contain granules. These can be stained histologically. They are the locus of storage of the zymogen precursor of α-amylase. If the gland is stimulated, the number of granules diminishes as the enzyme is released. The formation of new enzyme occurs rapidly in the acinar cell after stimulation, although it is the release, by exocytosis, not the synthesis, that is directly stimulated by the transmitter. It has been shown that after stimulation of the rat submandibular gland by feeding or by injection of acetylcholine, the content of α-amylase increases 10-fold.

The second messengers involved in the actions of the neurotransmitters on acinar cells are intracellular cAMP and Ca^{2+}. Activation of either β-adrenergic receptors or VIP receptors causes an increase in intracellular cAMP, while activation of α-adrenergic receptors, muscarinic acetylcholine receptors or substance P receptors results in increased Ca^{2+} influx into the cell. Substances that increase intracellular cAMP tend to produce a secretion that is richer in α-amylase than those that increase intracellular Ca^{2+} concentration, whilst those that increase intracellular Ca^{2+} concentration tend to produce a greater increase in the volume of acinar cell secretion. Mucins are also released by exocytosis as a consequence of influx of Ca^{2+} into the cell.

Blood flow

When the parasympathetic nerves are stimulated there is a rapid vasodilatation that can result in up to a five-fold increase in blood flow. This is followed by a slower vasodilatory effect. The immediate effect is probably due to a direct action of the transmitters acetylcholine and VIP released from parasympathetic nerve fibres that end on the arterioles in the glandular tissue. The two transmitters are probably released from the same nerve terminals. Stimulation of the sympathetic nerves causes vasoconstriction via the release of noradrenaline that acts on α-adrenergic receptors on the arteriolar smooth muscle.

The slower vasodilatory effect is an indirect consequence of stimulation of the parasympathetics. It is due to the formation of vasodilator metabolites, mainly bradykinin, by processes occurring following stimulation of the acinar cells that results in the release of proteolytic enzymes known as kallikreins, into the interstitial fluid. These enzymes catalyse the conversion of a precursor, bradykininogen, to bradykinin, the active vasodilator (Fig. 2.17).

Bradykinin acts on the arteriolar smooth muscle to cause vasodilatation. When the arterioles dilate the pressure drop across them diminishes and the pressure is transferred to the capillaries. The increased hydrostatic pressure and consequent increased transcapillary pressure result in increased filtration in the gland. The consequence is an increased flow of saliva. Furthermore saliva can actually be secreted at a pressure higher than the arterial pressure to the gland, as the triggering of active processes at the luminal surface of the gland by the parasympathetic nerves causes secondary water transport. Xerostomia can be treated by administration of pilocarpine, a partial cholinergic agonist that mimics the effect of stimulation of the parasympathetics (see Box 6).

Control of secretion by food

Saliva is secreted in response to the approach of food, and to the presence of food in the mouth. The effect is mediated via the parasympathetic nerves. Up to 50% of the secretion during a meal comes from the parotid glands. Two reflexes are involved: a conditioned reflex and an unconditioned reflex.

The conditioned reflex is due mainly to the sight and smell of food, although other sensory inputs such as sounds can trigger it. The reflex was first studied in dogs by Pavlov, a Russian physiologist who worked in St Petersburg. He usually fed the dogs at a time when the bells of the cathedral chimed. He discovered that they salivated when the bells chimed even on occasions when they

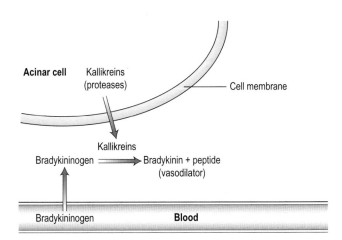

Fig. 2.17 Mechanism of vasodilation during stimulation of salivary secretion.

Case
2.1 **Xerostomia: 4**

Treatment and side-effects

The treatment of xerostomia depends on whether the patient can secrete saliva in response to a stimulus, i.e. whether he or she is a 'responder' who has functioning salivary gland epithelium, or a 'non-responder' who does not. Artificial salivas can be used in non-responders, but these are not wholly satisfactory. Low doses of pilocarpine are often used to treat the condition in individuals with residual salivary function. This drug is a partial agonist of muscarinic acetylcholine receptors. It mimics the effect of stimulation of the parasympathetic nerves, causing the acinar cells to secrete saliva and kallikreins, which in turn cause vasodilatation via bradykinin and hence increased secretion. However, systemic parasympathetic side-effects can occur, including bradycardia and decreased cardiac output, increased sweating and increased gut motility. If the dry mouth is a consequence of treatment with other medication, it is unwise to prescribe pilocarpine to treat the xerostomia. In these circumstances the possibility of treatment of the primary condition with an alternative drug that does not cause dry mouth should be explored. However, pilocarpine is often prescribed to treat xerostomia that occurs as a consequence of radiotherapy, although the side-effects can lead to its use being discontinued.

were not being fed, presumably in anticipation. Thus the conditioned reflex is a learned response because the first time the stimulus is presented it does not elicit a secretion.

The unconditioned reflex is due to the presence of food in the mouth. It occurs in response to activation of touch or taste receptors. Stimulation by food of taste receptors on the tongue, or pressure receptors in the mouth, results in impulses being set up in the afferent nerves to the brainstem. Figure 2.8 shows the arrangement of the neural pathways of the secretory reflex that occurs following stimulation of the taste buds. This involves afferent pathways from the tongue to the superior and inferior salivary nuclei. The afferent nerve fibres run in the chorda tympani and the glossopharyngeal nerves (see above). The efferent preganglionic parasympathetic nerves to the salivary glands also run in these nerves. The preganglionic fibres in the glossopharyngeal nerve synapse with postganglionic fibres in the otic ganglion and the postganglionic fibres innervate the parotid glands. The preganglionic fibres in the chorda tympani synapse with postganglionic fibres in the submandibular ganglion and the postganglionic fibres innervate the submandibular and the sublingual glands.

The precise role of the sympathetic nerves in stimulating saliva secretion in different physiological states is still unclear.

Oesophagus

Anatomical arrangements of the oesophagus

The structures associated with the oesophagus are shown in Figures 2.4, 2.18 and 2.21. The arrangement of the smooth muscle in the wall of the oesophagus is similar to that of the rest of the gastrointestinal tract in that there is an inner circular layer and an outer longitudinal layer (see Ch. 1). However, only the lower two-thirds of the oesophagus contain smooth muscle. The top-third contains skeletal muscle. The muscle tissue in an area in the middle of the oesophagus consists of a mixture of skeletal muscle and smooth muscle fibres, the skeletal muscle gradually being replaced by smooth muscle in the caudad direction. Both the skeletal muscle fibres and the smooth muscle fibres are under the control of the vagus nerve. The skeletal muscle is innervated directly by somatic motor neurones from the nucleus ambigus, whilst the smooth muscle is innervated indirectly by neurones in the vagus nerve that synapse with neurones in the myenteric plexus. The intrinsic nerves are in effect postganglionic autonomic nerves. Preganglionic parasympathetic neurones in the vagus nerve from the dorsal motor nucleus synapse with the cell bodies of these neurones.

The upper oesophageal sphincter (the hypopharyngeal sphincter or cricopharyngeus muscle) is composed of skeletal muscle. It is a thickening of the circular muscle layer. The lower sphincter comprises the last 1–2 cm of the oesophagus. It is not anatomically distinguishable as a discrete sphincter but the pressure is normally greater in this region than in the stomach.

Swallowing (deglutition)

The arrangement of the structures associated with swallowing is shown in Figure 2.4. The events involved are represented in Figure 2.18. The whole process lasts only a few seconds. It is initiated voluntarily but once initiated it cannot be stopped voluntarily, i.e. it becomes a classical 'all or none' reflex. The process can be divided into three phases: voluntary, pharyngeal, and oesophageal.

Phases of swallowing

Voluntary phase

In the voluntary phase, the tongue separates the food into a bolus and then moves it backwards and upwards

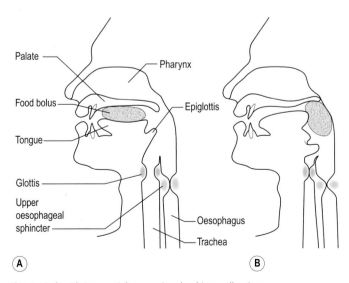
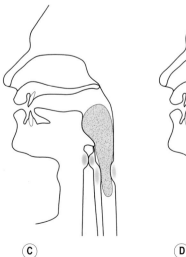
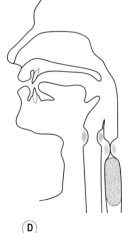

Palate — **Pharynx**

Food bolus — **Epiglottis**

Tongue

Glottis

Upper oesophageal sphincter — **Oesophagus**

Trachea

(A)　　　(B)　　　(C)　　　(D)

Fig. 2.18 (A–D) Sequential events involved in swallowing.

towards the back of the mouth. The lubricating properties of saliva are important for swallowing and individuals suffering from xerostomia have difficulty in swallowing (see Box 4).

Pharyngeal phase

As the bolus of food moves into the pharynx, it activates pressure receptors in the palate and anterior pharynx. This results in impulses in the trigeminal and glossopharyngeal nerves being transmitted to the swallowing centre in the brainstem. Each impulse serves as a trigger for the swallowing reflex. This causes the elevation of the soft palate that seals the nasal cavity and prevents food from entering it. The swallowing centre inhibits respiration, raises the larynx, and closes the glottis (the opening between the vocal chords). This prevents food from getting into the trachea. As the tongue forces the food further back into the pharynx, the bolus tilts the epiglottis backwards to cover the closed glottis. It is closure of the glottis, however, not the tilting of the epiglottis that is mainly responsible for preventing food from entering the trachea.

The upper oesophageal sphincter is closed at rest. It opens during swallowing, allowing the bolus of food to pass into the oesophagus. Immediately after the bolus has passed, it closes again, resealing the junction. The glottis then opens and breathing resumes. The skeletal muscle fibres of the upper oesophageal sphincter are so arranged that they contract when the sphincter opens and relax when it closes. This pharyngeal phase of swallowing lasts approximately 1 s. The relationship between the oesophagus and other thoracic structures is shown in Figure 2.19.

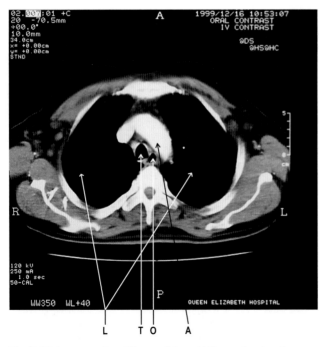

Fig. 2.19 A cross-section CT scan of the mid-thorax showing the anatomical relationship of the lungs (L), aortic arch (A), overlying the trachea (T), and the oesophagus (O).

Oesophageal phase

The food is moved along the oesophagus by peristalsis. A peristaltic wave consists of a wave of contraction of the circular muscle, followed by a wave of relaxation. The wave of contraction passes along the walls of the oesophagus and moves the food towards the stomach (Fig. 2.20). The wave of contraction takes about 9 s to travel the length of the oesophagus. The progression of the wave is controlled by autonomic nerves and is coordinated by the swallowing centre in the medulla. Thus it is not primarily gravity, but peristalsis that causes the food to move towards the stomach, although gravity assists the process. The importance of peristalsis to the process compared to that of gravity is seen by the fact that food can be swallowed and it will reach the stomach even in someone who is upside down. It is noteworthy that in other parts of the gastrointestinal tract the peristaltic waves are coordinated largely by the internal nerve plexi and the extrinsic nerves are less important, and can be sectioned without gastrointestinal function being dramatically affected.

As the peristaltic waves begin in the oesophagus, the muscle of the lower oesophageal sphincter relaxes, opening the sphincter and allowing the food bolus to enter the stomach. The sphincter muscle then contracts and reseals the junction. It remains closed in the absence of peristalsis, preventing reflux of the stomach's contents. Figure 2.21 shows the pressure changes in different regions of the oesophagus during swallowing.

Control of swallowing

Swallowing is coordinated by the 'swallowing centre' in the medulla oblongata. It involves efferent impulses from the medulla to 25 different skeletal muscles of the pharynx, the larynx, and the early oesophagus and the smooth muscles in the lower oesophagus.

Control of motility in the oesophagus

Swallowed food is propelled along the oesophagus to the stomach by the coordinated contraction of the muscle in the body of the oesophagus. This wave of contraction is due to a sequential activation of the muscles in the pharynx and oesophagus by neural impulses in the segmental efferent neurones of the vagus nerve that utilize acetylcholine as the neurotransmitter (Fig. 2.22).

The smooth muscle of the lower sphincter is innervated by both extrinsic and intrinsic nerves. Impulses in the cholinergic nerve fibres in the vagus are partly responsible for the maintained contraction of the muscle, i.e. its tone, when peristaltic activity is absent in the oesophagus. Stimulation of noradrenergic sympathetic nerves also causes contraction via activation of α-adrenergic receptors. However, if the extrinsic nerves are cut there is still some tone indicating that the intrinsic nerves are also important. An increase in the blood concentration of gastrin that is released from the stomach (see Ch. 4) can

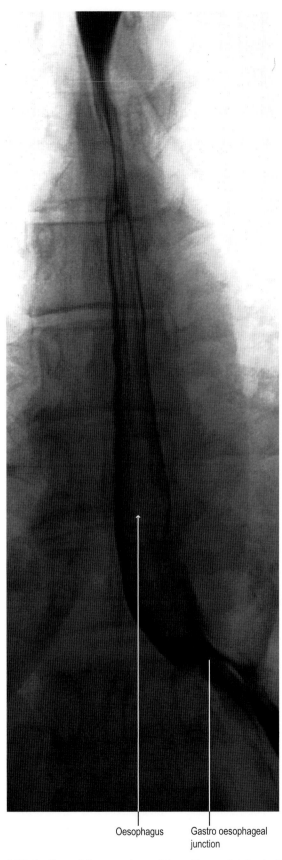

Fig. 2.20 An X-ray of the oesophagus taken after swallowing barium, showing a normal peristaltic wave.

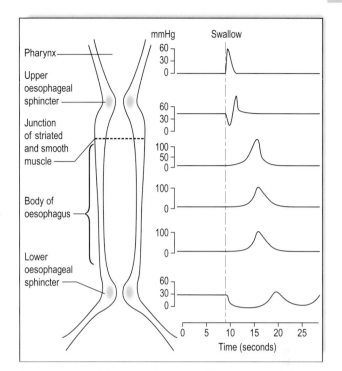

Fig. 2.21 Sequential pressure changes in different regions of the oesophagus during swallowing.

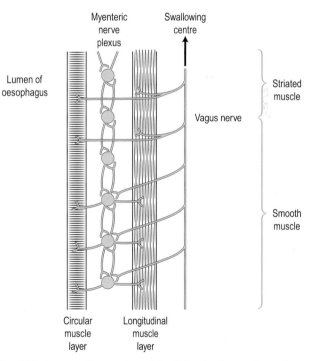

Fig. 2.22 Segmental innervation of the skeletal and smooth muscle of the oesophagus. Somatic motor neurones in the vagus nerve innervate the skeletal muscle directly. Autonomic nerve fibres in the vagus innervate the smooth muscle indirectly via the intrinsic nerves in the myenteric plexus. *Note*: The transition from skeletal muscle to smooth muscle in a region approximately one-third of the way down the oesophagus is gradual.

also increase the tone of the sphincter muscle. This mechanism may be important in preventing reflux of stomach contents into the oesophagus whilst the stomach is contracting. If the sphincter is incompetent, the reflux of stomach contents may damage the mucosa (Box 7).

Relaxation of the lower oesophageal sphincter is caused by impulses in inhibitory nerve fibres that innervate the circular smooth muscle. The transmitters involved may be VIP and nitric oxide. A decrease in cholinergic impulses also promotes relaxation of the sphincter.

Motor disease of the oesophagus can be due to disorders of the skeletal muscle or disorders of the smooth muscle. The various conditions are described in Box 7.

Box 2.1 Clinical conditions associated with the oesophagus

Disorders affecting skeletal muscle

In primary diseases of skeletal musculature (e.g. myasthenia gravis, myotonic dystrophy), or primary disease of the nervous system involving the somatic motor nerves (e.g. amyotrophic lateral sclerosis or poliomyelitis), the striated muscles affected include:

- The tongue
- Pharynx
- Upper oesophageal sphincter
- Wall of the upper oesophagus.

Difficulties in swallowing (dysphagia) are experienced and there is loss of propulsive force of the upper oesophagus.

Following a stroke, lesions in the brainstem can interfere with the coordination of the movements of the tongue and pharynx.

Disorders affecting smooth muscle

Cricopharyngeal spasm: characterized by swallowing difficulty, can be due to increased fibrosis of the cricopharyngeal muscle.

Achalasia (cardiospasm): a common condition caused by defective relaxation of the lower sphincter that impedes the flow of material into the stomach, and an abnormality of the function of the smooth muscle in the lower two-thirds of the oesophagus whereby the coordinated control of peristalsis is lost. These defects are due to defective innervation of the smooth muscle of the body of the oesophagus and the lower oesophageal sphincter.

Chaga's disease: prevalent in Latin America and caused by infection with the parasite *Trypanosoma cruzi* that destroys ganglion cells in the myenteric plexus, can be characterized by similar problems to those seen in achalasia, although defects in the function of the colon are probably more common in this condition (see Ch. 10).

Diffuse oesophageal spasm: a common condition in which prolonged contraction of the lower oesophagus occurs after swallowing (instead of a normal peristaltic wave). The aetiology of this condition is not known, but thickening of the smooth muscle of the oesophagus has been observed in many patients.

Reflux oesophagitis: gastric contents are refluxed into the oesophagus thus causing 'heartburn'. This may be accompanied by inflammation of the oesophagus. It is exacerbated by increased intra-abdominal pressure. Simple measures, such as weight loss and raising the head during sleep can prevent episodes of heartburn, which are often worse during the night in susceptible individuals. It is usually treated by administration of a proton pump inhibitor to inhibit acid secretion in the stomach (see Ch. 4). In many cases, reflux is due to dysfunction of the lower oesophageal sphincter. If the oesophageal sphincter is incompetent passive reflux of stomach acid into the oesophagus can result in damage to the unprotected oesophageal mucosa. An incompetent sphincter can be repaired surgically by wrapping the stomach around the lower oesophagus within the abdominal cavity (known as a stomach wrap). This effectively creates a one-way valve thereby preventing reflux of the gastric contents into the oesophagus, but can also prevent the process of vomiting by not allowing opening of the lower oesophageal sphincter.

THE STOMACH: BASIC FUNCTIONS

3

Chapter objectives

After studying this chapter you should be able to:

1. Understand the relationship between the structure of the stomach and its function in the process of digestion.

2. Understand the secretory processes of the stomach mucosa and how dysfunction may influence digestion, absorption and body homeostasis in terms of:

   a. Acid–base balance

   b. Red blood cell formation in the bone marrow.

3. Understand the protective functions of the stomach including those relating to:

   a. Mucosal structure and secretion

   b. Acid and pepsin secretion.

4. Understand the importance of stomach smooth muscle function in:

   a. The storage of food

   b. Mixing the food with the digestive secretions

   c. The regulation of the entry of the stomach contents into the small intestine.

5. Understand the process of vomiting.

Introduction

The primary function of the stomach is to store the food ingested during a meal and to regulate its release into the duodenum. Its other functions are to churn and mix the food with the gastric secretions producing a thick mixture known as 'chyme'. In addition it has a range of exocrine, paracrine and endocrine functions. The exocrine secretions, which are released into the stomach lumen are digestive juices, collectively known as gastric juice. The major paracrine secretion is histamine, a substance that stimulates gastric acid secretion. The major endocrine secretion is the hormone gastrin, which acts both locally on the stomach smooth muscle and mucosa to stimulate gastric motility and acid secretion, and distally on the intestines, pancreas and liver.

In this chapter, the secretory and emptying functions of the stomach will be considered in the light of a clinical problem concerning the consequences of partial gastrectomy, a condition in which these functions are compromised (Case 3.1: 1). Another clinical problem, the consequences of excessive vomiting, is also used to highlight the importance of the stomach for homeostasis. The control of stomach functions is the subject of Chapter 4.

Anatomy and morphology of the stomach

The stomach is a storage sac located between the oesophagus and the duodenum. Figure 3.1 indicates the major features of the stomach. It consists of three regions: the fundus, which is the upper region; the main body; and the antrum. Folds, known as rugae, are present on the inner surface of the empty stomach. The rugae can be clearly seen in Figure 3.2 which shows an X-ray of a stomach. The rugae flatten out as the stomach fills. A rare condition known as Ménétrièr's disease is characterized by giant gastric folds due to hypertrophy of the gastric epithelium (Box 3.1).

The wall of the stomach consists of various layers of tissue (Fig. 3.3). The inner lining is known as the mucosa. It comprises the lamina propria and the gastric glands (or pits). Beneath this lie the submucosa, the muscularis mucosae and the serosa which is covered by the peritoneum. The wall structure of the stomach is similar to that present throughout the rest of the gastrointestinal tract (see Ch. 1), except that the stomach has an oblique muscle layer in addition to the circular and longitudinal layers in the muscularis mucosae. This facilitates distension of the stomach and the storage of food. The muscle layers are not evenly distributed over the wall of the stomach. The external circular muscle layer is relatively thin in the fundus and body, and thick in the antrum, where strong muscular contractions aid the mixing of food. In addition, it is highly developed in the pylorus where it becomes a functional sphincter that regulates stomach emptying.

The lining of the stomach is covered with a protective layer of columnar epithelial cells. These have well developed tight junctions to protect the underlying

tissue from erosion by acid. In addition, the columnar cells secrete mucus and alkaline fluid to further protect the gastric mucosa from injury. The mechanisms of damage to the mucosal barrier are discussed in Chapter 4. Numerous gastric pits (approximately 3.5 million in the human) penetrate the surface. These are short ducts into which the more deeply lying gastric glands empty their secretions. The secretions enter the main compartment of the stomach via the necks of these ducts.

The stomach is separated from the duodenal bulb by the pyloric sphincter. Figure 3.1B shows the main structural features of the pylorus. It is not an anatomically discrete sphincter but a development of the circular smooth muscle layer. A ring of connective tissue separates the pylorus from the duodenum, enabling the contractions of the two regions to be independent. However, the myenteric nerve plexi of the pylorus and duodenum are continuous (see Ch. 7).

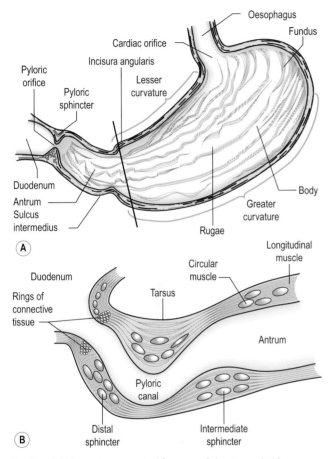

(A)

(B)

Fig. 3.1 (A) The main anatomical features of the stomach. The diagonal line shows the approximate division of the stomach into the two secretory regions; the oxyntic secretory area consisting of the fundus and the body, and the pyloric secretory area consisting of the pyloric antrum. (B) The structural features of the pylorus.

Secretory mucosa of the stomach

The secretory mucosa of the stomach can be considered as two separate regions (Fig. 3.1): the upper region comprising the fundus and the body of the stomach, known as the oxyntic glandular area, and the lower antral and pyloric region which secretes the hormone gastrin.

The secretory cells of the oxyntic glandular area produce most of the exocrine digestive juice known as gastric juice. The major secretory cells present in this area are oxyntic (or parietal) cells that secrete acid and intrinsic factor, and chief (or peptic) cells that secrete pepsinogen, the precursor of the proteolytic enzyme pepsin. The stomach also contains enterochromaffin (ECL)-like cells that secrete histamine, and D cells which secrete somatostatin. The gastrin-secreting cells, G cells, are restricted largely to the antral region. The secretions of these cells are involved in the control of many digestive functions including gastric secretion and motility (see Ch. 4).

Histology

The oxyntic cells and chief cells are located in deeper regions of the pits as are the endocrine cells. Mucus-secreting cells are located in the neck region providing a protective barrier to the deeper lying secretory cells. The location of endocrine cells in the deeper aspect of the gastric pits facilitates uptake of their secreted granules by the underlying capillaries (Fig. 3.4).

Figure 3.5 shows the three major exocrine cell types that produce secretions that enter the lumen of the stomach. These cells are all specialized in various ways to perform their secretory function. The oxyntic cell has a vast

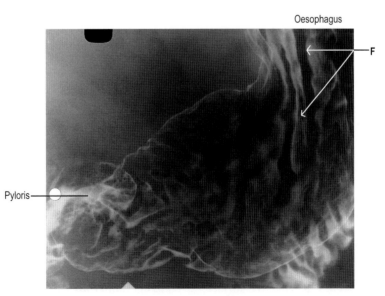

Fig. 3.2 An X-ray of the stomach taken after ingestion of barium. The thick mucosal folds (F) are clearly shown.

Box 3.1 Ménétrièr's disease

Ménétrièr's disease is a condition characterized by hypertrophy of the gastric epithelium that results in the secretion of abnormally large amounts of mucus, and loss of plasma proteins. This dangerous loss of protein can lead to reduction in the extracellular fluid volume, shock and dehydration. It can be treated by antisecretory drugs or enteral protein replacement, but these measures are not usually very effective.

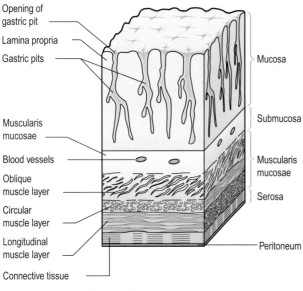

Fig. 3.3 Structure of the gastric mucosa.

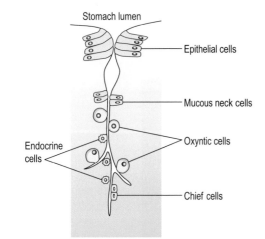

Fig. 3.4 Locations of different cell types in a gastric pit.

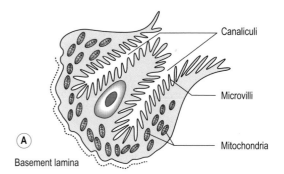

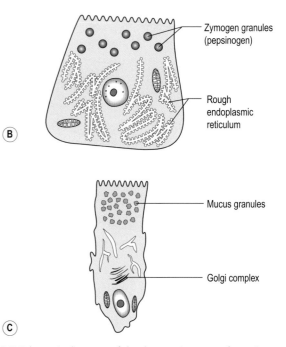

Fig. 3.5 Schematic diagrams of the three major types of exocrine secretory cell in the gastric mucosa (A) oxyntic cell, (B) chief cell, (C) mucus (goblet) cell. Note that each cell type has characteristic features associated with specialization for secretion.

surface area enabling it to produce large amounts of secretion. Invaginations of the luminal cell membrane form canaliculi (tubular passages) that penetrate deep into the cell. The canaliculi open on to the cell's free surface. They are lined with finger-like processes, known as microvilli, and these provide a large surface area for transport of secreted substances (see Ch. 1). When the cell is actively secreting, the canaliculi enlarge, as they fill with secreted juice. These cells are also rich in mitochondria that provide the energy in the form of ATP required for the secretory process.

The chief cell is specialized for the secretion of enzyme protein. It contains an extensive network of rough endoplasmic reticulum, the site of protein synthesis. Numerous dense zymogen granules, the loci of storage of the enzyme precursor protein, are located towards the luminal side of the cell.

The mucous cell also has a fairly extensive network of endoplasmic reticulum, and a prominent Golgi complex, a characteristic of cells which are specialized for the secretion of glycoproteins, in this case mucins. This cell contains numerous clear vesicles which are the sites of storage of mucins.

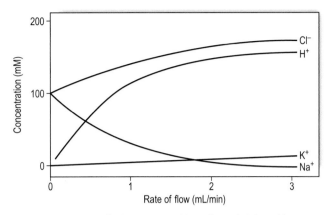

Fig. 3.6 Variation in the ionic composition of gastric juice with rate of flow.

Composition of gastric juice

The adult human secretes approximately 2 L of gastric juice per day. When a meal is being eaten, soluble substances in the food material stimulate the secretion of gastric juice. The stomach produces two different secretions: an acid secretion known as parietal juice which is released from the oxyntic (parietal) cells, and an alkaline juice released from the mucous cells. Gastric juice is isotonic with plasma but the concentrations of its various constituents vary with the rate of flow: the higher the rate the greater the acidity. During a meal therefore, the chyme becomes more acid; the acidity can reach pH 2.0. Maximum acid secretion can be induced by injection of histamine. Figure 3.6 shows the changes in concentration of some of the constituent ions in an individual in whom secretion was stimulated by injection of histamine. This procedure is used clinically to assess the secretory function of the stomach. It is known as the Gray and Hollander test after the physicians who first developed it in the early twentieth century. More recently, pentagastrin, a synthetic drug which contains the terminal tetrapeptide active site of gastrin, has been used instead of histamine, thereby avoiding the side-effects due to the action of histamine on H_1 receptors (e.g. hypertension, dizziness, headache, palpitations). However, intragastric pH-metry (for 12 or 24 h) has largely superceded the used of gastric secretory tests because this offers more accurate measurement of gastric acidity and is done under more natural conditions.

The concentration of H^+ ions increases with rate of flow, as does that of Cl^- and K^+ ions, while the concentration of Na^+ ions decreases. These changes in composition occur because when the stomach is stimulated during a meal it is only the rate of the acid parietal secretion that increases appreciably. The secretion of alkaline fluid is mainly a passive process and so its rate is relatively unaffected. Thus dilution of the chyme by the alkaline juice is therefore less at high flow rates and the H^+ and Cl^- ion concentrations increase. Both acid and alkaline secretions are isotonic with plasma.

Absence of HCl secretion (achlorhydria) is seen when the gastric pits are destroyed. It is usually associated with lack of intrinsic factor that results in vitamin B_{12} deficiency and pernicious anaemia (see below). However, when loss of HCl secretory capacity occurs, the first clinical manifestation is usually iron-deficiency anaemia because lack of acid results in ingested iron being retained in an unabsorbable form (see Case 3.1: 5).

Cellular mechanisms of secretion

Secretions of the oxyntic cell

Hydrochloric acid

The secretion of H^+ and Cl^- ions by the stomach are both active processes. The energy is derived from the hydrolysis of ATP. The H^+ ions are transported against an enormous concentration gradient: the concentration of H^+ ions in the blood is approximately 10^{-8} M while the concentration in the stomach lumen can be as high as 1.5×10^{-1} M.

The mechanism whereby the H^+ ions are generated within the cell is outlined in Figure 3.7. Carbon dioxide diffuses into the cell from the plasma. Inside the cell it combines with water to form carbonic acid. This reaction is catalysed by the enzyme carbonic anhydrase. The carbonic acid dissociates to give H^+ and HCO_3^- ions. The HCO_3^- ions are transported into the blood, down a concentration gradient, in exchange for Cl^- ions. The secretion of HCO_3^- ions into the blood when the stomach is secreting acid into the lumen results in the plasma becoming transiently alkaline. This phenomenon is known as the 'alkaline tide'.

Hydrogen ion secretion, across the apical surface of the oxyntic cell, into the canaliculus, is accomplished by proton pumps in the membrane of the canaliculus. The proton pump, which contains an ATPase, secretes H^+ ions in exchange for K^+ ions, in a ratio of 1:1. In the unstimulated cell the proton pumps are localized intracellularly in tubulovesicles. Upon stimulation of the cell to secrete, the vesicles travel to the luminal membrane and the vesicle membranes become incorporated into the plasma membrane, thereby causing a substantial increase in the 'secretory' area of the membrane. Drugs that inhibit the proton pump in the oxyntic cell are used to treat mucosal disorders such as duodenal ulcers that are potentiated by gastric acid (see Box 3.2 and Ch. 4).

Chloride ions are also secreted against a concentration gradient. The concentration of Cl^- ions in the blood is approximately 107 mM whereas in the lumen of the stomach it can reach 170 mM. Chloride is also secreted against an electrical gradient, as the apical surface of the resting cell is electronegative (-60 to -80 mV) with respect to the basolateral surface. Na^+/K^+ coupled pumps are present at the basolateral surface. The entry of Cl^- ions into the cell, down their concentration gradient, at the basolateral surface, occurs in exchange for HCO_3^- ions (see above

Box 3.2 Proton pump inhibitors

Drugs that reduce acid secretion in the stomach by inhibiting the proton pump are used to treat disorders such as duodenal ulcers and reflux oesophagitis that are potentiated by acid (see Chs 3 and 4). Omeprazole, the most commonly used, is a powerful proton pump inhibitor. It is a weak base which acts by blocking the H^+/K^+-ATPase activity of the proton pump. Omeprazole is inactive at neutral pH, but it is activated in acid conditions (pH 3.0). Such conditions exist only in the canaliculi of the oxyntic cell. The action of the drug is therefore restricted to this location in the gastrointestinal tract thereby avoiding the unwanted side-effects of disruption of Cl^- ion transport, which could occur in other organs such as the lungs, pancreas and skin (sweating) seen with use of other H^+ transport inhibitors which are active in less acid conditions. The treatment of peptic ulcer disease is discussed in more detail in Chapter 4.

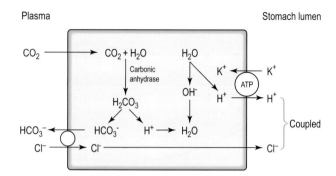

Fig. 3.7 Hydrochloric acid secretion by the oxyntic cell.

and Fig. 3.7). Cl^- ions are transported across the luminal surface via a chloride channel. This channel produces net transport of negative charges and operates without the exchange of an anion. Consequently when the cell is stimulated to secrete, the potential difference falls (to $-30\,mV$ and $-50\,mV$) and the apical surface becomes less electronegative. The proton and chloride pumps on the mucosal surface are coupled in the secreting cell so that H^+ and Cl^- ions are secreted in a ratio of 1:1. The coupling mechanism is not yet understood.

Acid–base disturbance of the body can follow gastrectomy as the ability to secrete acid is compromised. This topic is dealt with in Case 3.1: 2. It can also be a problem in an individual who vomits excessively as may be the case during chemotherapy. This is because a feedback mechanism operates whereby if the stomach contents become too acid, secretion is inhibited. If the stomach contents are lost, this feedback mechanism does not operate and acid secretion is not regulated in this way. The consequences of excessive vomiting for the acid–base balance of the body are addressed in Case 3.2: 2 below.

Intrinsic factor

Intrinsic factor is the only substance secreted by the stomach that is essential to life. It enables the absorption of vitamin B_{12} (which occurs in the ileum). It is a 55 000 kDa glycoprotein which complexes with vitamin B_{12} (cobalamin). The glycoprotein dimerizes and the dimer binds two molecules of vitamin B_{12}. The complex is resistant to digestion. There are four physiologically important forms of vitamin B_{12}. These cyanocobalamins bind to protein in the food, and are released from them by the action of acid and pepsin in the stomach. The vitamin is absorbed inefficiently by passive diffusion in the free, uncomplexed state, along the length of the intestine, but a specialized absorption mechanism exists in the distal ileum whereby vitamin B_{12} complexed to intrinsic factor can be

absorbed at a relatively rapid rate (see Ch. 8). Vitamin B_{12} deficiency leads to pernicious anaemia. This condition can result from disorders of the stomach mucosa that releases intrinsic factor, or from disorders such as Crohn's disease that affect the terminal ileum where vitamin B_{12} is absorbed (see Ch. 8). The consequence of vitamin B_{12} deficiency due to lack of intrinsic factor, after gastrectomy, are discussed in Case 3.1: 3 and the various causes of this condition are discussed in Chapter 8.

Role of the stomach in iron absorption

The body's stores of iron are small and need to be frequently replenished to promote adequate haemoglobin synthesis and red blood cell function. Iron is absorbed mainly as haem and as the ferrous (Fe^{2+}) ion. However, Fe^{2+} is oxidized to Fe^{3+} at physiological pH (i.e. pH 7.4). Ferric (Fe^{3+}) iron, which is the more abundant dietary form of non-haem iron, is absorbed very inefficiently. However, the acid environment in the stomach tends to maintain iron in its more soluble and absorbable ferrous form. Thus, individuals who take proton pump inhibitors such as omeprazole to reduce acid secretion may have a tendency to develop iron-deficiency anaemia.

There is a tendency for Fe^{2+} ions to form insoluble complexes with dietary PO_4^{3-} ions, phytate and oxalate in the duodenum and jejunum. Fe^{2+} ions are not absorbed when present in these insoluble complexes. However, if Fe^{2+} is chelated with dietary ascorbate (vitamin C) or citrate it is kept in an absorbable state. Thus vitamin C or citrate in the diet can protect against iron-deficiency anaemia. Iron-deficiency anaemia following gastrectomy is addressed in Case 3.1: 3.

Secretion of the chief cell

Pepsin, the proteolytic enzyme of the stomach is normally responsible for less than 20% of the protein digestion that occurs in the gastrointestinal tract. It is an endopeptidase that degrades proteins to peptides. It preferentially hydrolyses peptide linkages where one of the amino acids is aromatic. Pepsin, like other protease

Acid–base disturbance

Secretion of acid by the stomach during a meal is accompanied by transport of HCO_3^- ions into the blood (the alkaline tide). When the food reaches the duodenum it is mixed with the alkaline secretions from the pancreas, liver and walls of the intestines. The cellular mechanisms whereby these alkaline juices are secreted are in some ways the reverse of those whereby acid is secreted in the stomach (Fig. 3.7). Thus transport of HCO_3^- ions into the glandular ducts of these organs occurs simultaneously with the transport of an equal number of H^+ ions into the blood serving these organs. The consequent increase in blood H^+ concentration is normally neutralized by the HCO_3^- ions of the alkaline tide of the blood from the stomach. In addition the H^+ ions secreted by the stomach into the lumen are neutralized by the HCO_3^- ions present in the digestive juices (bile, pancreatic juice and intestinal juice) acting in the small intestine (Fig. 3.8). This balance can be upset by gastric resection that restricts acid production. Feedback control mechanisms normally regulate the secretion of H^+ and HCO_3^- ions to keep the pH values in the gut lumen within appropriate limits. Many metabolic functions in the body are extremely sensitive to pH change, and the pH of body fluids such as plasma, must therefore be maintained within a very narrow range.

Abnormalities can occur in the acid–base balance of the patient who has undergone partial gastrectomy but the body usually compensates for these disturbances. After removal of the stomach, the 'alkaline' tide obviously does not occur, but during a meal H^+ ions are still transported into the blood from the secreting pancreas, liver and intestines and the blood tends to become acidic. This 'metabolic' acidosis can be compensated in the short term by the respiratory system that responds with an increase in the rate and depth of breathing. This results in CO_2 being blown off from the blood. The reaction:

$$H^+ + HCO_3^- \rightarrow H_2CO_3 \rightarrow CO_2 + H_2O$$

is consequently driven to the right (the law of mass action) and the H^+ ion concentration in the blood falls towards normal.

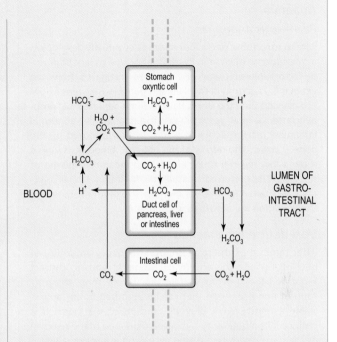

Fig. 3.8 Neutralization of acid in the blood and in the intestinal lumen.

However, full compensation of the acidosis takes longer and depends on processes in the renal tubules that conserve HCO_3^- and secrete acid. In the presence of impaired renal function, the patient's blood tests would show a low pH, low HCO_3^- concentration and a low $P\text{co}_2$. In a compensated patient, following a meal, acidotic urine would be excreted. A detailed explanation of the control of acid–base balance can be found in the companion volumes on the Respiratory and Renal systems.

---

enzymes, is formed from an inactive precursor, pepsinogen, which is stored in granules in the chief cells of the stomach and released by exocytosis. The synthesis and exocytosis of the enzyme protein is essentially similar to that described for pancreatic enzymes in Chapter 5. Pepsinogen is also secreted by mucous cells, and cells in the glands of Brunner in the duodenum. At least two immunologically distinct pepsinogens are secreted by the stomach, denoted pepsinogens I and II. Pepsinogen I, the major pepsin precursor, is secreted by the chief cells in the oxyntic glandular area, and pepsinogen II by cells throughout the stomach as well as in Brunner's glands. The role of pepsin in ulcer formation is described in Chapter 4.

Pepsinogen is activated in the stomach lumen by hydrolysis, with the removal of a short peptide:

$$\text{Pepsinogen} \atop (42\,500\,\text{kDa}) \xrightarrow[\text{pepsin}]{H^+} {\text{pepsin} \atop (35\,000\,\text{kDa})} + {\text{peptide} \atop (7\,500\,\text{kDa})}$$

H^+ ions are important for pepsin function because:

- Pepsinogen is initially activated by the H^+ ions. The activated enzyme then acts autocatalytically to increase the rate of formation of more pepsin.

- It provides the appropriate pH for the enzyme to act. The optimum pH for pepsin is approximately pH 3.5.

Anaemia

Pernicious anaemia

After gastrectomy, pernicious anaemia eventually develops as a consequence of vitamin B_{12} deficiency, due to lack of intrinsic factor, unless replacement therapy is instigated. However, vitamin B_{12} is stored in the liver and pernicious anaemia does not develop until the stores have become depleted, i.e. probably after several years. In pernicious anaemia, abnormal immature macrocytic (large) red cells are produced by the bone marrow. The results of the patient's blood tests would show a low red cell count and a high mean cell volume of the cells. The preferred treatment is by intramuscular injections of vitamin B_{12} every 3 months. The different causes of this condition are described in Chapter 8.

Iron-deficiency anaemia

After removal of the stomach, iron-deficiency anaemia can develop because the acid in the stomach tends to convert ferric iron (Fe^{3+}) in the diet to the ferrous form, the only form of non-haem iron that can be absorbed to any appreciable extent. Even if only the antrum of the stomach is removed, iron-deficiency can develop because of the removal of the gastrin-secreting G cells, as gastrin is a major stimulus for acid secretion in the stomach. The body's iron stores are more limited than those of vitamin B_{12}, and iron-deficiency anaemia can manifest itself within a few months of partial gastrectomy, while pernicious anaemia may not occur for 2 years or so. Iron-deficiency is characterized by the presence of small red blood corpuscles (microcytosis), although after gastrectomy, this may eventually be obscured by pernicious anaemia in which the red blood corpuscles are macrocytic. Iron-deficiency anaemia is discussed in more detail in Chapter 8.

- It denatures ingested protein; denatured protein is a better substrate for the enzyme than native protein.

The consequences of gastrectomy for digestion are discussed in Case 3.1: 4.

Secretions of the mucous cell

Mucus is a viscous sticky substance that contains glycoproteins known as mucins, which consist of about 80% carbohydrate, largely galactose and N-acetylglucosamine. The molecules are tetramers with a molecular weight of approximately 2 million. The carbohydrate chains protect the molecule from digestion by pepsin. Gastric mucus lubricates the pieces of food (in conjunction with salivary mucus) enabling them to be moved about and churned by the contractions of the stomach. The epithelial cells secrete an opaque alkaline mucus which has a high

Consequences for digestion

It can be assumed from the fact that gastrectomy is compatible with life, that the role of the stomach in the digestion of food is not indispensable. If the stomach is removed the lack of pepsin does not pose a problem as far as the overall digestion of protein is concerned. It is normally responsible for the digestion of only 10–20% of the protein present. In its absence, the proteases secreted by the pancreas, which act in the small intestine, can normally cope with the digestion of all the digestible protein present in the food. Chymotrypsin, an enzyme produced by the pancreas (see Ch. 5) has a similar substrate specificity to pepsin. However, pepsin and acid in the stomach have a further role in destroying aerobic bacteria that have been ingested with the food. Thus in a well-fed normal individual, infections such as cholera, for example, are rare. However, such infections are more likely to affect individuals who have undergone a gastrectomy, or who do not secrete acid (achlorhydria). As salivary amylase is normally inactivated by gastric acid in the stomach (see Ch. 2), this enzyme may remain active in the digestive tract for longer after gastrectomy, thereby theoretically increasing the rate of breakdown of starch.

bicarbonate content. This secretion increases when food is eaten. In addition, the mucus neck cells secrete a clear mucus in response to food. Mucus is released from the mucous neck cells and surface epithelium by exocytosis. It can also be released by desquamation of the epithelial cells from the surface.

Mucin tetramers form a dissolved gel when their concentration exceeds approximately $50\,mg/mL$. This gel forms a layer on the surface of the mucosa. Its stability depends on charged SO_4^-, COO^- groups and H^+ bonds, and dramatic changes in pH can cause precipitation of the mucus. The surface epithelial cells secrete non-parietal alkaline fluid (see above) and this fluid is entrapped in the layer of mucus. The alkaline mucus forms a barrier that lines the stomach and protects it from damage by acid and pepsin. Damage to the mucosal barrier results in the development of ulcers. This topic is addressed in Chapter 4.

Absorption in the stomach

Very few substances are absorbed in the stomach and the stomach is virtually impermeable to water. Aspirin and alcohol are the main substances that are absorbed at this location. Alcohol is lipid soluble and aspirin becomes more lipid soluble when it meets the acid pH present in the stomach (see Ch. 7). The consequences for absorption in the small intestine following gastrectomy are discussed in Case 3.1: 5.

Intestinal absorption

The sensations of dizziness, palpitations and sweating experienced by the gastrectomized patient after meals indicate activation of the sympathetic nervous system. We can now consider the explanations for these sensations and attempt to understand why the symptoms might be alleviated if the patient changed his eating habits.

If the stomach is removed, a normal-sized meal moves rapidly into the small intestine, due to the reduction in storage capacity. This results in the absorption of nutrients at an abnormally rapid rate. However, there may be insufficient time for the meal to be completely digested and absorbed before it is moved on along the intestines.

Hypoglycaemia

If the meal has a high carbohydrate content, the absorption of glucose can be so fast that the homeostatic mechanisms for attenuating the increase in blood glucose concentration during absorption are disturbed. Normally the blood glucose rises to a maximum level at 30–60 min after the meal has been ingested. An increase in blood glucose stimulates insulin secretion from the pancreas into the blood. This hormone lowers the blood glucose by promoting glucose uptake into muscle and adipose tissue. Normally the blood glucose returns to normal after 1.5–2 hours (Fig. 3.9). The insulin concentration also returns to normal. This is normally a finely tuned feedback control system (see Ch. 8). If the blood glucose concentration rises too rapidly however, the blood insulin concentration also rises rapidly to reach an abnormally high level in the plasma (Fig. 3.9). This results in rapid clearance of the blood glucose but it can overshoot to an abnormally low level (hypoglycaemia). Hypoglycaemia is associated with sweating and fainting, which are seen after meals in a patient who has undergone gastrectomy. Salivary amylase is normally inactivated by acid in the stomach (see Ch. 2), so after removal of the stomach, the concentration of active amylase in the small intestine can be abnormally high. This enhances the rate of glucose production in the lumen and uptake into the blood glucose. The hypoglycaemia that ensues could thereby be exacerbated. Sympathetic nerves are stimulated by low blood glucose and so hypoglycaemia causes symptoms associated with activation of the sympathetic nervous system; palpitations, sweating, vasoconstriction and pallor.

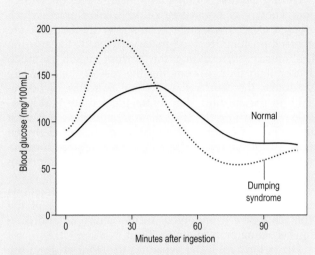

Fig. 3.9 Effect of eating an average-sized, high carbohydrate meal on the concentration of blood glucose in a normal adult (solid line) and in a patient who has undergone gastrectomy (dashed line).

Extracellular fluid volume

Another consequence of the rapid entry of material into the small intestine is a rapid loss of fluid into the gastrointestinal tract that results in a reduced intravascular volume. This happens because the contents of the intestinal lumen become hyperosmotic due to the breakdown of macromolecules in the food, being dissolved in an abnormally low volume of digestive juices. The presence of a hyperosmotic solution in the intestines results in the transport of water from the blood, down its osmotic gradient into the lumen. Other, unknown, factors may also be involved in fluid loss in this condition. The loss of water from the body can result in a dangerous fall in the extracellular fluid (ECF) volume. A concomitant fall in the intravascular volume results in hypotension that will exacerbate the fainting sensation caused by hypoglycaemia. Furthermore, the passage of hypertonic chyme through the small intestine into the large intestine will impair water absorption in the colon resulting in diarrhoea.

The symptoms that develop when a meal enters the small intestine too rapidly are collectively known as 'dumping syndrome'. All of these symptoms can be prevented by reducing the size of meals and so restricting the transit of food into the small intestine.

Motility in the stomach

The most important function of the stomach is its action to regulate the rate at which material enters the small intestine where digestion and absorption of most nutrients occurs. The stomach is responsible for churning the food and mixing it with gastric juice to produce a semi-liquid mass known as chyme. The empty stomach in the adult has a volume of approximately 50 mL and its lumen is only slightly larger than that of the small intestine. The surface interior of the stomach is highly folded into ridges. Upon being filled with food, the stomach expands and the folds diminish. Thus the wall tension and the intraluminal pressure change only slightly.

Mixing and emptying

The contractions of the stomach that are responsible for mixing the chyme and emptying it into the small intestine, depend on the activity of the smooth muscle in the wall. The stomach, like the rest of the gastrointestinal tract, is surrounded by layers of smooth muscle (Fig. 3.3).

During the first 30 min after a meal, waves of contraction, known as peristalsis, cause weak ripples which proceed at approximately 1 cm/s over the body of the stomach pushing the food material towards the antrum. The muscle surrounding the antrum region is much thicker than that surrounding the rest of the stomach. Gradually, the contractions become more intense, especially in the antrum. This contractile activity is responsible for churning the food material and mixing it with gastric juice. Eventually, a large part of the muscle in the terminal antrum undergoes an intense concerted contraction. This strong contraction is responsible for emptying material into the duodenum. Only a small spurt of material is emptied at any one time. The antral contractions force the rest of the chyme back into the body of the stomach where it undergoes further churning and mixing, becoming more and more fluid.

The pyloric sphincter separates the stomach from the duodenum. Although only a small amount of material is ejected through the sphincter each time the antrum contracts, immediately the food has entered the duodenum the back-pressure helps to close the sphincter. Thus, the function of the sphincter is to allow the carefully regulated emptying of gastric contents, and also to prevent regurgitation of the duodenal contents that contain bile into the stomach. The latter is important as the gastric mucosa is highly resistant to acid but may be damaged by bile. (The duodenal mucosa on the other hand, is resistant to bile but may be damaged by acid). Too rapid emptying of gastric contents can lead to duodenal ulcers, whereas regurgitation of duodenal contents may possibly contribute to gastric ulcers.

Vomiting

Vomiting is part of the protective role of the stomach as it protects the body from ingested toxic substances. Thus, it augments the other protective mechanisms of the stomach including acid and pepsin secretion that inactivate ingested aerobic bacteria, and mucin secretion that protects the columnar epithelium.

Vomiting or emesis is the forceful ejection of gastric contents, and sometimes, duodenal contents, through the mouth. It is a reflex that is usually preceded by a feeling of nausea. This can be accompanied by salivation, sweating, pallor, a fall in blood pressure, pupillodilation, increased heart rate and irregular breathing. It is usually also preceded by retching in which the gastric contents are forced into the oesophagus without entering the pharynx. A series of retches of increasing strength often precedes vomiting.

The vomiting reflex is controlled by the vomiting centre in the reticular formation in the medulla oblongata and the chemoreceptor trigger zone (CTZ) in the area

Box 3.3 Factors that can trigger vomiting

- Stimulation of sensory nerve endings in the stomach and duodenum (e.g. by solutions of copper sulphate and hypertonic sodium chloride)
- Drugs, such as cytotoxic drugs (e.g. cisplatin used in the treatment of cancer), and L-dopa used to treat Parkinson's disease
- Endogenous substances produced as a result of radiation damage, infections or disease
- Touch receptors at the back of the throat
- Disturbances of the vestibular apparatus (known as motion sickness)
- Stimulation of the sensory nerves of the heart and viscera (uterus, renal pelvis, bladder, testicles)
- A rise in intracranial pressure
- Nauseating smells, sights and emotional factors acting through higher central nervous system centres
- Endocrine factors (e.g. increase in oestrogen concentration in morning sickness)
- Migraine
- Circulatory syncope.

postrema that resides in the floor of the fourth ventricle near to the vagal nuclei that innervate the gastrointestinal tract. The reflex response involves stimulation of the respiratory and abdominal skeletal muscles as well as the smooth muscle of the gastrointestinal tract. A large number of different areas of the body have receptors that provide afferent inputs to the vomiting centre to trigger vomiting. Box 3.3 lists the major stimuli that can trigger vomiting.

Sequence of events

Vomiting starts with a deep inspiration. This is followed by closure of the glottis that protects the respiratory passages and holds the diaphragm down as the lungs cannot let air out. Air and saliva are drawn into the oesophagus that becomes distended. The soft palate is elevated to prevent vomit entering the nasopharynx. Then expiration occurs against a closed glottis with simultaneous contraction of the abdominal skeletal muscles. This increases both the intrathoracic and intra-abdominal pressures. The essential component of the vomiting reflex is relaxation of the lower oesophageal sphincter, without which the gastric contents cannot pass into the oesophagus. As the intrathoracic pressure is lower than the intra-abdominal pressure, relaxation of the lower oesophageal sphincter allows passive flow of gastric contents down the pressure gradient. The importance of the abdominal muscles in vomiting is demonstrated by the fact that vomiting can still be induced in an animal if the stomach has been replaced by a bladder.

Prior to vomiting, a number of cycles occur whereby the oesophagus is repeatedly filled and emptied, but as

Excessive vomiting: 1

A 55-year-old woman was being treated for ovarian cancer with a course of chemotherapy, using cisplatin, a cytotoxic anti-cancer drug. A few days after her first chemotherapy session, she became nauseous and could not stop vomiting. Nausea and vomiting is a side-effect of treatment with the anticancer drug cisplatin, which binds to receptors in the gastrointestinal tract and the Chemoreceptor trigger zone (CTZ). Persistent vomiting can become a chronic condition if the therapy has to be continued. The loss of acid can have serious consequences for the acid–base status of the patient unless antiemesis is instigated. On her next visit to the hospital, a sample of the patient's blood was tested to assess her acid–base status and electrolyte concentrations.

After consideration of the cellular mechanisms of hydrochloric acid secretion in the stomach and the disturbances of acid–base homeostasis following gastrectomy, some of the consequences of persistent vomiting can be predicted. These issues and the causes and treatment of chronic vomiting will be considered in Case 3.2: 2 and Case 3.2: 3.

Excessive vomiting: 2

Acid-base and electrolyte disturbance
Acid–base status

The measurements made on the patient's blood included pH, HCO_3^- concentration, $P{CO_2}$ and K^+ concentration. If the vomiting were not suppressed the patient's blood gas analysis would indicate a metabolic alkalosis; i.e. high pH, high $[HCO_3^-]$, $P{CO_2}$ normal or mildly elevated. The disturbance in acid–base balance is brought about because the HCO_3^- transported into the blood, from the secreting oxyntic cells in the stomach, would not be neutralized sufficiently by the H^+ ions transported into the blood as a result of the secretion of alkaline pancreatic juice, bile and intestinal juice (Fig. 3.8), which is not affected by persistent vomiting. Compensation for this alkalosis by the lungs and kidneys would become inadequate, due to the persistent loss of H^+ ions. (See the companion volumes on the Respiratory and Renal Systems for a discussion of these compensatory mechanisms.)

Electrolytes

Hypokalaemia (a low blood K^+ concentration) may also be present in this patient because K^+ would be exchanged for H^+ in the kidneys (to partially correct the blood pH) and lost in the urine. Hypokalaemia affects nerve function (of particular importance in the heart), and can lead to kidney damage. Alkaline K^+ salts, e.g. K^+ acetate, K^+ citrate or K^+ bicarbonate could be administered to correct the disturbance in plasma K^+ concentration.

the hypopharyngeal sphincter is closed, gastric contents cannot enter the mouth and they flow back into the stomach. Finally, a violent expulsive effort forces the material through the upper sphincter into the mouth. If the stomach still contains sufficient material, a second cycle can occur. Massive contractions of the duodenum can force intestinal contents into the stomach with the appearance of bile in the vomit. This is not due to reverse peristalsis but to the fact that when the stomach is relaxed, contractions of the duodenum will reverse the normal pressure gradient.

Excessive vomiting can occur as a side-effect of treatment with certain drugs, such as the anti-cancer drug cisplatin. Case 3.2: 1 and Case 3.2: 2 discuss the consequences of this problem for the acid–base and electrolyte balance of the blood.

Control of vomiting

Figure 3.10 summarizes the major pathways involved in the vomiting reflex. The final common pathway involves impulses from the vomiting centre to the skeletal and visceral smooth muscles. The vomiting centre is a functional rather than an anatomical entity. It receives impulses from the chemoreceptor trigger zone (CTZ) and the nucleus tractus solitarius (NTS) as well as from higher centres (which respond to repulsive sights, smells and emotional factors). The CTZ is 'functionally' outside the blood–brain barrier and it is affected directly by substances in the bloodstream such as the opioid analgesics morphine and apomorphine, and glycosides such as

digitalis, used in the treatment of cardiac conditions, and by high concentrations of urea (uraemia) associated with renal failure. It is also probably involved in motion sickness as removal of the area postrema in dogs has been shown to prevent motion sickness from being induced. Both the CTZ and the NTS also receive inputs from the visceral afferents (via the vagal nerves).

Transmitters involved in vomiting

The neurotransmitters in the areas of the brain that control vomiting are numerous. They include γ-aminobutyric acid, acetylcholine, noradrenaline, dopamine, 5-hydroxytryptamine, histamine, glutamate, substance P, endorphins and neurophysins, but their precise roles are still unknown. The main stimulatory factors and their pathways of action are indicated in Figure 3.10. In some clinical circumstances, for example after ingestion of a toxic substance, it is necessary to stimulate vomiting. The drug used is usually ipecacuanha. Its active ingredients are emetine and cephaeline that act locally on receptors in the stomach and stimulate vomiting via the NTS.

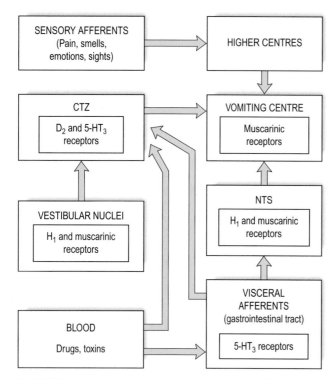

Fig. 3.10 The major peripheral and central areas involved in the control of vomiting and the receptors utilized. NTS, nucleus tractus solitarius; CTZ, chemoreceptor trigger zone.

Table 3.1 Antiemetic drugs and their actions

Receptor involved	Drug(s)	Used against vomiting by
Histamine H_1	Piperazine derivatives	Motion Morphine
Muscarinic	Hyoscine	Motion
		Copper sulphate
Dopamine	Phenothiazines	Apomorphine
		Gastrointestinal infections
		Radiation
		Cancer chemotherapy
		Oestrogen (morning sickness)
		Narcotics
5-Hydroxy-tryptamine (5-HT_3)	(Ondansetron)	Cancer chemotherapy
Cannabinoid	Nabilone	Cancer chemotherapy

Vomiting, which can be induced by a number of stimuli, can be treated with various drugs, depending to some extent on the particular stimulus that induces it. Table 3.1 lists the major antiemetic drugs and their uses against vomiting induced by different stimuli. All of these drugs can cause unwanted side-effects, especially drowsiness, as they all have an inhibitory effect on the central nervous system. The treatment of chronic vomiting which can be a side-effect of cancer chemotherapy is discussed in Case 3.2: 3.

Case 3.2

Excessive vomiting: 3

Mechanism and treatment

The receptors that respond to cisplatin to induce vomiting are present in the CTZ and the gastrointestinal tract. They include 5-HT_3 receptors and dopamine receptors in the chemoreceptor trigger zone (CTZ) and 5-HT_3 receptors in the gastrointestinal tract.

A very effective antiemetic drug to treat this condition is the 5-HT_3 antagonist ondansetron, which acts on the CTZ (Table 3.1). Dopamine antagonists such as phenothiazines and cannabinoids such as nabilone are also effective. These drugs probably act on the CTZ for their antiemetic effect.

THE STOMACH:
CONTROL

4

Chapter objectives

After studying this chapter you should be able to:

1. Understand the interplay of nervous and hormonal control of gastric function, and how this is coordinated by food in the gastrointestinal tract.

2. Understand how these control mechanisms result in coordinated function of the digestive system.

3. Understand how dysfunction can result in mucosal ulceration and how this can be diagnosed and treated.

4. Understand how dysfunction can result in secondary effects on the gastrointestinal tract and on systemic acid–base balance.

Introduction

Soluble substances in the food in the gastrointestinal tract and the mechanical pressure exerted by the food on the walls of the tract can stimulate or inhibit gastric secretion and motility. Nervous, paracrine and endocrine signals are involved. Peptic ulcer disease is a common condition in which gastric acid damages the mucosa of the duodenum or the stomach. In this chapter, the pathology and complications of this disease are used to emphasize the importance of the proper control of the functioning of the stomach (Case 4.1: 1).

A leading role in the coordination of gastrointestinal functions is played by the hormone gastrin that is released from the stomach into the bloodstream during a meal. It stimulates both secretion and motility in the stomach. It also stimulates the blood supply and growth of the gastric mucosa. In addition, it controls many functions of other regions of the gastrointestinal tract and its associated glandular organs. Gastrin is released from G cells located mainly in the mucosa of the pyloric antrum, and so these cells are ideally placed to respond to the presence of ingested material in the stomach. Tumours of ectopic G cells, known as gastrinomas, can give rise to the Zollinger–Ellison syndrome. This rare disease is characterized by over-secretion of gastrin, which results in excessive secretion of acid, and hypermotility of the gastrointestinal tract. In this chapter the physiological and clinical importance of this hormone is illustrated by discussion of the functional abnormalities that arise in Zollinger–Ellison syndrome (Case 4.2: 1).

Control of gastric secretion

The control of secretion of gastric juice involves extrinsic and intrinsic nerves, hormones and paracrine mediators.

Hormonal control

Gastrin

Gastrin is a hormone that is secreted from the G cells in the stomach. It stimulates gastric juice secretion, and has a general role in the preparation of the gastrointestinal tract for the digestion and absorption of food. It was the first hormone to be discovered (Box 4.1).

Biologically active forms of gastrin

In the normal human, gastrin is produced mainly in the gastric antrum, although small amounts are produced in the proximal small intestine. Two major forms of gastrin exist, gastrin-34 (G34, composed of 34 amino acids) and gastrin-17 (G17, composed of 17 amino acids). In humans, over 90% of the gastrin present in the antral mucosa is the G17 form. Gastrin-17 has a half-life in the circulation of approximately 6 min and G34 a half-life of approximately 36 min. Both peptides stimulate gastric acid secretion. The short half-life of the G17 form is consistent with its main influence being via local receptors in the stomach. The active part of the molecule is the carboxy-terminal tetrapeptide sequence.

The active sequence is contained in the pentapeptide drug pentagastrin, a synthetic drug that consists of the C-terminal tetrapeptide to which a substituted β-alanine has been added to stabilize the molecule. It exhibits all the physiological actions of gastrin. Clinically, it is administered as an alternative to histamine (see Ch. 3) to test gastric secretion.

G cells and gastrin secretion

In normal individuals, most of the G cells, which secrete gastrin, are found in the mucosa of the gastric antrum, although some (<20%) are present in the duodenal mucosa. The G cells comprise less than 1% of the mucosal cells. In the human, these cells, together with other endocrine cells, are found between the basal and neck regions of the gastric glands (see Ch. 3). The mature cells are replaced from immature precursor cells located in the isthmus of the antral glands. The turnover of the G cells is slow (unlike that of the epithelial cells). It is stimulated by gastrin. G cells (Fig. 4.2) are 'open' APUD endocrine cells (see Ch. 1). In these cells, microvilli are present along their apical surfaces, which are in contact with the lumen of the stomach. This structural feature of the cell enables it to sample the gastric contents. Receptors present on the luminal surface membrane sense chemical substances in food, known collectively as 'secretogogues', which regulate the release of gastrin (see below). Gastrin is stored in secretory granules present along the basolateral border of the cell which lies in close proximity to the blood vessels. It is released into the circulation at the basolateral membrane in response to neural, endocrine or paracrine stimuli, and by local factors in the lumen of the stomach.

Gastrin receptors

A variety of cell types possess specific surface receptors for gastrin. The oxyntic cell is the type that has been most studied. Interestingly, gastrin and cholecystokinin (CCK, a hormone secreted by the duodenal mucosa) have the same active carboxy-terminal tetrapeptide and act on the same receptors. There are two such receptors, the CCK-A receptor, present in the pancreas and the gall bladder, and the gastrin-CCK-B receptor, present on the ECL cell and the oxyntic cell. The two hormones exhibit different potencies at these receptors. CCK has a 10-fold higher potency than gastrin at the CCK-A receptor, and gastrin is the more potent at the CCK-B receptor. This difference in binding affinities between gastrin and CCK at the two CCK receptors is the main reason for their different patterns of biological activity. CCK exerts its main physiological effects on the biliary tree and the pancreas where CCK-A receptors predominate, whereas gastrin is more potent in the stomach.

Case
4.1

Peptic ulcer disease: 1

A 45-year-old man, from a family with a history of peptic ulcer disease, visited his general practitioner and complained of dull burning pain in his upper abdomen. This was associated with periodic nausea, vomiting, heartburn and loss of appetite. He was a heavy drinker and smoker. Upon examination, the pain was found to be localized to the epigastric region. The patient said that the pain was worse when his stomach was empty and was eased by eating a meal. He also complained of symptoms of hypersecretion of acid during the night. He often woke in the early hours with a burning sensation behind his lower sternum. He had been taking antacids that afforded him some relief. The doctor sent him for an endoscopy. This showed the presence of an ulcer in the proximal duodenum. He was advised to stop smoking and not to drink alcohol. He was initially prescribed ranitidine, an H_2 blocker, the preferred treatment for ulcers at the time. However after 6 weeks, the symptoms from the ulcer had not resolved. He was then prescribed omeprazole, and symptomatic relief was quickly obtained. Unfortunately, the symptoms returned after approximately 8 months. Omeprazole treatment was started again, but this time it was prescribed in combination with a course of antibiotics. His symptoms disappeared, and by 2 years later he had suffered no further relapse.

After considering the details of this case you should be able to answer the following questions:

- Why did the general practitioner suspect from what the patient said that he might have a duodenal ulcer rather than a gastric ulcer?
- Which is the most common location for ulcers in the duodenum? Why do they usually occur at that location?
- Which is the most common site for ulcers in the stomach and why do they occur at that location?
- What is the mechanism of action of H_2 receptor antagonists such as ranitidine? Why are these drugs usually effective in relieving the symptoms of peptic ulcer disease? Why should they be administered at night in this patient?
- What is the mechanism of action of omeprazole?
- Why was the patient given a course of antibiotics?

Case
4.2

Gastrinomas (Zollinger–Ellison syndrome): 1

A 40-year-old woman who had been suffering, for several years, from intermittent abdominal pain and diarrhoea, visited her general practitioner. She had previously been diagnosed (by endoscopy) as having peptic ulcer disease, and had been prescribed omeprazole and a short course of antibiotics, but with no long-term relief of her symptoms. Consequently, she had undergone surgical division of the vagal nerves to the stomach (a selective vagotomy). Surprisingly, her symptoms persisted following the surgery. Further tests were initiated to investigate the possibility that they were due to a gastrinoma. Her basal acid secretion and her acid secretion in response to an injection of pentagastrin were investigated. This involved aspiration of gastric juice. A radioimmunoassay for gastrin was performed on a blood serum sample. She was restarted on a high dose of omeprazole to protect against further ulceration, and arrangements were made for her to have a further endoscopy. Hypertrophy of the gastric rugae, and ulceration extending into the second part of the duodenum, were seen. In the light of these observations, and the abnormal plasma gastrin level found, a computerized tomogram (CT scan) of her upper abdomen was performed. This demonstrated a mass in the pancreas (fig. 4.1).

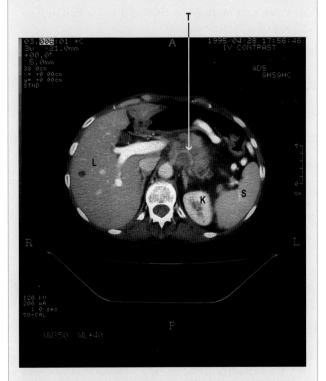

Fig. 4.1 A CT scan showing a cross-section of the upper abdomen. A large swelling in the head of the pancreas can be seen, suggestive of a tumour (T). The normal liver (L), spleen (S) and left kidney (K) are seen on the same image.

Cellular actions of gastrin on acid secretion

Oxyntic cell

In the healthy individual the secretion of acid and intrinsic factor by the oxyntic cell are regulated in parallel, so that stimulation of acid secretion is accompanied by increased secretion of intrinsic factor. Gastrin stimulates acid secretion by two mechanisms: it stimulates the oxyntic cell directly, and it stimulates it indirectly through stimulation of the ECL cell to release histamine which in

Case 4.2 Gastrinomas (Zollinger–Ellison syndrome): 1 (continued)

A laparotomy (abdominal operation) was performed and the surgeon confirmed that a tumour was present in the pancreas, and the tumour was removed. Subsequent histological analysis of the resected specimen demonstrated that the tumour was a gastrinoma. Removal of the tumour cured the patient's symptoms and her serum gastrin concentration declined to within the normal range.

After studying the details of this case we can consider the following:

- What abnormalities in blood gastrin levels, gastric acid secretion, and pepsinogen secretion, might we expect to see in this patient? What changes might we expect following surgical vagotomy?
- Why was hypertrophy of the gastric mucosa present?
- Why was ulceration seen in the second part of the duodenum? Which other sites in the gastrointestinal tract are likely to be ulcerated in this condition?
- Which of the diagnostic tests used would have given indications that the condition was Zollinger–Ellison syndrome and not simple gastric or duodenal ulceration?
- What is the rationale for treating this condition with a high dose of omeprazole?
- What are the explanations for the patient's diarrhoea?
- What are the physiological consequences of excessive gastrin and acid production?

Box 4.1 Gastrin: the first hormone

Gastrin was the first hormone to be discovered. The existence of a substance that is released into the blood in response to food in the stomach, and which circulates to stimulate acid secretion, was first proposed by Edkins in 1905. However, when it was realized that histamine, a substance present in abundance in gastric mucosa, stimulated acid secretion, it was assumed that this was the main mediator. It was not until 30 years later that Grossman and his colleagues demonstrated the existence of a blood-borne factor that stimulated acid secretion. They isolated a pouch from the body of the stomach in a dog and transplanted it into the neck region. They showed that food placed in the antrum, which remained *in situ*, stimulated acid secretion in the transplanted pouch. Increased secretion occurred even if the antrum was denervated, indicating that the stimulus was a blood-borne factor released from the gastric antrum; that is, a 'hormone'. In 1964, Gregory and Tracey isolated the pure peptide hormone from hog stomach. It was subsequently called gastrin.

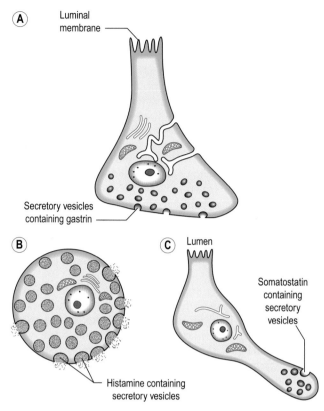

Fig. 4.2 (A) Gastrin-secreting (G) cell. (B) Histamine secreting (ECL) cell. (C) Somatostatin secreting cell.

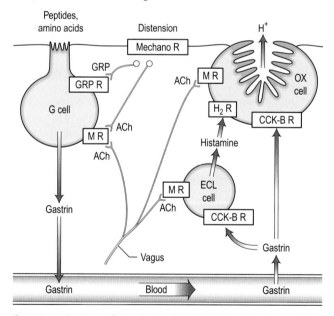

Fig. 4.3 Mechanisms of stimulation of acid secretion from the oxyntic cell by gastrin, histamine and neurotransmitters. ACh, acetylcholine; GRP, gastrin–releasing peptide; CCK-BR, cholecystokinin B receptor; H_2R, histamine H_2 receptor; MR, muscarinic receptor; OX, oxyntic.

turn stimulates the oxyntic cell (Fig. 4.3). It binds to CCK-B receptors on the cell membranes in both types of cell. The result of this stimulation is the incorporation of proton pumps into the canalicular membrane of the oxyntic cell (see Ch. 3). Gastrin also stimulates the expression of the gene for the proton pump in the oxyntic cell, thereby increasing its synthesis.

Gastrin also has trophic actions. It controls the growth and proliferation of a variety of cell types in the gastric mucosa, including ECL cells and the precursors of oxyntic cells. Hyperplasia of ECL cells and oxyntic cells occurs in conditions where hypergastrinaemia is present (see Case 4.2: 2).

ECL cell and histamine

Gastrin binds with a high affinity to CCK-B receptors on ECL cells, to cause the release of histamine (Fig. 4.3). Histamine acts in a paracrine manner on the oxyntic cell to release acid. The binding of gastrin to the ECL cell also stimulates histamine synthesis from histidine (see below).

It is produced in large amounts by the gastric mucosa. It is produced by decarboxylation of histidine:

$$\text{Histidine} \xrightarrow{\text{histidine decarboxylase}} \text{histamine} + CO_2$$

Histamine acts on H_2 receptors on the oxyntic cells to release acid (Fig. 4.3) via a cyclic AMP-mediated mechanism. Its presence is necessary for the secretion of normal amounts of acid. Thus inhibition of the enzyme histidine decarboxylase reduces acid secretion.

Neural control of gastric secretion

The functions of the stomach are controlled by intrinsic nerves in the internal nerve plexi of the enteric nervous system and by extrinsic nerve fibres in the vagus nerve and sympathetic nerves (see Ch. 1). Axons of nerve fibres (in the intramural plexi) innervate both secretory cells and smooth muscle cells. In general activation of cholinergic fibres stimulates gastric secretion and motility. Cases 4.1 and 4.2: 2 shows the arrangement of the vagal cholinergic nerve trunks that innervate the stomach. Activation of adrenergic fibres generally inhibits secretion and motility.

It should also be noted that a number of sensory nerves leave the stomach and travel in the vagus nerve and the sympathetic nerves. Sensory nerves in the stomach also provide afferent paths of intrinsic reflex arcs, which travel in the intramural plexi of the stomach. This provides some intrinsic control of smooth muscle contractions and gastric juice secretion.

Acetylcholine and gastrin-releasing peptide

Acetylcholine released from cholinergic nerve fibres in local nerves can stimulate oxyntic cells to release acid, or G cells to secrete gastrin. Some fibres in the vagus nerve also contain gastrin-releasing peptide (GRP), which exists as two major forms, in which the active site is a nonapeptide. The structurally similar peptide bombesin that has been extracted from the skin of the frog *Bombina bombina* has similar actions. GRP released from nerves in

the stomach stimulates gastrin release from the G cells (Fig. 4.3). It probably also stimulates acid release by a gastrin-independent mechanism. This interaction of the neural and gastrin control mechanisms facilitates a rapid response to food ingestion.

Inhibitory control of acid secretion

Feedback control via acid

Gastric acid secretion is blocked if the contents of the stomach become too acid (pH 3.0, or lower). This is a negative feedback mechanism that prevents the gastric contents (and probably more importantly the duodenal contents) from becoming too acid. When the acidity of the stomach reaches pH 2.0 it is virtually impossible to stimulate gastrin release by any means. The inhibition is indirect and is exerted via inhibition of gastrin release. In conditions where achlorhydria (lack of acid secretion) is present (such as some types of pernicious anaemia), there are usually high levels of gastrin in the blood because this feedback mechanism cannot operate. The inhibitory action of acid on gastrin secretion is due to its action to stimulate the release of the hormone somatostatin from D cells in the mucosa. Somatostatin is a potent inhibitor of acid secretion; it inhibits gastrin secretion from G cells and histamine secretion from ECL cells. Furthermore, the D cells exhibit gastrin-binding sites, and gastrin itself can stimulate somatostatin release from these cells. However these binding sites are probably CCK-A receptors which are more sensitive to CCK than to gastrin. Stimulation of somatostatin release via these receptors is therefore probably normally due mainly to circulating CCK (see below).

In both peptic ulcer disease and in Zollinger–Ellison syndrome, acid secretion is increased but gastrin levels are only increased in Zollinger-Ellison syndrome (Cases 4.1: 2 and 4.2: 2).

Somatostatin

Somatostatin exists predominantly as the 14-amino-acid peptide somatostatin-14 in D-cells in the fundic and antral mucosa. It is released from cytoplasmic processes on the D cells in the antrum in the vicinity of its target cell, the G-cell (Fig. 4.5). It binds to somatostatin-2 (ST-2) receptors on the G cells. It acts primarily in a paracrine manner via diffusion in the intercellular spaces, but it also acts systemically through its release into the local mucosal circulation. Somatostatin also acts on ECL cells to inhibit histamine release. These interactions are outlined for the antrum region in Figure 4.5. Somatostatin also acts upon the oxyntic cells in the fundus to inhibit the release of acid directly.

Fundic D cells are 'closed' APUD cells (see Ch. 1) and do not respond to luminal acidity. Somatostatin appears to exert a tonic inhibition of acid release in the fundus. However, antral D cells are 'open' APUD cells, and they respond to changes in H^+ concentration in the stomach

Causes and diagnosis

Individuals with duodenal ulcer disease often have a family history of the condition. The duodenum is the most frequent site for ulcer formation, the duodenal cap being the most vulnerable area. Excessive secretion of acid and pepsinogen are directly implicated in chronic ulceration of the duodenum. High H^+ concentration can lead to the breakdown of the protective mechanisms of the mucosal barrier (see Box 4.3). Patients with simple duodenal ulcer usually have a high basal acid output with normal levels of serum gastrin. In contrast, patients with gastric ulcer appear to have normal or slightly low acid secretion (Table 4.1). In gastric ulcer the primary defect may be a reduced ability of the mucosa to withstand damage by acid and pepsin (see Cases 4.1 and 4.2: 1).

An endoscopy can be carried out on patients with suspected peptic ulcer to locate an ulcer and confirm that it is not a tumour (which can present with similar symptoms).

The patient described in Case 4.1 demonstrated hypersecretion of acid which is more typical of a duodenal ulcer than a gastric ulcer. He also complained of heartburn and pain when his stomach was empty. Eating provided relief because food buffers the acid. Symptoms of hypersecretion at night are supposedly more usually seen with a duodenal rather than a gastric ulcer but in practice there is often overlap of symptoms between the two types. In the case of a duodenal ulcer the symptoms usually last for a few weeks followed by a remission.

Gastric ulcer

Although a family history is often present in duodenal ulcer inheritance appears to be unimportant in gastric ulcer. In a patient with gastric ulcer the pain is poorly localized but may be perceived in the midline area. It occurs at any time but is often worse during or after a meal. Physical examination does not usually demonstrate epigastric tenderness. There is not usually nausea or vomiting and food does not ease the pain. In practice,

however, the differential diagnosis between gastric and duodenal ulcer cannot be ascertained on the basis of symptoms alone.

Figure 4.4 shows an X-ray of the stomach of a patient with a chronic gastric ulcer.

An endoscopy would demonstrate a gastric ulcer. In the case of a suspected gastric ulcer it is important to ask whether the patient has lost weight and to take a biopsy of the ulcerated mucosa because there is a risk of malignancy, which is not seen in the case of a duodenal ulcer.

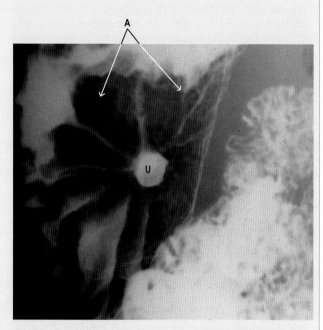

Fig. 4.4 An X-ray of the stomach taken after ingestion of barium. The normal folds of the antrum (A) have been disrupted by the chronic ulceration, giving rise to linear scarring around the ulcer (U).

Table 4.1 Acid and gastrin secretion in peptic ulcer disease and Zollinger–Ellison syndrome

Acid	Rate of acid secretion			Blood gastrin (pmol/L)
	Basal day (mmol/h)	Basal night (mmol/12 h)	Maximum (mmol/h)	
Normal	1–5	18	25	30
Gastric ulcer	1–5	8	25	30
Duodenal ulcer	4–10	60	40	30
ZES	45	120	55	650

Typical mean values are given for acid secretion and blood gastrin levels in normal subjects, and patients with simple gastric ulcer, duodenal ulcer or Zollinger–Ellison (ZES) syndrome. Maximum acid output is elicited by injection of pentagastrin (6 μg/kg).

| Case 4.2 | Gastrinomas (Zollinger–Ellison syndrome): 2 |

Causes and diagnosis

In 40% of patients with Zollinger–Ellison syndrome familial inheritance has been recorded. The syndrome can be inherited in an autosomal dominant fashion, so relatives may be affected. For this reason it is important to obtain a family history from patients diagnosed with the disease.

The gastrinomas present may be ectopic, commonly presenting in the pancreas. They may be small and difficult to locate. In 60% of patients, the tumours are malignant. The gastrinoma tumours secrete excessive amounts of gastrin into the portal blood stream. The high serum gastrin levels elicit massive secretion of acid from the oxyntic cells. It is the basal acid secretion (which occurs between meals) that is stimulated to the greatest extent by the high gastrin levels. The secretion of gastrin from the gastrinomas (as with many other secretory tumours) is independent of secretogogues such as peptides in the stomach. Thus secretion of acid during a meal is not abnormally affected. Table 4.1 shows typical values for the basal and maximum acid secretion (induced by injection of pentagastrin), and serum gastrin levels in normal individuals, and in patients with gastric ulcer, duodenal ulcer, or Zollinger–Ellison syndrome. The basal acid output is usually considerably elevated in Zollinger–Ellison syndrome. However, the maximum acid output measured after pentagastrin injection is not increased proportionately, unlike in normal individuals or patients with peptic ulcer disease. The basal acid output is usually not less than 60% of the maximum output, and is often the same as the maximum output.

In normal individuals, a low pH in the stomach lumen inhibits acid secretion by inhibiting gastrin secretion from the antral G cells (see below) but secretion by gastrinomas is independent of this feedback control.

Pepsinogen secretion is also stimulated by gastrin, so its secretion is also usually abnormally high in Zollinger–Ellison syndrome.

Diagnosis

The diagnosis of Zollinger–Ellison syndrome requires consideration of the results of a number of different procedures. Basal acid secretion is dramatically elevated, and serum gastrin levels are often elevated over 10-fold, as a consequence of the uncontrolled secretion (Table 4.1). However, high basal acid production by the stomach and high levels of gastrin in the blood are merely suggestive of the condition.

The 'secretin test' has been used in the past to assist the diagnosis of Zollinger–Ellison syndrome, but now that gastrin levels can be measured directly and accurately by radioimmunoassay, it is no longer often employed. The basis of the test depends on the fact that whereas secretin infusion normally inhibits acid secretion during the intestinal phase of digestion (by acting on the oxyntic cell directly and on the G cell), and normally has little effect on basal acid secretion between meals, it stimulates secretion of gastrin from ectopic gastrinomas; the so-called 'paradoxical' effect of secretin in Zollinger–Ellison syndrome.

Radiological imaging (Fig. 4.4), particularly magnetic resonance imaging (MRI) can detect lesions as small as 1 cm in diameter. When malignant lesions are present, metastases are usually visible in the liver. Exploratory surgery is required to confirm the lesion (and to remove benign tumours). Malignant tumours are usually treated with proton pump inhibitors to simply control the symptoms of excessive acid secretion.

Note: Gastrin has trophic actions on the mucosa of the gastrointestinal tract. It is a growth factor for the stomach mucosa and in Zollinger–Ellison syndrome the high levels can stimulate hypertrophy of the mucosa. The rugal folds may become extremely thick. This can sometimes be seen in medical imaging procedures such as the barium meal test.

---

lumen. During a meal, as the contents of the stomach become increasingly acid, secretion from the oxyntic cell declines, due to the action of somatostatin. The release of somatostatin is inhibited when the luminal acid is neutralized.

Other inhibitory factors

Numerous peptides inhibit gastric acid secretion. Some of these peptides are released from APUD cells by the presence of chyme in the duodenum (see below). Importantly, CCK, which is secreted in response to fat, causes inhibition of acid secretion in two ways:

- It competitively inhibits gastrin-mediated stimulation of acid release by binding to CCK-B receptors on the oxyntic cell and the ECL cell. A high level of CCK in the blood (if gastrin levels are high) results in displacement of gastrin from its receptors, but as it is less potent than gastrin this results in reduced acid secretion, when gastrin is present in the circulation

- It is a potent antagonist of gastrin-stimulated acid secretion, by its action on CCK-B receptors on D cells, to release somatostatin, which in turn inhibits acid secretion.

The duodenal hormone secretin also produces a profound inhibition of gastrin release and gastric acid secretion. It is released in response to the presence of food in the duodenum. It is a 27-amino-acid peptide which has structural similarities to the pancreatic hormone glucagon. The most potent stimulus for secretin release is acid in the duodenum. Secretin inhibits the secretion of gastrin from G cells and the secretion of acid from oxyntic cells. Other peptides which inhibit gastric acid release, include gastric inhibitory peptide (GIP, a 43-amino-acid peptide) released in response to fat in the duodenum or ileum, and the 28-amino-acid peptide vasoactive intestinal peptide (VIP), which is released into the circulation from nerve endings in the enteric nerves of the submucosal and myenteric plexi. VIP and GIP have considerable sequence homology (14 amino-acids) with secretin, and they act on the same receptors as secretin on oxyntic cells and G cells to inhibit acid release. The receptors for all these hormones are denoted VIP receptors. Although the primary effect of these peptides is to reduce gastric juice secretion, tumours of APUD cells, such as VIPomas, cause increased motility, and consequently diarrhoea. Table 4.2 summarizes the actions of some of the endogenous peptides which inhibit acid production, and indicates their sites of release, and the likely mechanisms involved.

Finally, prostaglandins synthesized in the gastric mucosa inhibit acid secretion. They function to protect the deeper mucosal layers from damage by acid (as discussed below).

Control of pepsinogen secretion

Pepsin is a proteolytic enzyme which is responsible for only 15% of dietary protein digestion in the gastrointestinal tract and this role is dispensable (see Ch. 3). It is important clinically however, because it exacerbates the acid-induced ulceration of the stomach and duodenum (Cases 4.1 and 4.2: 1).

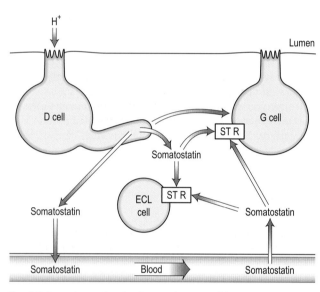

Fig. 4.5 Paracrine and endocrine mechanisms of feedback inhibition of acid secretion by somatostatin released in response to low pH in the antrum. STR, somatostatin receptor.

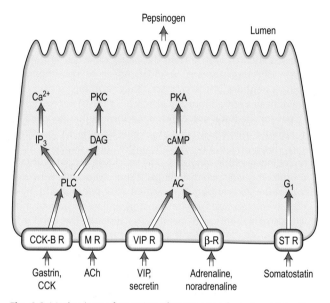

Fig. 4.6 Mechanisms of secretion of pepsinogen from the chief cell. CCK, cholecystokinin; ACh, acetylcholine; MR, muscarinic receptor; VIP, vasoactive intestinal peptide; R, receptor; PKC, protein kinase C; PKA, protein kinase A; DAG, diacylglycerol; AC, adenyl cyclase; IP$_3$, inositol trisphosphate; β-R, β-adrenergic receptor; STR, somatostatin receptor; G$_1$, G protein.

Table 4.2 Gastrointestinal peptides that inhibit acid production in the stomach

Peptide	Main stimulus	Location	Mechanism of action
Somatostatin	Acid	D cells (Stomach)	inhibition of heritance and gastrin release
CCK	Fat	APUD CELLS (duodenum)	Somatostatin release (CCK-B receptors) Competes with gastrin (CCK-A receptors)
		Enteric nerves	
Secretin	Acid	APUD cells (duodenum)	Inhibition of gastrin and acid release
GIP	Fat	APUD cells	Inhibition of gastrin and acid release
		Enteric nerves	
VIP	Distension of stomach	Enteric nerves	Somatostatin

CCK, cholecystokinin; GIP, gastric inhibitory peptide; VIP, vasoactive intestinal peptide; ACh, acetylcholine.

Pepsinogen, the precursor of pepsin, is released from the chief cell by acetylcholine, as well as by a number of gastrointestinal hormones. Figure 4.6 illustrates the various secretogogues and their receptors and the second messenger systems involved in their actions. Acetylcholine released upon stimulation of the vagus nerve and local nerves is probably the most potent stimulus. It acts on muscarinic receptors on the chief cell membrane. H^+ ions trigger the local cholinergic reflex that stimulates the chief cells. They also enhance the effects of other stimuli on the chief cell. In addition H^+ ions stimulate the release of secretin in the duodenum (see below) and secretin also stimulates pepsinogen secretion. These effects of H^+ may account in part for the correlation between acid and pepsin secretion. Gastrin stimulates pepsinogen secretion directly via CCK receptors, but the most potent effect of gastrin on pepsinogen secretion is its indirect action via acid secretion.

Activation of muscarinic receptors, and CCK (CCK-A and CCK-B receptors) on the chief cells, results in the generation of inositol trisphosphate and diacylglycerol. The relative importance of these two intracellular messengers has not yet been elucidated. Receptors for secretin, VIP, cholera toxin and prostaglandins are also present but these are linked to the adenyl cyclase-cAMP second messenger system. Pepsinogen secretion is decreased by somatostatin, which inhibits adenyl cyclase in the chief cell.

Protective mechanisms in the mucosa

The mucosal barrier

The mucosa of the stomach and duodenum is protected from acid damage by:

- Secretion of alkaline fluid

- Secretion of mucus. Surface mucous cells secrete mucus in response to chemicals such as alcohol, and in response to contact with roughage in the food. Mucus neck cells are also stimulated by gastrin to secrete mucus

- Adequate blood flow

- The presence of growth factors which promote the replacement of damaged cells

- Prostaglandins, which maintain mucosal integrity and cause decreased acid secretion and increased bi-carbonate and mucin production and increased blood flow, all of which modify the local inflammatory response caused by high acidity. Non-steroidal anti-inflammatory drugs (NSAIDs) inhibit prostaglandin synthesis (see Box 4.2).

In peptic ulcer disease the protective mechanisms are inadequate. The mechanisms of ulcer formation in the stomach and the duodenum are described in Cases 4.1 and 4.2: 1.

Acid reduction therapy

A variety of different classes of drugs can be effective in the treatment of peptic ulcer disease and other conditions such as gastrinomas and acid reflux. Figure 4.8 shows the sites of action of the different drugs which can inhibit acid secretion in the stomach. The treatment of peptic ulcer disease and gastrinomas with such drugs is discussed in Cases 4.1 and 4.2: 1. Reduction of acid secretion by drug therapy will increase the pH of the chyme and thereby reduce the activity of pepsin, and so also protect the mucosa from its action.

Antacids

Antacids are weak bases that act by neutralizing gastric acid (Fig. 4.8). Raising the pH of the stomach contents results in suppression of the action of pepsin that exacerbates ulceration due to acid. Thus, antacids can be used to relieve gastric pain caused by excessive acid secretion. Compounds that are commonly used include magnesium hydroxide, magnesium trisilicate, aluminium hydroxide. Sodium bicarbonate is a rapidly acting antacid, but it should not be used for long-term treatment in peptic ulcer disease as it is absorbed in the intestines and may cause metabolic alkalosis. The release of CO_2 from bicarbonate dissolved in the stomach chyme can also be a problem as it causes belching (eructation).

H_2 receptor antagonists

Histamine H_2 receptor antagonists competitively inhibit the actions of histamine at H_2 receptors on the oxyntic cell,

---

Box 4.2 Non-steroidal anti-inflammatory drugs and ulceration

Ingestion of non-steroidal anti-inflammatory drugs (NSAIDs) such as aspirin (acetylsalicylate) can cause ulceration of the gastric mucosa because they inhibit prostaglandin synthesis by inhibiting the enzyme cyclooxygenase. Indeed a deficiency of prostaglandins may be a contributing factor in peptic ulcer formation. Aspirin is a weak acid and at low pH values it tends to exist in the unionized form. The unionized acid is lipid soluble and it is readily absorbed across the lipid membranes of the stomach. Because prostaglandins inhibit acid secretion, inhibition of prostaglandin synthesis by aspirin results in increased acid secretion. This may result in ulceration in some individuals. The mechanism probably also involves disruption of the normal body repair mechanisms including cell turnover, which prevents healing of small abrasions in the mucosa.

Interestingly however, this reduction in cell turnover by aspirin is protective against cancer in the mucosa of the colon (see Ch. 11).

thereby reducing acid secretion (Fig. 4.8). These drugs are usually effective in relieving the symptoms of peptic ulcer disease (Cases 4.1 and 4.2: 2). These drugs can inhibit acid secretion by up to 90% and promote healing of the ulcers. The drugs used are cimetidine, ranitidine, famotidine and nizatidine. Long-term maintenance with these drugs was widely used until effective treatment with proton pump inhibitors and antibiotics became available.

Proton pump inhibitors

Proton pump inhibitors block the hydrogen ion pumps in the oxyntic cell. They include omeprazole and lansoprazole (Fig. 4.8 and Cases 4.1 and 4.2: 2). These powerful drugs block the H^+/K^+ ATPase proton pump, markedly inhibiting both basal and stimulated secretion of gastric acid. Omeprazole is a powerful proton pump inhibitor. It is a weak base which acts by blocking the H^+/K^+ ATPase activity of the proton pump. It is inactive at neutral pH, but it is activated in acid conditions (pH 3.0 and below). Such conditions exist only in the canaliculi of the oxyntic cell. The action of the drug is therefore restricted to this location in the gastrointestinal tract thereby avoiding the unwanted side-effects of disruption of Cl^- ion transport, which could occur in other organs such as the lungs, pancreas and skin (sweating) with use of other H^+ transport inhibitors which are active in less acid conditions.

Cases 4.1 and 4.2

Peptic ulcer disease and gastrinomas: 1

Ulceration of the mucosa

Peptic ulcers can occur in the stomach or duodenum. However, the most common location for ulcers is in the duodenum. There are differences in the mechanisms of ulcer formation depending on their location. In the duodenum, the primary defect appears to be hypersecretion of acid, but in the stomach the main defect is probably a deficiency in the protective mucosal barrier.

Duodenum

Duodenal ulcers usually occur at the duodenal cap, where the acidic chyme meets the duodenal mucosa, before it mixes with the alkaline secretions of the duodenum. The duodenum does not have the same protective mechanisms as the stomach mucosa. In individuals with duodenal ulcers there is often a higher than normal basal secretion of acid, and an abnormally high rate of maximum secretion in response to histamine stimulation.

Individuals with duodenal ulcer may have twice the average normal number of oxyntic cells in their mucosae. In addition pepsinogen secretion is also usually high. The sensitivity to gastrin, the hormone that stimulates acid secretion is also usually increased in these individuals. If acid concentrations are high, local vasodilation initially allows mucus and bicarbonate production to be maintained.

The eventual consequence is that chyme with an abnormally high level of acid and pepsin is passed into the duodenum where the mucosa is not protected, resulting in the formation of ulcers.

Helicobacter pylori (*H. pylori*) has high urease activity. This causes increased NH_4^+ production from urea. This allows the bacteria to colonize in the acid environment. The bacteria also release cytokines that are involved in the inflammatory response. *H. pylori* has been implicated in causing hypersecretion of gastric acid in duodenal ulceration. It does this by inhibiting the secretion of somatostatin that inhibits acid secretion. The inhibition of somatostatin release results in removal of its inhibitory effect on gastrin release and consequently increases the rate of gastrin secretion. This stimulates more acid production. The trophic effect of gastrin to stimulate proliferation of the oxyntic and peptic cells in the gastric mucosa could exacerbate the condition as this would result in increased acid and pepsin secretion.

Stomach

The most common site in the stomach for ulcers to occur is the antrum, where the oxyntic mucosa meets the pyloric mucosa, i.e. the acid acts on the mucosa that does not have the same protective mechanisms as the body and fundus.

The stomach normally has a low permeability to acid due to the presence of the protective mucosal barrier. The barrier is partly due to the presence of mucins but other factors such as adequate blood flow and the presence of growth factors, which promote the replacement of damaged cells, are also important. However, it should be noted that mucus does not form a continuous layer and the protection is due to a great extent to the fact that the rate of acid production keeps pace with the buffering capacity of the food. Peptic ulcers (Fig. 4.4) form in the stomach due to the action of acid when the mucosal barrier is damaged and the stomach is unable to protect itself and replace the damaged cells. Thus ulcers in the stomach are not usually due to an increased rate of acid secretion but rather to a defect in the ability of the mucosa to withstand damage (which may be caused by substances such as aspirin, ethanol and bile salts). In fact in some individuals with peptic ulcers, the rate of acid secretion may be lower than normal. The decreased rate of acid secretion is caused in part by H^+ ions leaking into the mucosa in exchange for Na^+. The H^+ ions accumulate and the pH of the cells falls. This results in cellular injury and cell death. The H^+ ions also damage mucosal mast cells causing them to release histamine.

This exacerbates the condition by acting on the mucosal capillaries causing ischaemia and vascular damage. A small amount of blood loss (occult) is usually associated with the ulcer, and in chronic ulcers this will result in anaemia. Occasionally, the ulceration can erode into a major vessel (commonly the gastroduodenal artery behind the first part of the duodenum) and life-threatening bleeding can occur.

H. pylori has been implicated in gastric ulcer as well as duodenal ulcer disease. It is responsible for breaking down the gastric epithelial barrier in gastric ulcer disease. It penetrates the barrier and releases digestive enzymes that digest the stomach wall. Local vasodilation initially allows mucus and bicarbonate production to be maintained. The entry of acid into the mucosa damages mast cells, causing increased release of histamine that results in inflammation. Other factors (PAF, leukotrienes, etc.) that cause a reduction in blood flow may be produced. *H. pylori* also increases gastric acid secretion by the mechanism described above. Thus, although an increase in acid secretion cannot be measured in gastric ulcer disease it is probably increased, but in this case the acid leaks back across the defective epithelium.

Role of pepsin in ulceration

The presence of pepsin is implicated in acid-induced ulceration. This enzyme can digest damaged mucosa in the oesophagus, stomach, and duodenum, when activated by the presence of acid. Disruption of the mucosal barrier will provide the opportunity for pepsin to digest the columnar epithelium and promote ulceration. Thus, pepsin potentiates (rather than initiates) ulcer formation.

Gastrinomas

The massive secretion of acid and pepsinogen in Zollinger–Ellison syndrome (Table 4.1) leads to widespread ulceration of the upper gastrointestinal tract. In this disease, ulcers may occur in the oesophagus, the stomach and the duodenum. In the duodenum they occur at the same sites where they are seen in simple duodenal ulcers, in which the first part of the duodenum is the typical site. However, they may also occur at more distal sites in the duodenum, because of the very low pH, and the high pepsin content, of the chyme leaving the stomach.

Treatment

Drug therapy

A variety of different classes of drugs can be effective in the treatment of peptic ulcer disease. Currently antacids, H_2 receptor blockers, proton pump inhibitors and antibiotics all have a role to play.

Long-term treatment with antacids can produce healing of duodenal ulcers but they are ineffective for healing gastric ulcers.

Patients often self-medicate with H_2 blockers as they are available without prescription and are effective in controlling the symptoms. They are most effective if taken at night because the hypersecretion of acid from the empty stomach at night and its entry into the empty duodenum may be the most important factor in duodenal ulcer formation. When the stomach contains food, buffering of acid, by proteins for example, and the mixing of acid in the chyme reduces the exposure of the mucosa to the acid. These drugs can inhibit acid secretion by up to 90% and promote healing of the ulcers. However, if treatment is withdrawn in patients with duodenal ulcers the ulcers are likely to reoccur.

Proton pump blockers, such as omeprazole, are very powerful drugs for reducing acid secretion. They are usually the first-line therapy in controlling the symptoms of peptic ulcer disease

as well as reflux oesophagitis and gastrinomas. However, if the treatment is withdrawn the ulcers usually reoccur.

Triple therapy

Combinations of omeprazole (see below) and antibiotics have proved to be extremely effective in the treatment and often the cure of duodenal ulcers. In practice, 'triple therapy' consisting of a proton pump inhibitor and the antibiotics amoxicillin and either metronidazole or clarithromycin is often instigated. *H. pylori* is generally eradicated after 2 weeks of this regimen.

Surgery

Treatment with H_2 antagonists or proton pump inhibitors and antibiotics is highly effective for duodenal or gastric ulcers but surgery is sometimes necessary. Most bleeding ulcers require endoscopy to stop bleeding with cautery, or injection. Surgery for peptic ulcer disease is usually restricted to patients with complications such as haemorrhage from a blood vessel at the base of an ulcer (usually the gastroduodenal artery which passes behind the first part of the duodenum), and erosion through the stomach into the peritoneal cavity which results in perforation and peritonitis due to leakage of duodenal contents into the cavity. If a peptic ulcer perforates, air leaks into the peritoneal cavity. If the patient stands erect the air will float to a position under the diaphragm. This can be detected by a chest X-ray.

(Continued)

Prior to the development of effective drug treatment, surgery was the main treatment for chronic peptic ulcer disease. It involved either division of the vagus nerve (vagotomy), or antrectomy (resection of the stomach antrum). Vagotomy was performed to reduce vagal stimulation of acid secretion in the stomach. Unfortunately, this also resulted in impairment of gastric motility and emptying. To overcome this problem, division of the pyloric muscle (pyloroplasty) was also performed. In the 1970s highly selective vagotomy, which preserved the function of the pyloric muscle, was developed (Fig. 4.7). This circumvented the need for a pyloroplasty.

A more radical approach sometimes used was surgical removal of the antrum (antrectomy) that was performed in order to remove the G cells and so reduce gastrin stimulation of acid secretion. As gastrin has trophic actions to maintain the gastric mucosa, patients who have undergone resection of the antrum have low circulating gastrin concentrations and may display atrophy of the oxyntic glandular mucosa.

Gastrinomas

The recognized treatment for Zollinger–Ellison syndrome is first to control the overproduction of acid by treatment with a proton pump inhibitor, such as omeprazole. This enables the ulcers to heal and controls the diarrhoea. Patients usually survive for many years with pharmacological treatment alone. When the ulcers are under control, surgery to remove a gastrinoma can be attempted to try to effect a cure.

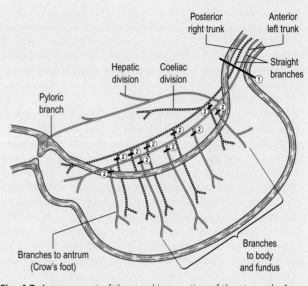

Fig. 4.7 Arrangement of the vagal innervation of the stomach. 1. Site of vagus nerve in a vagotomy; 2. sites of nerve section in a highly selective vagotomy.

However, many patients with Zollinger—Ellison syndrome (approximately 25%) have multiple endocrine neoplasia type 1 (MEN 1), which may preclude surgical intervention.

Omeprazole has few unwanted side-effects, although there remains concern about lowering acid secretion too drastically, because of the resultant elevation of serum gastrin levels, which in theory could be mitogenic (and therefore tumour-promoting) because acid is a potent inhibitor of G cell proliferation, and because of this, the chronic administration of a proton pump blocker such as omeprazole results in proliferation of G cells and ECL cells. For this reason, if omeprazole treatment is suddenly discontinued, rebound hyperacidity can result.

Muscarinic receptor antagonists

Anticholinergic drugs that bind to muscarinic M_2 receptors on the oxyntic cell and the ECL cell can antagonize the effects of vagal nerve stimulation and reduce gastric acid secretion (Fig. 4.8). Most muscarinic M_2 antagonists are less effective than H_2 receptor antagonists or proton pump blockers, although they can have beneficial antispasmodic effects on gut smooth muscle. Furthermore muscarinic receptors are present at many locations within the gastrointestinal tract and outside it, and for this reason, parasympathetic side effects, including effects on the cardiovascular system, are common with these drugs.

However, the drug pirenzepine is a relatively specific M_1 receptor antagonist that probably acts on postsynaptic nerves in parasympathetic ganglia, to block the stimulation of oxyntic cells.

Antibiotics

Over the last few years, evidence has accumulated that chronic infection of the gastric mucosa by the bacterium *Helicobacter pylori* is causally involved in potentiating peptic ulcer disease. These bacteria are present in the stomach in many individuals but only a minority develop peptic ulcer disease. The reasons for this are unknown. Over 80% of patients with gastric or duodenal ulcers are infected with it. It is a spiral Gram-negative bacterium which can survive in the low pH environment in the stomach. The action of this organism leads to impairment of the function of the protective mucosal barrier. It is sensitive to a large number of antibiotics but those that penetrate the submucosa where the microorganisms reside, such as clarithromycin and metronidazole, are the most effective. Eradication of *H. pylori* by antibiotic therapy prevents ulcer recurrence and so prevents the need for long-term treatment.

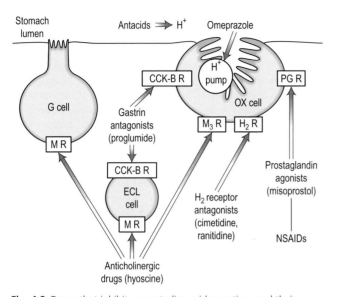

Fig. 4.8 Drugs that inhibit or neutralize acid secretion, and their targets. OX, oxyntic cell; M R, muscarinic receptor; H_2 R, histamine H_2 receptor; CCK-B R, cholecystokinin-B receptor; PG R, prostaglandin receptor; NSAIDs, non-steroidal anti-inflammatory drugs.

Box 4.3 *H. pylori* and peptic ulcers: history

The role of bacterial infection in peptic ulcer disease was disputed for many years, in spite of some compelling evidence. The first recorded use of antibiotics to treat peptic ulcers was by Lykoudis, a Greek general practitioner, in 1958. In 1982 Warren and Marshall, two Australian doctors, rediscovered this role for bacteria. They proposed that peptic ulcer disease and gastritis were caused by colonization with *H. pylori*. This hypothesis was not well-received by the drug companies, so Marshall performed an experiment upon himself to demonstrate the role of *H. pylori*. He drank a culture of organisms extracted from a patient and soon developed gastritis. His symptoms disappeared after 2 weeks but he treated himself with antibiotics to kill the remaining bacteria at the urging of his wife, as halitosis is one of the symptoms of infection. In 1997, a campaign was launched to educate healthcare providers about the link between *H. pylori* and peptic ulcer disease. In 2005, Warren and Marshall were awarded the Nobel Prize for their discovery.

Short-term treatment with antibiotics combined with symptomatic relief by a proton pump inhibitor is now the standard treatment for peptic ulcer disease (Box 4.3).

Other possible drug treatments

Prostaglandins, which are synthesized in the gastric and intestinal mucosa, can also be effective in reducing acid secretion. In particular, prostaglandins of the E (PGE) and I (PGI) series can be administered to protect the deeper mucosal cells from damage. PGE1 and PGE2 and stable analogues such as misoprostol also inhibit the histamine-mediated stimulation of acid secretion (Fig. 4.8). In practice, their use has been superceded by proton pump inhibitors in the prevention of gastric damage from chronic use of non-steroidal anti-inflammatory drugs (NSAIDs), such as aspirin (see Box 4.2).

Antagonists of gastrin have been developed (Fig. 4.8). An example is proglumide. However, these compounds are not potent enough for clinical use. Finally, agonists of somatostatin and duodenal peptides such as secretin could theoretically be useful in peptic ulcer disease, but at the present time suitable stable analogues of such drugs are not yet available.

Control of motility in the stomach

In the stomach, the pacemaker cells are located in the longitudinal muscle in the greater curvature region of the fundus. The basal electrical rhythm (spontaneously oscillating membrane potential) generates action potentials in the pacemaker cells and these are transmitted through the sheets of smooth muscle. The muscle therefore exhibits contractile activity even in the resting state (see Ch. 1). This contractile activity can be increased or decreased in amplitude and frequency by factors that control the electrical activity of the smooth muscle cell membranes.

The electrical changes are of different shape and amplitude in different regions of the stomach. The membrane potential is relatively stable in the fundus region, but a slow wave can be recorded in the rest of the stomach. This slow wave is of relatively small amplitude in the body of the stomach but its amplitude progressively increases in regions closer to the pylorus. The frequency of the slow waves remains the same, approximately 3/min, in the different regions because they are driven by the same pacemaker cells (see Ch. 1). In gastric smooth muscle, there is a threshold potential for action, potential generation and contraction of the muscle. When the membrane potential during the slow wave exceeds the threshold, contraction occurs (Fig. 4.9). The greater the depolarization and the longer the membrane potential remains above the threshold, the more action potentials are generated and the greater the tension developed.

In the antrum the action potentials exhibit an initial rapid depolarization phase, followed by a long plateau phase (Fig. 4.9). The rapid depolarization phase is caused by Ca^{2+} entry into the cells through voltage-gated channels and the plateau phase is due to entry of both Ca^{2+} and Na^+ through slower voltage-gated channels. The influx of Ca^{2+} leads to muscle contraction (see Ch. 1). In the terminal antrum, action potential spikes occur on the plateaus of the slow waves. Trains of action potentials that occur during the plateau phase elicit vigorous contractions in the antrum and these can lead to gastric emptying.

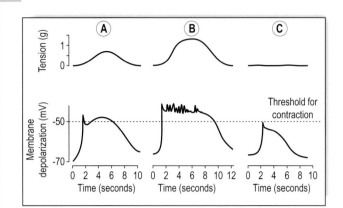

Fig. 4.9 Control of smooth muscle contraction in the stomach antrum. (A) Electrical recordings of the membrane potential in the absence of chemical mediators. (B,C) Effects of gastrin and noradrenaline, respectively, on the membrane electrical changes and the contractile force.

Table 4.3 Endogenous factors which control smooth muscle tension

Factor	Location	Stimulus	Receptor
Depolarization (increased muscle tension)			
Stretch	Stomach	Distension	
Ach	Nerves	Distension, peptides	Muscarinic
Gastrin	Stomach	Peptides, distension	CCK-B
Hyperpolarization (decreased muscle tension)			
NA, adrenaline	Nerves	Stress (e.g. exercise)	β-adrenergic
ATP	Nerves	Chewing, taste, smells, etc.	Purinergic
CCK	Duodenum	Fat	CCK-A?
Secretin	Duodenum	Acid	VIP
VIP	Enteric nerves	Distension	VIP
GIP	Duodenum	Fat	VIP

ACh, acetylcholine; NA, noradrenaline; VIP, vasoactive intestinal peptide; GIP, gastric inhibitory peptide; CCK, cholecystokinin.

Box 4.4 Postoperative gastric stasis

After surgical procedures, motility in the stomach is inhibited. This is known as gastric stasis. If severe, it can result in acute gastric dilatation (Fig. 4.10). It is a condition that can last for several days. It may be due to activation of the sympathetic nervous system, i.e. excessive release of noradrenaline (Fig. 4.9). Biopsies of the human antrum of such patients have been investigated electrophysiologically. The action potentials recorded have a shorter plateau phase during repolarization. This leads to less tension being generated, and the stomach dilates. Because the pylorus is closed, the gastric juice accumulates in the stomach. It can be easily relieved by passing a fine tube (a nasogastric tube) into the stomach via the oesophagus, which allows free drainage of the gastric juice and air from the stomach. The condition is self-limiting and usually resolves over 48 h.

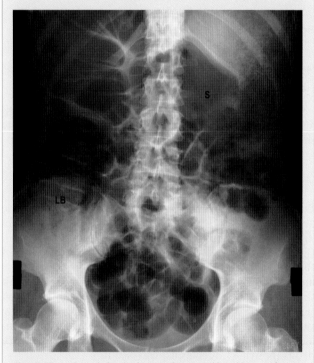

Fig. 4.10 A plain abdominal X-ray showing dilated loops of large bowel (LB) and a massively dilated stomach (S) containing food residue.

Stretch or distension of the stomach walls increases the tension (the myogenic reflex, see Ch. 1). Increased levels of circulating gastrin or stimulation of the vagus nerve also lead to a greater force of contraction. This effect is due to an increase in the amplitude and duration of the slow wave depolarization (Fig. 4.9).

Stimulation of the adrenergic sympathetic nerves to the stomach or increasing levels of CCK, secretin or GIP (see below) in the blood results in hyperpolarization of the membrane, fewer action potentials, and relaxation of the muscle (Fig. 4.9). Sympathetic nerves are activated during exercise and therefore the motility of the gastrointestinal tract is decreased. Stimulation of purinergic fibres in the vagus during the cephalic phase of gastric control (see below) also inhibits muscle contraction. These nerves release ATP which hyperpolarizes the smooth muscle membranes. Table 4.3 summarizes the effects of endogenous factors on smooth muscle electrical potential and muscle tension.

After stomach surgery, the motility of the stomach is reduced, a phenomenon which may be attributed to catecholamine release (Box 4.4).

Control of the pyloric sphincter

The mucosal and muscle layers of the stomach and duodenum are discontinuous due to the presence of a ring of connective tissue on the duodenal side of the pyloric sphincter, but the myenteric plexi of the pylorus and duodenal bulb are continuous. The basal electrical rhythm of the duodenum is faster (approx. 10/min) than that of the stomach. The duodenal bulb contracts rather irregularly because it is influenced by the basal electrical rhythm of both the stomach and the duodenum. However, the activity in the antrum and duodenum is coordinated, and when the antrum contracts, the duodenal bulb is relaxed. The pylorus is densely innervated by parasympathetic (vagal) and sympathetic nerve fibres. The sympathetic nerves release noradrenaline, which acts on adrenergic receptors to increase the constriction of the sphincter. Relaxation of the sphincter is due to impulses in peptidergic fibres in the vagus that release VIP. After non-selective vagotomy this constriction is unopposed, and the outlet of the stomach can be obstructed. Interestingly there are also excitatory (cholinergic) fibres in the vagus nerve, activation of which increases constriction of the sphincter. However, as the sphincter relaxes when the stomach empties, activation of the inhibitory fibres predominates during stomach emptying. Finally, CCK causes constriction of the pyloric sphincter in physiological concentrations that cause gall bladder contraction. Therefore, CCK is probably also one of the physiological regulators of the sphincter.

Control of gastric function by food

Motility in the stomach is controlled partly by blood glucose levels. When the blood glucose concentration falls during fasting, gastric smooth muscle is stimulated. Peristaltic contractile activity increases, but not gastric emptying. These contractions can be strong enough to cause 'hunger pains'. They are due to impulses in the vagus nerve that is sensitive to low blood glucose.

Acid is secreted at a low rate even when the stomach is empty. The basal rate is approximately 10% of the maximum rate. However, the basal rate is not constant as it shows a diurnal variation: it is lowest in the morning and highest in the evening.

When a meal is eaten, the mechanisms which control the secretion of gastric juice and the motility and emptying of the stomach interact in a complex manner to coordinate the functions of this organ. The control of gastric function during a meal can be conveniently divided into three main phases depending on the location of the food:

1. The cephalic phase: occurs before the food reaches the stomach. It is a response to the approach of food (i.e. smell, sight of food), or food in the mouth.
2. The gastric phase: occurs in response to food when it reaches the stomach.
3. The intestinal phase: due to food material in the intestines, mainly the duodenum and upper jejunum.

In practice of course, for much of the time during a meal, ingested material is present at different locations at the same time.

The effects of hypersecretion of acid in peptic ulcer disease and gastrinoma on gastrointestinal functions are described in Cases 4.1 and 4.2: 3.

The cephalic phase

Secretion

During the cephalic phase, gastric acid and pepsinogen secretion is activated by the thought, sight or smell of food, and by food in the mouth. The mechanisms of control of gastric secretion during the cephalic phase are summarized in Figure 4.11. Emotions also influence gastric secretion. The response to the sight and smell of food is a conditioned reflex; a learned response based on previous experiences of eating food. The release of acid at the sight and smell (approach) of food was first demonstrated by sampling of the gastric contents through a gastrostomy (fistula) in subjects who could not swallow food and had therefore been provided with a permanent fistula so that food could be placed directly in the stomach. Emotions were found to elicit increased or decreased acid secretion. This was shown by Wolff and Wolff, physicians who studied a patient with a closed oesophagus who was provided with a gastrostomy. They showed that hostility and resentment tended to increase gastric secretion whilst depression tended to reduce it.

The taste and the touch of food in the mouth also elicits secretion of gastric juice (before the food reaches the stomach). This is a non-conditioned reflex. It was studied by the physician Janowics, in a patient who had had a gastrostomy because she could not swallow food. It was found that if the patient placed some food in her mouth and chewed it, there was an increased secretion of gastric juice. Furthermore, food that the patient enjoyed elicited a more copious secretion than food which she merely tolerated. The secretion in response to palatable food is known as 'appetite juice'. This gives some physiological justification for starting a meal with a savoury course (hors d'oeuvre).

The gastric juice secreted during the cephalic phase is rich in pepsinogen, but also contains some acid. The secretion of both pepsinogen and acid is due to impulses in the vagus nerve. Stimulation of the nerves releases acid both directly from the oxyntic cell and indirectly via the release of gastrin (Fig. 4.11). Less than half the acid produced in response to a meal is secreted during the cephalic phase. Vagotomy (section of the vagus nerve, see Cases 4.1 and 4.2: 1) reduces the secretion of gastric juice mainly because its effect during the cephalic phase is abolished. When acid is secreted during the cephalic phase, that is while the stomach is still empty, there is very little protein present in the stomach to buffer the

Effects on gastrointestinal function

Peptic ulcer disease

Stomach function

High acidity in the stomach normally causes the release of somatostatin that inhibits the release of gastrin to reduce the secretion of acid in the stomach. In peptic ulcer disease *H. pylori* inhibits somatostatin secretion and the rate of gastrin secretion could consequently increase. This would stimulate more acid production. Gastrin also has a trophic effect to stimulate proliferation of the oxyntic and chief cells in the gastric mucosa which exacerbates the condition by causing increased acid and pepsinogen secretin.

Excess acid in the duodenum normally causes the release of secretin, which inhibits the secretion of gastric acid, but these effects are overwhelmed by the high acid secretion in peptic ulcer disease.

Gastrinomas

Digestion and absorption

In the patient with gastrinomas diarrhoea is a frequent symptom. This is due to hypersecretion and hypermotility, secondary to chronic gastrin stimulation. Such patients can also suffer from steatorrhoea; fat in the faeces. Normally, almost all neutral fat ingested is digested and absorbed in the small intestine (see Ch. 8). Therefore steatorrhoea is an indication of malabsorption of fat. The excessive acid production in Zollinger–Ellison syndrome can lead to fat malabsorption for two reasons:

1. Pancreatic lipase (and other enzymes) are active at neutral or slightly alkaline pH values and are reversibly inactivated at acid pH values, so digestion of food is reduced.
2. Effective absorption of the monoacylglycerol and long-chain fatty acid products of lipid digestion, and lipid-soluble vitamins (A, D, K and E), depends on them being sequestered in micelles (see Ch. 8). Micelle formation will only take place at neutral or alkaline pH values, so again, fat absorption is reduced.

Thus, in Zollinger–Ellison syndrome, the excessive acid secretion may lead to defective absorption of lipids and other nutrients. The consequences are defective lipid absorption, deficiency of essential fatty acids required for healthy nerves and deficiency of vitamin A (required for night vision), vitamin D, required for Ca^{2+} absorption (see Ch. 8) and Ca^{2+} homeostasis, and vitamin K, required for effective blood clotting.

Pernicious anaemia

Vitamin B_{12} is poorly absorbed in the ileum at low pH values for reasons that are not yet understood. As a consequence of this, pernicious anaemia can develop in Zollinger–Ellison syndrome.

Diarrhoea

Diarrhoea is usually a prominent symptom in Zollinger–Ellison syndrome. It is present in approximately 65% of cases. There are a number of causes:

- Elevated gastrin concentrations in the blood cause massive volumes of secretion from the stomach, pancreas, liver and intestines. The absorptive capacity of the small intestines and colon is consequently overwhelmed, and diarrhoea results. This is probably the major mechanism involved in causing diarrhoea in this condition
- Impaired digestion and malabsorption of nutrients (see above) results in the chyme becoming highly concentrated and therefore hyperosmotic. In the colon, undigested nutrients ferment to produce a further increase in osmotic particles. Water is consequently transported from the blood into the lumen of the intestines, down the osmotic gradient, and 'osmotic diarrhoea' results
- As gastrin increases, smooth muscle contractility and high circulating levels can result in increased gastrointestinal motility. This will reduce intestinal transit time and cause diarrhoea.

The mechanisms involved in diarrhoea are discussed more fully in Chapter 7.

---

acid. Therefore a small amount of acid will produce a marked fall in pH. This results in the feedback control mechanism coming into operation, whereby acid secretion is inhibited. The secretion of pepsinogen during the cephalic phase is due both to direct stimulation of the chief cells by the vagal impulses, and to the release of gastrin, which also stimulates the chief cells.

Motility

Motility in the stomach smooth muscle is reduced during the cephalic phase. The sight, smell, taste and touch of food in the mouth all inhibit gastric emptying. Pain, depression, fear and sadness also inhibit it. The mechanism is probably via impulses in inhibitory purinergic fibres in the vagus nerve. The activity in these nerve fibres causes relaxation of stomach smooth muscle and inhibits gastric emptying. At the same time, the pyloric sphincter is constricted. The latter effect is probably also due to impulses in cholinergic fibres in the vagus nerve. This delay in the emptying of the stomach permits the stomach initially to store a greater volume of material, and so allows time for the digestive processes to operate. Interestingly, aggression and anger increase gastric motility but the mechanisms involved have not yet been elucidated.

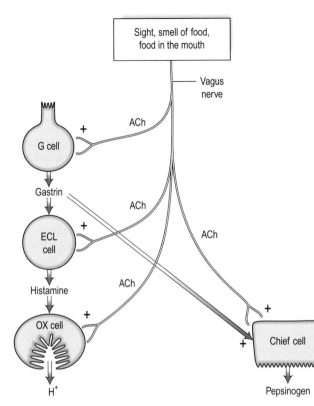

Fig. 4.11 Cephalic phase of control of gastric secretion.

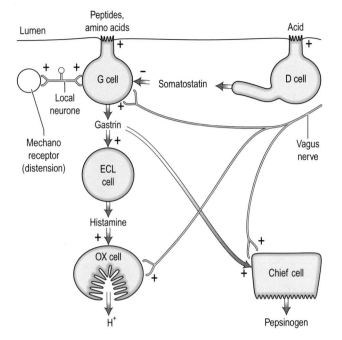

Fig. 4.12 Gastric phase of control of gastric secretion, OX, oxyntic cell, ECL, enterochromaffin-like cell.

The gastric phase

Secretion

Food placed directly into the stomach through a gastric fistula (gastrostomy) elicits an increase in both acid and pepsinogen secretion. The gastric phase accounts for more than 50% of the acid secreted during a meal. The control of secretion during the gastric phase is summarized in Figure 4.12. The amount of secretion depends on the chemical content of the food, and its volume. Secretion of gastric juice is in response to chemicals in the food and to distension of the walls of the stomach by food. The products of protein digestion, especially peptides and amino acids (in particular tryptophan and phenylalanine), and caffeine (present in tea, coffee, coca cola), and alcohol, stimulate gastric secretion. These chemical substances in the food, or 'secretogogues', are sensed by APUD cells which behave as chemoreceptors or 'taste' cells. The G cells sense peptides and amino acids. Distension, another stimulus that increases acid secretion, is detected by pressure receptors or nerve endings in the mucosa. Distension is not as powerful a stimulant as the chemical constituents of food. A low pH in the stomach causes inhibition of acid secretion, although pepsinogen secretion is stimulated. The D cells sense H^+ ions. The regulation of gastric secretion in this phase is via coordinated neural, hormonal and paracrine mechanisms. The neural signals are conducted in extrinsic nerves of the vagus nerve, and in intrinsic nerves of the enteric nerve plexi.

Motility

During the gastric phase, the stomach empties at a rate that is proportional to the volume of material within it. This is due partly to the effect of distension; the chyme stimulates pressure receptors in the wall of the stomach, which trigger impulses in nerves in the internal nerve plexi. It is probably also due to the direct effect of stretching the smooth muscle (the myogenic reflex, see Ch. 1). There is also a vagal mechanism involved in the response to distension, but in the gastric phase (unlike the cephalic phase), impulses in the vagus nerve increase peristalsis and gastric emptying. In this case it is the cholinergic nerve fibres in the vagus that are activated. However, excessive distension inhibits contractility (see Ch. 1) thereby allowing a longer time for the digestive processes to operate. Gastrin release into the blood in response to peptides and amino acids also causes potentiation of peristalsis.

Gastric emptying is brought about by strong periodic contractions of the antrum, potentiated by gastrin, and acetylcholine in the vagus nerve. The pyloric sphincter relaxes when the antrum contracts and allows a portion of the gastric chyme into the duodenum. The relaxation of the sphincter is probably due to impulses in peptidergic nerve fibres which release VIP, in the vagus nerve.

The intestinal phase

The intestinal phase of gastric function is largely inhibitory. Gastric secretion and motility are both inhibited. In the duodenal phase, the food is mixed with the digestive secretions of the pancreas and liver. The inhibition of

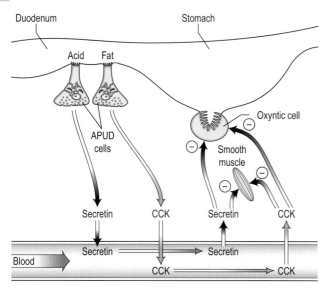

Fig. 4.13 Intestinal phase of gastric control.

Cases
4.1
and
4.2

Peptic ulcer disease and
gastrinomas: 4

Acid–base balance
Peptic ulcer disease

Acid secretion in the stomach is accompanied by secretion of bicarbonate into the blood that makes the blood alkaline (the 'alkaline tide', see Ch. 3). This is normally neutralized by the acid secreted into the blood when alkaline bicarbonate secretions (pancreatic juice, bile, intestinal secretions) are produced. The acid secretions are increased in duodenal ulcer disease and the consequent raised blood pH will take longer to be neutralized by respiratory and renal compensatory mechanisms. However, these mechanisms usually maintain the pH within normal parameters.

Gastrinomas

In Zollinger–Ellison syndrome there is excessive secretion of acid, due to the high levels of circulating gastrin, which can lead to a pronounced alkaline tide. Gastrin not only stimulates acid secretion in the stomach, it also stimulates the production of alkaline juices from the duct cells of the liver and pancreas. Furthermore, acid in the duodenum stimulates alkaline pancreatic juice and bile secretion via secretin (see Chs 5 and 6), which would normally result in an 'acid tide'. However, the exaggerated alkaline tide resulting from the copious acid secretion seen in Zollinger–Ellison syndrome may overwhelm these homeostatic mechanisms. The respiratory and renal mechanisms may be inadequate to compensate for this effect, so metabolic alkalosis occurs.

gastric emptying by food in the duodenum enables the duodenal contents to be processed before more material enters it from the stomach.

Secretion

Although food in the duodenum is largely inhibitory as far as gastric secretion is concerned, there is an early stimulatory phase in response to slight distension of the duodenum, probably due to the release of gastrin from APUD cells in the walls of the duodenum. However, appropriate stimulation of the duodenum inhibits gastric secretion. Inhibitory stimuli include distension of the duodenum, fats and peptides in the chyme, increased acidity, and hypertonic solutions. All of these stimuli cause the release of hormones from APUD cells. This phase of control of secretion is summarized in Figure 4.13.

Acid in the duodenal chyme causes the release of secretin, and fat in the duodenal chyme causes the release of CCK and GIP into the blood, and these hormones all inhibit secretion of gastric juice (see above). This is a feedback mechanism that prevents the duodenal contents becoming excessively acid. It is important for several reasons:

- Digestive enzymes, which act in the small intestine require neutral or acid pH values for optimum activity

- Micelle formation, which is necessary for fat digestion and absorption in the small intestine (see Ch. 8) will only take place at a neutral or slightly alkaline pH

- The duodenum is the most common site for ulcer formation in the digestive tract and acid is the prime cause of ulceration in this region. The reduction of acid secretion begins when the pH of the duodenal contents falls to 5.0, and it is complete at a pH value of approximately 2.5.

Control of the pH of the gastrointestinal tract helps to maintain the pH of the blood within normal limits (see Ch. 3). The effects of hypersecretion of acid on acid–base balance are described in Cases 4.1 and 4.2: 4).

Motility

Motility in the stomach can be influenced by food in the duodenum, food in the ileum and food in the colon. Distension of the duodenum inhibits gastric motility via two mechanisms:

1. A quick enterogastric reflex which employs nerve fibres in the vagus nerve and an unknown neurotransmitter.

2. A slower humoral mechanism involving the release of hormones from the walls of the duodenum into the blood. These hormones are collectively known as enterogastrones. They include CCK and secretin (Fig. 4.13).

When food material reaches the ileum, the emptying of the stomach is delayed. This is a neural reflex initiated by activation of mechanoreceptors in the walls of the ileum, which trigger action potentials in nerve fibres in the internal nerve plexi. Interestingly, when food enters the stomach the motility of the ileum is increased. Thus the ileogastric reflex operates in both directions.

There is also a neural reflex response when the chyme enters the colon; distension of the colon activates pressure receptors which triggers impulses in internal nerves to delay gastric emptying.

PANCREAS: EXOCRINE FUNCTIONS

5

Chapter objectives

After studying this chapter you should be able to:

1. Describe the macroscopic and microscopic anatomy of the pancreas and relate these to its function.

2. Describe the components of exocrine function of the pancreas and apply this knowledge in understanding the pathological conditions of acute and chronic pancreatitis and cystic fibrosis.

Introduction

The pancreas contains exocrine tissue that secretes pancreatic juice, a major digestive secretion, and endocrine tissue that secretes the hormones insulin and glucagon. The hormones are important in the control of metabolism and their roles in the absorptive and postabsorptive metabolic states will be discussed in Chapter 9. This chapter will be mainly concerned with the exocrine secretions of the pancreas, their functions, and the mechanisms whereby the secretory processes are controlled.

Pancreatic juice finds its way into the duodenum via the pancreatic duct that opens into the duodenum at the same location as the common bile duct (Fig. 5.1). Entry of both pancreatic juice and bile into the duodenum is controlled by the sphincter of Oddi. The smooth muscle of the sphincter is contracted between meals so that the junction is sealed. When a meal is being processed in the gastrointestinal tract, the sphincter muscle relaxes and allows the pancreatic juice and bile into the small intestine. The control of the sphincter of Oddi is discussed in Chapter 7. Pancreatic exocrine dysfunction may be due to disorders of the pancreas itself, or to blockage of the ducts which prevents the exocrine secretions reaching the duodenum. Duct blockage may also result in impaired bile flow from the liver, which can result in jaundice.

In the small intestine, pancreatic juice, bile and the juices secreted by the walls of the intestines, mix with the fluid (chyme) arriving from the stomach (see Fig. 7.1). Pancreatic juice provides most of the important digestive enzymes. In addition, by virtue of its bicarbonate content, it helps to provide an appropriate neutral or alkaline pH in the intestinal lumen for the enzymes to act on their nutrient substrates. The functional importance of the pancreas to the digestive processes can be illustrated by the problems arising in chronic pancreatitis (Case 5.1: 1) and cystic fibrosis (Case 5.2: 1) conditions in which pancreatic tissue is destroyed.

Anatomy and morphology

The pancreas is an elongated gland that lies in the abdominal cavity. It can be divided into three regions: the head, the body and the tail (Fig. 5.1). The head is an expanded portion that lies adjacent to the C-shaped region of the duodenum to which it is intimately attached by connective tissue, and to which it is connected by a common blood supply. The body and tail extend across the midline of the body toward the hilum of the spleen. The pancreatic duct (duct of Wirsung) extends through the long axis of the gland to the duodenum. Pancreatic juice empties from this duct into the duodenum via the ampulla of Vater. In some individuals, there is also an accessory pancreatic duct. Bile in the common bile duct from the liver also enters the duodenum at the ampulla of Vater, by passing through the head of the pancreas. This is why inflammation (pancreatitis) and tumours (pancreatic cancer) involving the head of the pancreas are commonly associated with jaundice, as a consequence of blockage of the common bile duct.

Exocrine tissue

The exocrine units of the pancreas are tubuloacinar glands that are organized like bunches of grapes (Fig. 5.3), in a similar manner to the units in the salivary glands. The exocrine units surround the islets of Langerhans, the endocrine units of the pancreas. For this reason, destructive diseases such as chronic pancreatitis involve impairment of both exocrine and endocrine function. A thin layer of loose connective tissue surrounds the gland. Septa extend from this layer into the gland, dividing it into lobules and giving it an irregular surface. Larger areas of connective tissue surround the main ducts and the blood vessels and nerve fibres that penetrate the gland. Small mucous glands situated within the tissue surrounding the pancreatic duct secrete mucus into the duct.

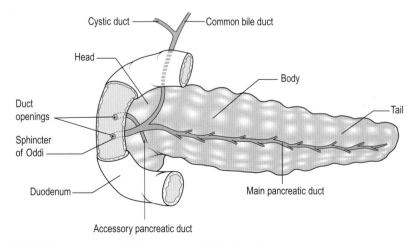

Fig. 5.1 The pancreas and its innervation and blood supply.

Case 5.1 | Chronic pancreatitis: 1

A 40-year-old man who had been a heavy drinker for many years, went to see his general practitioner. He had made two previous visits over the past year complaining of recurrent episodes of abdominal pain. Although the pain had been intermittent at first, it was now continuous. The doctor ascertained that the pain originated in the epigastrium, and radiated through to the back. The patient had lost a considerable amount of weight since his last visit. The doctor noticed that he was mildly jaundiced. Arrangements were made for the patient to be admitted to hospital for tests.

An X-ray examination, and serum and urine analyses were performed. The patient's stools were collected over 3 days. These were pale-coloured and bulky, indicating a high fat content (steatorrhoea). He was told to abstain from food the next morning so that a glucose tolerance test (see Chapter 9) could be performed.

The blood tests showed increased bilirubin and alkaline phosphatase. The glucose tolerance test showed an abnormally high and prolonged rise in serum glucose, and urine analysis confirmed the presence of glucose (glycosuria), indicating that the patient was diabetic. The presumptive diagnosis was chronic pancreatitis. The patient was prescribed pethidine to control the pain. He was advised to abstain completely from alcohol, and to eat regular meals. Figure 5.2 shows a CT (computerized tomography) scan of the abdomen of an individual with chronic pancreatitis. The swollen pancreas can be clearly seen. Examination of the details of this case gives rise to the following questions:

- Is the primary defect in chronic pancreatitis known?
- What might the X-ray have revealed?
- What could be the cause of the condition in this patient?
- How are the exocrine and endocrine functions of the pancreas impaired in chronic pancreatitis?
- What did the high faecal fat content indicate?

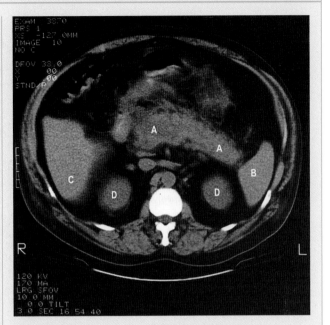

Fig. 5.2 CT scan: cross-section of the abdomen showing a swollen pancreas caused by pancreatitis (A) lying posteriorly on the abdominal wall. The spleen (B), lower border of liver (C) and kidneys (D) are also seen.

- What is the basis of the glucose tolerance test and why has diabetes mellitus developed in this patient?
- Why did the patient appear jaundiced?
- Why were the patient's serum bilirubin and alkaline phosphatase abnormally high?
- What are the main physiological consequences of this disease and how can the condition be treated or managed?

These questions will be addressed in this chapter.

Endocrine tissue

The endocrine units, or islets of Langerhans, are most numerous in the tail region of the pancreas. They consist of clusters of cells which are surrounded by the pancreatic acini (Fig. 5.3). The islets vary considerably in size. As with all endocrine tissue, the hormones they produce are secreted into the blood. The major endocrine cell types present are: α, β, D and PP cells, which secrete glucagon, insulin, somatostatin, and pancreatic polypeptide, respectively (for more information, see Ch. 9). Different types of endocrine cells can be distinguished under the electron microscope by the different appearance of the granules within them. The islet cells have the general features of APUD cells (see Ch. 1). In addition, there are a few (<5%) small 'clear' cells with as yet no clearly defined function.

Glucagon and insulin, the hormones produced by the α and β cells, respectively, are taken up by the local blood vessels to act systemically. Somatostatin acts locally in a paracrine manner to inhibit the secretion of the α and β cells, as well as the exocrine secretions of the acinar and duct cells. Pancreatic polypeptide acts in a paracrine manner to inhibit the exocrine secretions of the pancreas.

Oxygenated blood is supplied to the pancreas by branches of the coeliac and superior mesenteric arteries. The pancreatico-duodenal artery lies between the duodenum and the head of the pancreas. The close proximity of these structures means that it would be hazardous to remove the pancreas without the duodenum, because the main arterial supply would inevitably be damaged. The blood drains from the pancreas via the portal vein to the liver. This arrangement is important for the transport of pancreatic hormones to the liver where they contribute

A 12-year-old boy who was suffering from cystic fibrosis was taken to the outpatient clinic for his regular check-up. Cystic fibrosis is an inherited autosomal recessive disorder. The primary defect is a mutation in the gene that encodes the cystic fibrosis transport regulator (CFTR). The CFTR is responsible for cyclic-AMP-regulated Cl^- conductance in the membranes of secretory cells of epithelia. The defect causes impaired Cl^- transport that is predominantly a problem in the wet surfaces of the respiratory tract, but also causes severe problems in the pancreas. It is also manifest in the reproductive tract and sweat glands. The boy's condition had been diagnosed soon after birth and he had both respiratory tract and pancreatic involvement. He had been asked to bring a sample of his stool. This was pale-coloured, poorly formed and oily in appearance. It was sent to the laboratory for analysis to assess his pancreatic function. His exocrine pancreatic insufficiency was being treated with a pancreatic enzyme preparation and the anti-ulcer drug ranitidine.

After studying the above details, we can attempt to answer the following questions:

- How is the inherited defect manifest in the pancreas?
- Which abnormalities of pancreatic function result from this pathology?
- Why was the boy's stool pale coloured?
- Which tests would be performed on the stool sample?
- Would there be any abnormalities in the acid–base status of this patient?
- Why was the child being treated with an enzyme preparation and would there be any problem with giving such a preparation by mouth?
- Why is the boy being treated with ranitidine?

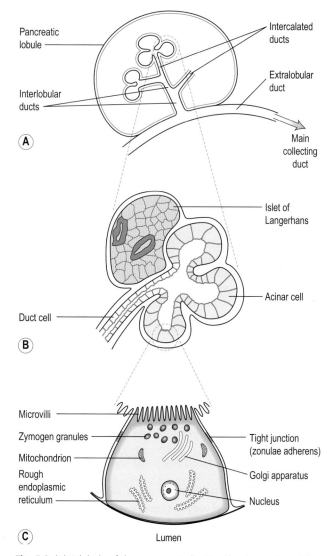

Fig. 5.3 (A) A lobule of the pancreas indicating the duct system. (B) The relationship of an exocrine unit and an islet of Langerhans. (C) An acinar cell.

to the control of energy metabolism, a topic discussed in Chapter 9. The acini and ducts are surrounded by separate capillary beds. Some of the capillaries that supply the islets converge to form efferent arterioles which then enter further capillary networks around the acini. This arrangement is important for the paracrine control of pancreatic exocrine secretion.

Cholinergic preganglionic fibres of the vagus nerve enter the pancreas. These synapse with postganglionic cholinergic nerve fibres which lie within the pancreatic tissue and innervate both acinar and islet cells. Postganglionic sympathetic nerves from the coeliac and superior mesenteric plexi innervate the pancreatic blood vessels as well as the acinar and duct cells.

Histology of the exocrine tissue

Figure 5.3 shows the structure of a pancreatic lobule. The exocrine units of the pancreas, or pancreatins, each consist of a terminal acinar portion and a duct (Fig. 5.4).

The duct that drains the acinus is known as an intercalated duct. These empty into larger intralobular ducts. The intralobular ducts in each lobule drain into a larger extralobular duct that empties the secretions of that lobule into still larger ducts, and the latter converge into the main collecting duct, the pancreatic duct.

The acinus is a rounded structure consisting of mainly pyramidal epithelial cells (Fig. 5.4). These cells secrete the digestive enzymes of the pancreatic juice. They display polarized features that are common to secretory cells (Fig. 5.3). The nucleus of the acinar cell is situated at the base of the cell. The cytoplasm in the basal region can be stained with haematoxylin or basic dyes due to the presence of rough endoplasmic reticulum, the site of production of the digestive enzymes. Small mitochondria are situated throughout the cell. The apical portion of the cell contains the Golgi apparatus, and numerous zymogen

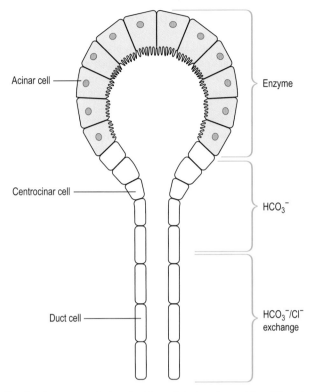

Fig. 5.4 Secretory unit showing the cellular locations of the different secretions.

Labels: Acinar cell, Centrocinar cell, Duct cell, Enzyme, HCO_3^-, HCO_3^-/Cl^- exchange

from the spaces. They also have gap junctions that permit the transmission of membrane electrical changes between the cells. These ducts lead into the intralobular ducts that are lined with cuboidal or low columnar epithelium. Larger ducts contain interlobular connective tissue cells and APUD cells.

Pancreatic juice

The pancreatic juice entering the duodenum is a mixture of two types of secretion: an enzyme-rich secretion from the acinar cells and an aqueous alkaline secretion from the ducts. Thus, if the ducts are ligated near the acini, which results in acinar cell degeneration, the secretion of the alkaline component of the juice is largely unaltered, but the secretion of enzymes is markedly reduced. The alkaline secretion originates largely from the centroacinar cells and the duct cells of the intralobular and small interlobular ducts. These relationships are illustrated in Figure 5.4.

Alkaline secretion

Composition

The cells of the upper ducts secrete an isotonic juice which is rich in bicarbonate but contains only traces of enzymes. There is a continuous resting secretion of this juice, but it can be stimulated up to 14-fold during a meal. It contains Na^+, K^+, HCO_3^-, Mg^{2+}, Ca^{2+}, Cl^- and other ions present in concentrations similar to those of plasma. It therefore resembles an ultrafiltrate of plasma, but is alkaline by virtue of its high HCO_3^- content.

Functions

The pancreatic juice arriving in the duodenum is mixed with the chyme by contractions of the smooth muscle of the small intestine. The function of the alkaline pancreatic secretion, together with the other alkaline secretions (bile and intestinal juices) that act in the small intestine, is to neutralize the acid chyme arriving from the stomach. This is important for several reasons:

- The pancreatic enzymes require a neutral or slightly alkaline pH for their activity

- The absorption of fat depends on the formation in the intestinal lumen of micelles, a process which only takes place at neutral or slightly alkaline pH values

- It protects the intestinal mucosa from excess acid which can damage it, leading to the formation of ulcers. This (peptic) ulceration most commonly occurs in the first part of the duodenum, before the acidic chyme has mixed with the alkaline pancreatic juice.

granules that contain the pancreatic enzymes or their precursors. The apical region therefore stains with acid dyes such as eosin. Microvilli extend from the apical surface of the acinar cell into the lumen. The apical poles of neighbouring cells are joined by tight junctions, known as zonulae adherens. These junctions separate the fluid in the lumen of the acinus from the fluid in the intercellular spaces that bathes the basolateral surfaces of the cells. The tight junctions are impermeable to macromolecules, such as digestive enzymes, in the luminal fluid, but permit the exchange of water and ions between the interstitial spaces and the lumen of the acinus. Disruption of these junctions may be an aetiological factor in the development of chronic pancreatitis. Gap junctions between neighbouring cells allow rapid changes in membrane potential to be transmitted between the cells. They also permit the exchange of low molecular weight molecules (<1400 kDa mass) between cells.

The intercalated duct begins within the acinus. This is a unique feature of secretory glands. The upper duct cells within the acinus are known as centroacinar cells (Fig. 5.4). These stain lightly with eosin. They are squamous cells with a centrally placed nucleus. These cells are continuous with those of the short intercalated duct that lies outside the acinus and drains it. The intercalated ducts are lined by flattened squamous epithelial cells. The neighbouring duct cells are joined by tight junctions, as in the acinus. These separate the duct lumen from the intercellular spaces and function to exclude large molecules

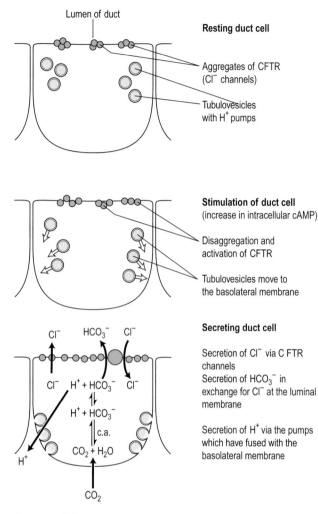

Resting duct cell

Aggregates of CFTR
(Cl⁻ channels)

Tubulovesicles
with H⁺ pumps

Stimulation of duct cell
(increase in intracellular cAMP)

Disaggregation and
activation of CFTR

Tubulovesicles move to
the basolateral membrane

Secreting duct cell

Secretion of Cl⁻ via CFTR
channels
Secretion of HCO₃⁻ in
exchange for Cl⁻ at the luminal
membrane

Secretion of H⁺ via the pumps
which have fused with the
basolateral membrane

Fig. 5.5 Cellular mechanisms involved in the production of HCO_3^- and H^+ in a duct cell. c.a., carbonic anhydrase; CFTR, cystic fibrosis transport regulator.

Cellular mechanisms of secretion

The mechanisms involved in the production of intracellular HCO_3^- in the centroacinar and upper duct cells are illustrated in Figure 5.5. The initial intracellular step involves the reaction of CO_2 with water. Secreted H^+ ions react with HCO_3^- ions in the blood perfusing the gland and this generates CO_2, some of which diffuses into the duct cell. More than 90% of the HCO_3^- in pancreatic juice is derived from blood CO_2. In the cell, the CO_2 combines with intracellular water to generate carbonic acid, in a reaction catalysed by carbonic anhydrase II, an enzyme present in the centroacinar and upper duct cells. The carbonic acid dissociates to give HCO_3^- and H^+. Whilst bicarbonate is being secreted the partial pressure of CO_2 (pCO_2) in the cells is lower than in the blood as it is being used up in the production of HCO_3^- ions, and the higher the rate of secretion the greater the downhill gradient for diffusion of CO_2 into the cell.

The HCO_3^- ions are secreted across the luminal membrane by Cl^-/HCO_3^- exchange, and the H^+ ions are secreted into the blood. Thus for every HCO_3^- ion that is secreted into the duct lumen one H^+ ion is secreted into the blood. Therefore the blood flowing through the pancreas becomes transiently acid when it is secreting HCO_3^-. The H^+ ions in the blood help to neutralize the 'alkaline tide' produced during a meal by the secreting stomach (see Ch. 3), by combining with plasma HCO_3^- to produce CO_2. In conditions where a patient is provided with a pancreatic fistula, loss of HCO_3^- must be carefully monitored (Box 5.1).

The exchange mechanism in the centroacinar and upper duct cells, whereby HCO_3^- is secreted in exchange for Cl^-, obviously depends on the presence of Cl^- in the fluid in the lumen. This is achieved by flux of Cl^- ions out of the cell into the lumen via a chloride conductance channel known as the cystic fibrosis transmembrane conductance regulator (CFTR) which is regulated by cyclic AMP. It is a defect in the CFTR that results in impairment of the secretory process and disruption of pancreatic function in cystic fibrosis (Case 5.2: 1). Immunocytochemical studies using fluorescent antibodies against the CFTR have shown that it is localized to the apical region of centroacinar and intralobular duct cells. The CFTR is coupled to the HCO_3^-/Cl^- exchanger.

The CFTR Cl^- channel is present in clusters in the apical plasma membranes. When the gland is stimulated (by secretin or by an increase in cAMP), the channel clusters disaggregate (Fig. 5.5) increasing the number of open channels. The channel is regulated in two ways:

1. Via phosphorylation and dephosphorylation by protein kinase A and a phosphatase respectively, serving as a molecular switch involved in the gating of the channel.

2. Via activation of the channel by hydrolysis of ATP and other nucleotides.

The main features of the ion transport relationships in the pancreatic duct cell are shown in Figure 5.5. It has been observed, using electron microscopy, that when the cell is not being stimulated it contains numerous tubulo-vesicles in its apical cytoplasm. The membranes of these vesicles contain proton pumps that are ATPases. When the cell is stimulated, the tubulovesicles are translocated to the basolateral surface and their membranes fuse with the basolateral plasma membrane. Thus, the proton pumps are incorporated into the membrane. Then H^+ ions are actively pumped out of the cell into the intersti-tial fluid in the lateral spaces, and from there they dif-fuse into the plasma. Electron microscope studies have shown that stimulation of secretion involves a change in the shape of the cell. This is associated with expansion of the basolateral plasma membranes as the membrane of the vesicles fuse with it. The fusion of the membranes is an active process that derives its energy from the breakdown of ATP that is catalysed by the ATPase of the pumps.

Cl^- ions are secreted by the cells into the lumen via the CFTR (Fig. 5.5). Na^+ and K^+ ions reach the pancreatic juice by the paracellular route (between the cells), trav-elling down the electrochemical gradient. Water flows down the osmotic gradient (created by the ion transport) either transcellularly or paracellularly, from the lateral spaces. A Na^+/K^+-ATPase pump in the lateral borders of the cell transports Na^+ out of the cell and this maintains a low intracellular concentration and high extracellular concentration of Na^+ ions. A Na^+/H^+ exchange mecha-nism also operates at the basolateral pole of the cell to keep the intracellular pH stable, but this mechanism is probably not activated during secretion.

Failure of the secretory mechanism is seen in chronic pancreatitis (Case 5.1: 2) and in cystic fibrosis, in which there is an inherited defect in the gene which encodes the CFTR (Case 5.2: 2). As water transport would normally follow the ion transport (down the osmotic gradient), the defective ion secretion in these conditions results in a vis-cous fluid in the ducts with a high concentration of pro-tein in the pancreatic ducts which can block the lumen. This results in secondary pancreatic damage.

Variation in composition with rate of flow

The concentration of bicarbonate in the pancreatic juice that enters the duodenum ranges from 25 to 150 mM. The electrolyte composition of the juice varies with the flow rate. Figure 5.8 shows the changes in concentrations of

HCO_3^- and Cl^- ions with increasing rates of flow. There is a reciprocal relationship between the concentrations of the two ions. The concentration of HCO_3^- increases with increasing flow rate and the concentration of Cl^- decreases. The sum of the concentrations of the two ions is kept constant by the action of the ion exchange pumps. As the HCO_3^- concentration increases, the juice becomes more alkaline.

The changes in the ionic composition of the juice with rate of flow are due to the presence of transport systems in the membranes of the duct cells. The primary alkaline juice secreted at the tops of the ducts is modified as it passes down the ducts by transport systems in the cells lower down in the extralobular ducts, and in the main ducts. At high flow rates, the time the juice spends in contact with the cells is not sufficient for appreciable modification via HCO_3^-/Cl^- exchange and other processes to take place. Therefore the composition of the juice produced at high flow rates resembles that of the primary secretion more closely than juice secreted at low flow rates.

Pancreatic enzymes

The enzymes released from the pancreatic acinar cells comprise the major enzymes involved in the digestion of foodstuffs. Many of these are secreted as inactive precur-sors. The acinar cells contain zymogen granules, which are the locus of storage of enzyme or enzyme precursor protein. The enzyme precursors produced by the acinar cells include those of the proteolytic enzymes, trypsin, chymotrypsin, carboxypeptidase and elastase, and that of phospholipase A. Lipase, α-amylase, ribonuclease, and deoxyribonuclease are secreted as active enzymes. The release of enzymes as inactive precursors ensures that the activated enzymes do not autodigest the pancreatic tissue.

The importance of the pancreatic enzymes for nutri-tion can be illustrated by consideration of the impairment of function and the treatments employed in chronic pan-creatitis and cystic fibrosis (Case 5.1: 3 and 4 and Case 5.2: 3 and 4).

Secretion of enzymes and precursors: cellular mechanisms

The mechanism of secretion in the acinar cell is illus-trated in Figure 5.9. This scheme was first discovered by Palade in the 1970s. He was awarded the Nobel Prize for the work. The enzymes or precursors are synthesized on the rough endoplasmic reticulum of the cell. The mole-cules are then released into the cisternae of the endoplas-mic reticulum. Buds containing the enzymes or enzyme precursors break off the cisternal membranes and the buds coalesce in the region of the Golgi complex to form 'condensing vacuoles'. The vacuoles migrate towards the luminal membrane. If the cells are stained for zymogen the vacuoles can be seen to be more and more densely

Defect and causes

The primary malfunction in chronic pancreatitis is defective ductal secretion of bicarbonate and water, which results in a high protein concentration in the pancreatic juice in the ducts. The protein precipitates and forms plugs, with consequent dilatation of the proximal ducts. A high pressure is generated behind the blockages causing pain. Secondary back-pressure may lead to disruption of the ductal epithelium and result in destruction of the pancreatic tissue. This can lead to an inflammatory and fibrotic process in and around the pancreatic tissue. This in time leads to pancreatic insufficiency due to destruction of islet cells and acinar glands. The pancreas lies in close proximity to the coeliac plexus and inflammation around these autonomic nerves results in chronic back pain.

Chronic pancreatitis is characterized by progressive damage to the pancreas with permanent destruction of pancreatic tissue. Exocrine and endocrine pancreatic insufficiency usually follow. However, owing to the tremendous reserve of pancreatic tissue, the insufficiency may be subclinical and tests of pancreatic function may be necessary to reveal it. The histopathology indicates irregularly distributed fibrosis, reduced number and size of islets of Langerhans, and variable obstruction of pancreatic ducts of all sizes. Protein precipitation initially occurs in the lobular and interlobular ducts, leading to the formation of plugs that calcify by surface accretion. Concentric lamellar protein precipitates appear in the major pancreatic ducts and these also calcify to form stones. A specific protein, called stone protein, a normal constituent of pancreatic juice, which has a high affinity for Ca^{2+}, is the major protein present in the stones. The calculi contain calcium bicarbonate or hydroxyapatite (calcium phosphate and calcium bicarbonate). The stones can be seen in X-rays (Fig. 5.6). The chronic inflammation may extend to adjacent organs, including the duodenum, common bile duct, stomach antrum and transverse colon.

In up to 80% of patients with chronic pancreatitis, there is a history of excessive alcohol intake but rare autosomal dominant inherited forms of the disease have been described. The incidence of the disease is low, being approximately 30/100 000 in the UK. Onset is usually in middle age. The disease is approximately three times more common in males than females. Most alcoholic patients already have sustained permanent structural and functional damage to the pancreas by the time of their first attack of abdominal pain. Moreover, morphological changes are evident at post-mortem examination in many alcoholics who had no symptoms of pancreatic disease during life.

It is not known how alcohol causes chronic pancreatitis. It may promote the precipitation of proteins in the pancreatic secretion.

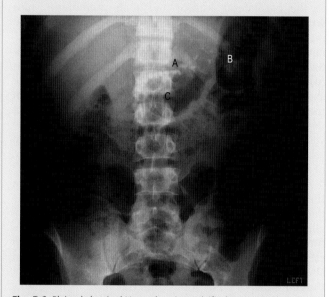

Fig. 5.6 Plain abdominal X-ray showing calcified stones in the pancreatic duct (A), from a patient with chronic pancreatitis secondary to alcoholism. Gas in the left colon (B) and overlying stomach (C) are also seen.

stained as they approach the surface. At the luminal membrane the membranes that surround the 'zymogen' granules fuse with the cell membrane and the vesicles break open to release their contents, a process known as exocytosis. The different enzymes are packaged together in each zymogen granule and they are probably released together in constant proportions. The zymogen granule membrane is rapidly recycled from the surface membrane.

It is exocytosis, rather than the synthesis or sequestration of the enzyme proteins that is under physiological control by hormones and neurotransmitters. Exocytosis is triggered by an increase in intracellular Ca^{2+}. The rise in intracellular Ca^{2+} when the cell is stimulated is via influx from the extracellular spaces or release from intracellular stores.

Activation of enzyme precursors

The enzyme precursors secreted by the acinar cells are activated in the lumen of the duodenum and jejunum. Trypsinogen is converted to trypsin plus a short peptide, in a reaction catalysed by enterokinase, an enzyme present in the brush border of the epithelial cells of the small intestine. Once a small amount of activated trypsin has been formed it can catalyse the conversion of more trypsinogen to trypsin. Trypsin is a powerful proteolytic enzyme that can convert chymotrypsinogen, procarboxy-peptidase, proelastase and prophospholipase A to their activated forms. Thus once a small amount of trypsin is formed a catalytic chain reaction occurs (Table 5.1).

In acute pancreatitis, a condition which can be life-threatening, activated enzymes are present in the pancreatic ducts leading to destruction of the pancreatic tissue (Box 5.2). Various mechanisms exist to prevent this:

- The pancreas normally secretes a polypeptide known as Kazal inhibitor that inhibits any small amounts

of activated trypsin which may find its way into the ducts, by complexing with it

- Another pancreatic factor, enzyme Y, which is activated by traces of active trypsin degrades zymogen, thus exercising a protective function

- The alkaline pH (8.0–9.5) and low Ca^{2+} concentration in pancreatic secretions promote the degradation rather than the activation of trypsinogen.

Table 5.1 Activation of enzyme precursors in the small intestine

Precursor		Active enzyme
Trypsinogen	*enterokinase, trypsin* →	trypsin + peptide
Chymotrypsinogen	*trypsin* →	chymotrypsin + peptide
Proelastase	*trypsin* →	elastase + peptide
Procarboxypeptidase	*trypsin* →	carboxypeptidase + peptide
Prophospholipase A	*trypsin* →	phospholipase A + peptide

Case 5.2 Cystic fibrosis: 2

Defect and diagnosis

In the pancreas, the defect in the CFTR is associated with defective secretion of chloride into the ducts, and therefore reduced water transport so that the fluid in the ducts becomes viscous. This leads to the formation of protein-rich plugs which can obstruct the proximal intralobular ducts, resulting in secondary pancreatic damage (a process similar to that which occurs in chronic pancreatitis, see Case 5.1: 2). Thus, the digestive enzymes do not reach the duodenum. The tests performed on the stool sample would show a high fat content. Chymotrypsin or trypsin content would also be high. Over 80% of patients have steatorrhoea due to pancreatic dysfunction and meconium ileus (obstruction of the small intestine by impacted material) is common in the newborn (Fig. 5.7).

The same process of mucous plugging results in blockage of the bronchioles. This leads to recurrent respiratory infection and eventually to respiratory failure. These bronchopulmonary and gastrointestinal manifestations usually alert the clinician to the possibility that the child has cystic fibrosis. The condition can be diagnosed by DNA analysis or the presence of a high Na^+ concentration (over 60 mmol/L) in sweat. The latter is due to the impaired Cl^- transport in the secretory cells of the sweat glands as water transport into the sweat depends on the setting up of an osmotic gradient.

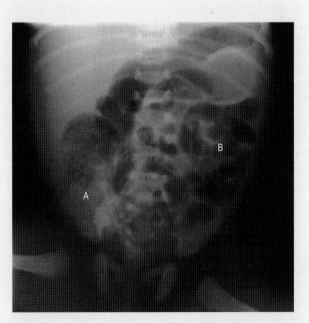

Fig. 5.7 Plain abdominal X-ray taken from a baby with cystic fibrosis. The meconium stool has obstructed the bowel and can be seen in the caecum (A). The proximal small bowel loops have dilated (B) and are filled with gas.

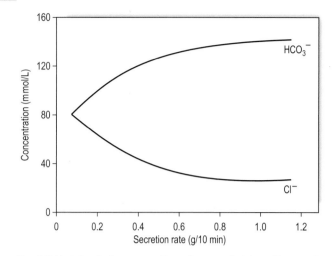

Fig. 5.8 Variation in the composition of pancreatic juice with respect to Cl^- and HCO_3^-, with rate of flow.

Control of secretion

The control of the exocrine secretion of the acinar and duct cells of the pancreas is via peptides such as the hormones secretin, cholecystokinin (CCK) and vasoactive intestinal peptide (VIP), and somatostatin which acts mainly as a paracrine factor, and neurotransmitters.

Hormonal control

The major hormones involved in stimulating secretion are secretin, which stimulates the secretion of the alkaline aqueous component, and cholecystokinin (CCK) that stimulates the secretion of the enzyme component. These hormones are produced by the APUD cells in the duodenal mucosa (see Ch. 1) in response to food constituents in the duodenal chyme (see below). As secretion of the two components of pancreatic juice is controlled by separate regulatory mechanisms, the composition of the juice entering the duodenum can vary with respect to its enzyme protein content. It can contain between 1% and 10% protein.

CCK and gastrin compete for the same receptor on the acinar cell (Fig. 5.12). CCK, gastrin and acetylcholine all increase enzyme protein synthesis and secretion via:

- Increase in phosphatidylinositol turnover
- Increase in intracellular Ca^{2+} concentration.

Secretin and VIP act on the acinar cell to increase the intracellular levels of cAMP (Fig. 5.12). This increase in cAMP by secretin and VIP potentiates the effect of CCK, gastrin and acetylcholine. Thus the enzyme secretion is greater when the two types of secretogogue are acting together.

Somatostatin

Somatostatin, which is present in D cells in the islets of Langerhans of the pancreas, is a powerful inhibitor

Impairment of functions

Both exocrine and endocrine secretions of the pancreas are impaired in chronic pancreatitis.

The blockage of the secretory ducts and loss of acinar tissue lead to a decrease in both alkaline juice and enzymes. The reduced alkaline secretion leads to: (1) reduced activity of enzymes in the small intestine which results in malabsorption and weight loss; (2) impaired micelle formation (essential for adequate lipid absorption) which leads to steatorrhoea (high fat content in the stools); (3) possibly duodenal ulceration as a consequence of the high acidity.

Destruction of islet tissue can lead to decreased secretion of the hormones insulin and glucagon, which are both involved in the control of glucose metabolism. Insulin lowers the blood glucose by increasing the uptake of glucose into tissues whilst glucagon increases blood glucose by stimulating glucose release from the liver (see Ch. 9). Thus, the two hormones have opposite effects on blood glucose concentration, although the effect of insulin is dominant.

Insulin is normally released from the pancreas in response to an increase in blood glucose concentration during a meal. The glucose tolerance test measures the insulin response to ingestion of a glucose solution (see Fig. 9.4). The insulin response is impaired early in chronic pancreatitis, i.e. the time taken for the increased blood glucose to return to normal is prolonged. Overt diabetes eventually develops in many patients.

Chronic progressive jaundice may also occur in chronic pancreatitis. This is due to fibrosis around the lower end of the common bile duct as it passes through the head of the pancreas. The fibrosis prevents the access of bile to the small intestine resulting in a raised serum bilirubin due to reflux of bile constituents into the systemic circulation. Raised serum alkaline phosphatase is also seen as this enzyme is released by damaged cells lining the biliary tree.

In chronic pancreatitis, there may also be coexisting alcoholic liver disease, making it difficult to determine whether the jaundice is primarily due to disease of the pancreas or to cirrhosis of the liver. Thus a liver biopsy and histological assessment of the tissue may also be required.

of pancreatic secretion. It acts in a paracrine manner to inhibit the release of the exocrine alkaline and enzyme secretions, as well as the pancreatic hormones insulin and glucagon. In addition, it inhibits the release of a number of gastrointestinal hormones, including CCK, secretin and gastrin. Circulating somatostatin probably augments the actions of locally released somatostatin. It originates from a number of sites in the body, including various locations in the gastrointestinal tract. Pancreatic somatostatin is predominantly the tetradecapeptide form, S-14. The release of this hormone is stimulated by CCK, gastrin and secretin. Analogues of somatostatin

Case 5.2
Cystic fibrosis: 3

Impairment of functions

In cystic fibrosis, the primary defect in the pancreas is a lack of Cl⁻ secretion leading to defective bicarbonate secretion. The secretion of enzymes is not initially affected but the blockage of the ducts prevents them reaching their site of action in the small intestine. Thus digestion and absorption are impaired leading to malnutrition if the condition remains untreated. Undigested fat is passed out of the intestines and appears in the stools, accounting for their pale colour (steatorrhoea).

Although the secretion of bicarbonate is impaired abnormalities in the patient's acid–base status may not be present as secretion of both alkaline and acid digestive juices are affected.

Later in the disease, the pancreas may become damaged and there may be a deficiency of the pancreatic hormones insulin and glucagon. As insulin is the dominant hormone, diabetes mellitus may develop (as in chronic pancreatitis, see Case 5.1: 3).

Case 5.1
Chronic pancreatitis: 4

Physiological consequences, treatment and management

The main consequences of malabsorption and diabetes mellitus are malnutrition and weight loss. Lack of alkaline secretion can lead to alkalosis because the 'alkaline tide' in the blood which results from gastric acid secretion during a meal (see Ch. 3) is normally partially neutralized by the 'acid' tide resulting from the secretion of alkaline juice by the pancreas. However, in chronic pancreatitis, the alkalosis is normally compensated by respiratory and renal mechanisms (see the companion volumes: *The Respiratory System* and *The Renal System*).

Treatment is usually non-surgical in uncomplicated chronic pancreatitis. The need for complete abstention from alcohol is emphasized. Pain relief is initially via treatment with a non-steroidal anti-inflammatory drug (NSAID) such as aspirin, and then, if necessary, via opiates. Nutritional support in the form of simple nutrients (amino acids, glucose, fatty acids) may be advised. Oral pancreatic extract can be prescribed to replace the pancreatic enzymes. Usually, the extract is enriched with lipase as the secretion of this enzyme tends to decrease more rapidly than that of proteolytic enzymes. The enzyme preparation can be administered together with an anti-ulcer drug (proton pump inhibitor) to reduce acid production by the stomach, as this inactivates the enzymes. Alternatively, the enzymes can be administered in the form of granules within which the enzymes are enclosed in a pH-dependent polymer. The protective coating dissolves only when the pH is more alkaline than 6.0, i.e. not in the stomach, but hopefully in the duodenum or upper jejunum.

The metabolic complications of diabetes are discussed in Chapter 9. If diabetes is present, it is treated with insulin.

Case 5.2
Cystic fibrosis: 4

Treatment

There is currently no cure for this condition. Genetic screening is usually offered to couples with a family history of the condition. Some 90% of affected individuals survive into their teens and most will now survive into middle age. Lung or heart–lung transplantation can be successful in prolonging and improving the quality of life. Genetic engineering offers hope for a cure in the future. However, even if the CFTR gene could be stably transfected into the secretory epithelial cells, there would be a need for repeat treatment as the cells are continuously being shed and replaced by new ones. This problem might one day be overcome if the gene could be transfected into the progenitor (stem) cells.

Although the pulmonary problems dominate the condition in most cases, the management of the pancreatic insufficiency is necessary to maintain overall nutrition and growth. The treatment is the ingestion of a pancreatic enzyme preparation by mouth. This should be done throughout a meal to ensure optimum mixing of the enzymes with the food. The dosage is determined by the level of fat in the stools (steatorrhoea). The enzymes are usually administered in enteric-coated form that renders them resistant to degradation by acid in the stomach. The coating is susceptible to degradation in the alkaline environment of the small intestine, the enzymes consequently being released at their usual site of action. Degradation of the enzymes by gastric acid can still be a significant problem but this can be minimized by concomitant treatment with an H₂ receptor antagonist such as ranitidine or a hydrogen pump inhibitor such as omeprazole.

such as octreotide are used clinically to inhibit pancreatic enzyme secretion (Box 5.3).

Nervous control

The nervous control of pancreatic secretion is via both parasympathetic and sympathetic nerves. Stimulation of cholinergic fibres in the vagus nerve enhances the rate of secretion of both enzyme and alkaline fluid. Stimulation of the sympathetic nerves inhibits secretion, mainly by reducing the blood flow to the gland (via vasoconstriction of the arterioles) that decreases the volume of juice secreted. However, stimulation of the sympathetic nerves to the pancreas depresses the enzyme content of the secretion as well as the volume of juice secreted.

Control of secretion during a meal

The control of the secretion of pancreatic juice during a meal depends on the volume and composition of the food. Ingested material present at different locations within the gastrointestinal tract affects the control of the

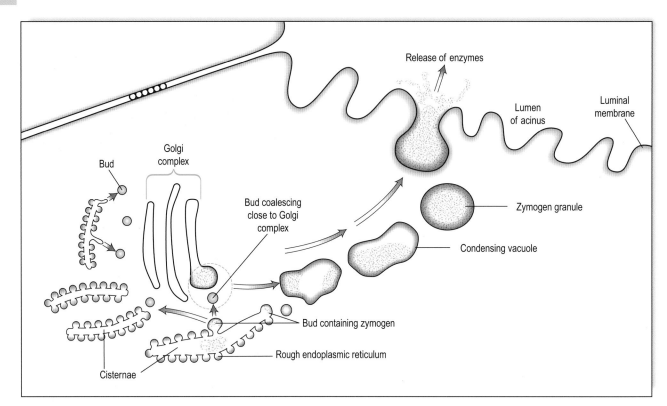

Fig. 5.9 Mechanism of enzyme secretion in the acinar cell.

secretions in different ways. The control during a meal can accordingly be divided into three phases (see Ch. 1), according to the location of the food or chyme:

1. The cephalic phase: due to the approach of food or the presence of food in the mouth.
2. The gastric phase: when food is in the stomach.
3. The intestinal phase: when food material is in the duodenum.

Cephalic phase

The sight and smell of food, or other sensory stimuli associated with the impending arrival of food, elicit increased pancreatic secretion via a 'conditioned' reflex. The presence of food in the mouth stimulates secretion via a 'non-conditioned' reflex. The control during this phase is therefore nervous. It is mediated by impulses in cholinergic fibres in the vagus nerve. The juice secreted is mainly the enzyme-rich secretion, containing very little HCO_3^-.

In response to vagal stimulation, the acinar cells also secrete kallikreins, which catalyse the production of bradykinin, a vasodilator. This results in increased blood flow to the pancreas, and increased volume of secretion. The mechanism involved in this effect is similar to that

which occurs in the control of salivary secretion that is described in Chapter 2.

Gastric phase

The presence of food in the stomach stimulates the secretion of pancreatic juice via a hormonal mechanism. Activation of chemoreceptors in the walls of the stomach by peptides, and the activation of mechanoreceptors, causes the release of the hormone gastrin from G cells, into the local circulation. Stimulation of cholinergic nerves is also involved in this phase of control. During the gastric phase the secretion of both the enzyme-rich and the alkaline components of pancreatic juice is increased.

Intestinal phase

The intestinal phase of control is the most important phase of the response to food. Food material in the duodenum stimulates both the alkaline and the enzyme-rich components of pancreatic juice. The alkaline component of pancreatic juice is secreted in response mainly to acid in the duodenal contents. Acid stimulates the release of secretin from APUD cells in the walls of the intestine and this hormone stimulates the duct cells to secrete the alkaline fluid. This is a feedback control mechanism that helps to control the pH of the duodenal contents.

Box 5.2 Acute pancreatitis

Acute pancreatitis is a condition in which the pancreatic tissue is destroyed by digestive enzymes. Most attacks of this acute disease (approximately 75%) are mild but in some more severe cases the condition can result in haemodynamic instability and multi-organ failure. The physiological mechanisms underlying acute pancreatitis are not completely understood. It is characterized by the presence of activated enzymes in the pancreatic ducts. The consequence of this is autodigestion of the pancreatic tissue.

In acute pancreatitis activated trypsin in the ducts of the pancreas proteolytically activates more trypsinogen and other proteolytic enzyme precursors (chymotrypsinogen, proelastase and procarboxypeptidase) and prophospholipase A.

The active enzymes digest the pancreatic tissue. When the walls of the acini on the surface of the pancreas are digested, the enzymes leak into the abdominal cavity and a generalized peritonitis results. In 5% of cases, the condition is extremely serious and the blood vessels are digested by pancreatic elastase resulting in internal bleeding, and eventually ischaemia (due to hypotension) and anaemia. The condition is then known as haemorrhagic necrotizing pancreatitis, which has an 80% mortality rate.

It is not known how activated digestive enzymes appear in the pancreatic ducts in acute pancreatitis, but one possibility is that it is due to reflux of intestinal chyme containing activated enzymes, into the pancreatic duct. The condition is often associated with the presence of gallstones in the bile ducts. It is likely that small gallstones lodge at the ampulla of Vater and prevent the closure of the sphincter of Oddi. This process may allow duodenal juice containing activated enzymes to reflux into the pancreatic duct. Alcohol abuse, infections, pancreatic tumours and treatment with certain drugs may also have a causative role in acute pancreatitis.

The diagnosis of acute pancreatitis depends on the presence of high concentrations of α-amylase in the blood. This enzyme, together with others, leaks from the lysed pancreatic cells into the blood. α-Amylase may also be present in the urine because it is not adequately reabsorbed in the kidney tubules. An ultrasound scan (Fig. 5.10) of the abdomen may reveal the presence of biliary gall stones. CT scanning (Fig. 5.11) enables the extent of necrosis to be assessed.

Hypocalcaemia may also be present. This is partly due to loss of albumen, with bound Ca^{2+}, in the protein-rich exudates from the pancreas. This exudation also causes a rise in the haematocrit due to loss of plasma volume.

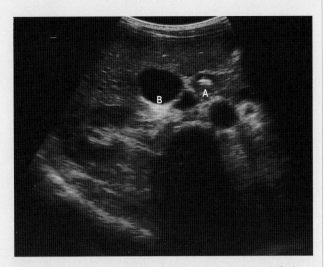

Fig. 5.10 Ultrasound scan of the biliary tree, showing a calcified stone in the common bile duct (A) which is dilated around the stone. The adjacent gallbladder is also seen (B).

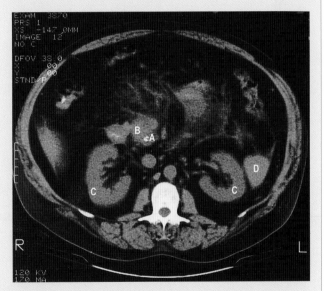

Fig. 5.11 CT scan of the same patient as Fig. 5.10, showing the calcified stone at the lower end of the common bile duct (A) lying within a swollen head of the pancreas (B). The kidneys (C) and spleen (D) are also visible.

The enzyme-rich juice is released during the intestinal phase in response to fat and peptides in the food. The fats and peptides cause the release of CCK from the walls of the duodenum into the blood. CCK stimulates the acinar cells to secrete enzymes. Trypsin in the duodenum inhibits the release of enzymes via inhibition of CCK release. This is another feedback control mechanism, which limits the quantity of enzymes present in the intestines, and may have some protective function.

Secretin exerts a permissive effect on the secretion of enzymes; it does not stimulate enzyme secretion on its own, but it enhances the effect of CCK. Similarly, CCK exerts a permissive effect on the secretion of the alkaline fluid by secretin. Stimulation of the vagus nerve causes the

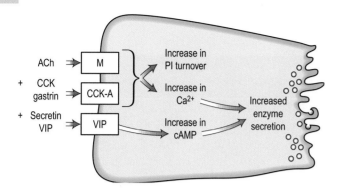

Fig. 5.12 Cellular mechanisms of control in the acinar cell. M, muscarinic receptor; PI, phosphatidylinositol.

release of mainly the enzyme-rich secretion, but if the vagi are sectioned, the alkaline secretion elicited in response to secretin is reduced by 50%, indicting a functional overlap between the effects of vagal stimulation and secretin. Thus the vagal mechanism may enhance the effect of secretin.

Box 5.3 Somatostatin analogues

Analogues of somatostatin such as octreotide are used clinically to inhibit pancreatic enzyme secretion in acute pancreatitis, and following pancreatic surgery. Reducing the secretion of digestive enzymes allows the pancreas to heal more safely following injury (whether due to inflammation or surgery). Octreotide is an octapeptide which contains the tetrapeptide sequence which is known to be essential for somatostatin activity. Somatostatin itself, when injected, has a short half-life (<4 min). However, octreotide injected subcutaneously, has a half-life of approximately 100 min and its action is therefore relatively long-lasting. This is important in the clinical setting as somatostatin is only effective if given as a continuous infusion, whereas analogues such as octreotide are effective if given as a bolus two or three times per day.

LIVER AND BILIARY SYSTEM

6

Chapter objectives

After studying this chapter you should be able to:

1. Understand the role of the liver in the digestive process and the excretion of waste metabolites and toxic substances.

2. Understand the relationship between the structure of the hepatobiliary tract and its function in the secretion and storage of bile.

3. Understand the mechanisms of secretion of the important components of bile, and their recycling via the enterohepatic circulation.

4. Understand the mechanisms of control of bile secretion and its release into the duodenum.

Introduction

The numerous functions of the liver can be divided into two broad categories:

1. Those concerned with the processing of absorbed materials and synthetic reactions

2. Those concerned with secretion and excretion.

This chapter is concerned with the secretory and excretory roles of the liver. The processing of absorbed nutrients and the role of the liver in the control of energy metabolism are discussed in Chapter 9.

The most important exocrine functions of the liver are:

- The provision of bile acids and alkaline fluid for the digestion and absorption of fats, and for the neutralization of gastric acid in the intestines

- The degradation and conjugation of waste products of metabolism

- The detoxification of poisonous substances

- The excretion of waste metabolites and detoxified substances in bile

- Detoxified substances and waste metabolites are eliminated from the body either in the bile, via the gastrointestinal tract, or via secretion from the liver into the blood for subsequent excretion by the kidneys.

The liver has enormous reserves of function, and normal homeostasis can be maintained even after three quarters of it have been removed. Clinical manifestation of liver disease therefore implies considerable damage to the organ.

Gallstones form in the gall bladder and biliary tract as a consequence of various derangements of the hepatobiliary system. The problems encountered in a patient with gallstone disease are given in this chapter to illustrate many of the roles of the liver in secretion and excretion. A second case history involving a patient who had taken an overdose of paracetamol is used to emphasize the important role of the liver in the detoxification of drugs.

Overview of the functioning of the hepatobiliary system

The anatomical arrangement of the liver, gall bladder and biliary tract is shown in Figure 6.1. The liver is continually secreting substances both into the blood, and into the bile. Bile is both a secretory fluid and an excretory medium. In the human, it is stored between meals in the gall bladder, where it is concentrated. During a meal it is released from the gall bladder and enters the cystic duct that in turn drains it into the common bile duct. The bile enters the small intestine at the level of the duodenum. Its entry into the small intestine is controlled by a smooth muscle sphincter: the sphincter of Oddi.

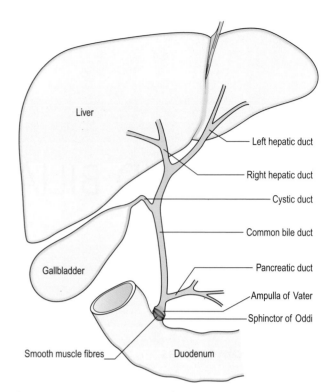

Fig. 6.1 Anatomical arrangement of the liver, gall bladder and biliary tract.

The gall bladder is surrounded by smooth muscle. Between meals, when the gall bladder smooth muscle is relaxed, the sphincter of Oddi is closed, preventing the bile from entering the small intestine. Consequently, the bile passes into the gall bladder where it is stored and concentrated. Contraction of the gall bladder forces the bile into the common bile duct. At the same time the smooth muscle in the sphincter of Oddi relaxes, and the sphincter opens to allow the bile to enter the duodenum. Food in the duodenum is the main stimulus for gall bladder contraction.

Anatomy and morphology of the liver

The liver is the largest single organ in the body. In the adult it comprises approximately one-fiftieth of the body weight. In the infant it is proportionately even larger. It consists of right and left lobes (Fig. 6.2A), the right lobe being six times the size of the left in the adult.

The liver is composed of lobules (Fig. 6.2B). In the centre of each lobule is the central canal, in which lies a hepatic vein, which is a tributary of the inferior vena cava. Columns of liver cells (hepatocytes) and sinusoids radiate out from the central canal. Several portal tracts lie at the periphery of each lobule. Each tract (or 'portal triad') contains a bile duct, a branch of the portal vein, and a branch of the hepatic artery.

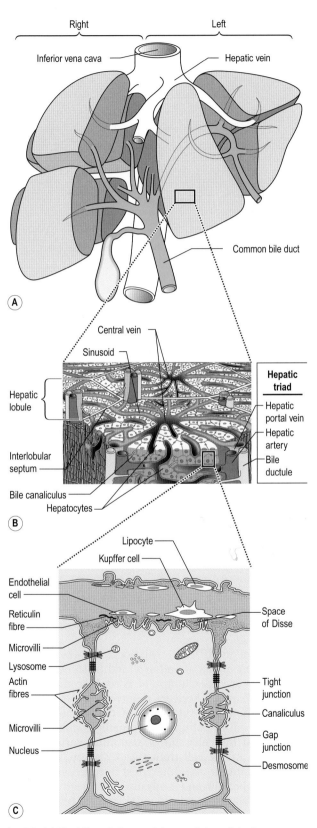

The liver has a double blood supply: the hepatic artery supplies the liver with oxygenated blood from the lungs, and the portal vein supplies it with nutrient-rich blood from the intestines (see Ch. 1). The arterial blood comprises approximately 20% of the total blood supply of the liver and the portal venous blood, approximately 80%. The arterial blood and the portal venous blood mix together in the liver sinusoids. The sinusoidal blood drains away via the hepatic veins to the vena cava. This direction of flow is determined by the relatively higher pressure of the blood in the portal vein compared to the central vein.

In liver cirrhosis, scar tissue replaces normal healthy tissue. This scar tissue distorts the normal structure and regrowth of liver cells and blocks the flow of blood through the organ. This disease is described in Box 6.1.

The liver is covered by a fibroconnective tissue capsule known as the capsule of Glisson, from which thin connective tissue septa enter the organ to divide it into lobes and lobules. The capsule is covered by peritoneum, except in an area known as the 'bare area' which is in direct contact with the diaphragm.

The secretory system of the liver begins with minute tubules, the canaliculi. These are formed by oppositely aligned grooves in the contact surfaces of adjacent hepatocytes (Figs 6.2C, 6.3). The membrane of each liver cell contributes to several bile canaliculi. Bile secreted into the canaliculi flows in the opposite direction to the flow of blood in the sinusoids. The canaliculi drain into terminal bile ductules. The ductules converge to form intralobular ducts, and these converge to form interlobular ducts, which in turn converge to form the right and left hepatic bile ducts. These converge outside the liver to form the common hepatic bile duct.

Histology

The major type of cell in the liver is the hepatocyte that is an epithelial parenchymal cell. The hepatocytes are arranged in plates which branch and anastomize to form a three-dimensional lattice (Fig. 6.2). Between the plates are the blood-filled sinusoids. In this respect the liver resembles an endocrine gland. There is usually only one layer of hepatocytes between the sinusoids.

The sinusoidal spaces differ from blood capillaries in that they are of greater diameter and their lining cells are not typically endothelial. The basal lamina around the sinusoids is incomplete and this enables direct access of the plasma to the surface of the hepatocyte. This allows active metabolic exchange between the blood and the cells (Fig. 6.2C). The perisinusoidal space is an interstitial space that contains reticular and collagenous fibres. A few mesenchymal cells called lipocytes produce the fibres. Two main cell types are present in the sinusoidal lining. These are endothelial cells and Kupffer cells. They lie in a mesh of fine reticular fibres. The endothelial cell has small elongated nuclei and greatly attenuated cytoplasm. The cytoplasm may interdigitate with cytoplasmic

Fig. 6.2 (A) The biliary drainage of the two lobes of the liver. (B) Lobular structure of the liver, illustrating the biliary secretory system and the dual blood supply. (C) Features of the hepatocyte, and its relationship to adjacent cells and the sinusoid.

Box 6.1 Liver cirrhosis

In cirrhosis of the liver scar tissue replaces normal healthy tissue and blocks the flow of blood from the portal vein through the organ. This leads to reduced synthesis of proteins and other molecules by the liver and reduced oxidative capacity. Metabolism of bile constituents, and drug detoxification, and secretion and excretion of bile constituents become inadequate to maintain health.

Liver cirrhosis has many causes, including:

- Chronic alcoholism. Cirrhosis does not usually develop until after more than 10 years of alcohol abuse. This is a major cause of liver cirrhosis in the western world
- Chronic hepatitis C, B or D. Hepatitis C virus causes low-grade damage, which over the course of many years can lead to cirrhosis. This is a major cause of liver cirrhosis. It was commonly transmitted by blood transfusion before routine testing for hepatitis C virus was available. Hepatitis B virus is the most common cause of liver cirrhosis in the third world but is less common in more developed countries
- Autoimmune disease: the immune system attacks the liver causing inflammation and tissue damage which can eventually lead to cirrhosis
- Inherited diseases including α1-antitrypsin deficiency, haemachromatosis, Wilson's disease, galactosaemia and glycogen storage diseases
- Drugs, toxins and infections. Severe reactions to prescription drugs, prolonged exposure to environmental toxins, parasitic infection (with schistosomes) can also cause liver cirrhosis.

The signs and symptoms of liver cirrhosis include fatigue, weight loss, nausea, abdominal pain, spider-like blood vessels on the skin, oedema of the legs and abdomen (ascites), jaundice (see Box 6.2), gallstones (see Case 6.1: 1–6), itching (due to bilirubin being deposited in the skin) and a tendency to bleed easily (due to reduced clotting factor synthesis in the liver).

The treatment of liver cirrhosis depends on the cause of the condition and the complications experienced. The damage cannot be reversed but the progression of the disease can be arrested or delayed by, for example cessation of alcohol abuse or medication to treat infections and other causes. When liver damage is so pronounced that the liver stops functioning, a transplant is necessary. The survival rate after liver transplantation is over 90% now that effective immune-suppression drugs are available.

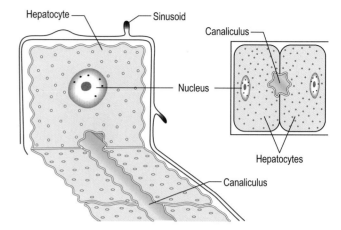

Fig. 6.3 Early secretory system of the liver. Inset: canaliculus (in cross-section) formed by adjacent hepatocytes.

extensive cytoplasm, with processes that extend into, and sometimes across, the sinusoidal space. They increase in number when required for phagocytosis, possibly by differentiation of the endothelial type of cell.

Hepatocytes

The hepatocyte is a polygonal cell with a clearly defined cell membrane, which is closely apposed to the cell membranes of adjacent hepatocytes (Figs 6.2C, 6.3). The membranes of adjacent cells are partially separated to form a bile canaliculus. The plasmalemma of adjacent hepatocytes shows irregularities with tight junctions, spot desmosomes and gap junctions. These separate the canaliculus from the rest of the intercellular space (Fig. 6.2C).

The plasma membrane of hepatocytes is specialized in certain regions. Adjacent to a sinusoidal blood space the hepatocyte is separated from the wall of the sinusoid by the perisinusoidal space (the space of Disse) and at this location the plasma membrane of the hepatocyte has numerous long microvilli. Vesicles and vacuoles are present in the subadjacent cytoplasm (Fig. 6.2C). The microvilli provide a large surface area for absorption and secretion.

The nuclei in different hepatocytes show considerable variation in shape and size and in some cases the cells are binucleate. Clumps of basophilic material are present in all cells. There are numerous small mitochondria throughout the cytoplasm of the hepatocyte. The structure of all hepatocytes is broadly similar but the cytoplasm of the cells shows a gradual variation with the distance of the cell from the periphery. The differences are related to the differences in functional activity of the peripherally and centrally positioned cells. The hepatocytes closest to the afferent blood supply, the 'periportal' cells, are exposed to the highest concentrations of nutrients and oxygen and those in the central region, the 'perivenous' cells, near to the efferent outflow, are exposed to the lowest concentrations. The periportal

processes from adjacent cells of the same type or another type. They contain few organelles but numerous pinocytotic vesicles. They also contain large fenestrae that are not closed by a diaphragm. Kupffer cells are phagocytic and often contain degenerating red cells, pigment granules, and iron-containing granules. They have large nuclei and

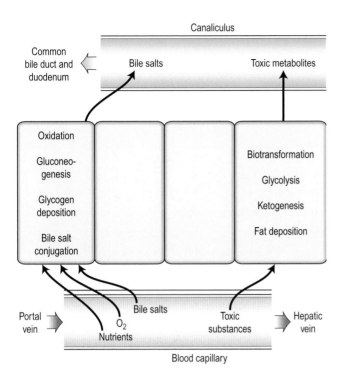

Fig. 6.4 Major functions of periportal and perivenous hepatocytes.

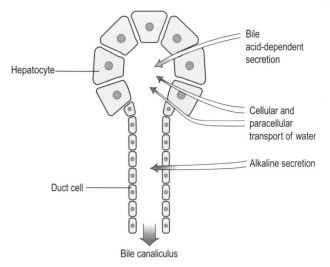

Fig. 6.5 Sites of secretion of the two component secretions of bile.

cells are the most active in the uptake from the blood of bile salts and in the secretion of many bile constituents into the canaliculi as well as in oxidative metabolism and gluconeogenesis (Fig. 6.4). After feeding, glycogen is deposited first in the periportal cells. It is only after a heavy carbohydrate meal that the more centrally located perivenous cells store glycogen. Moreover, when the blood sugar concentration falls, glycogen is removed first from the perivenous cells. The perivenous cells, which are exposed to depleted plasma, are the more active in biotransformation reactions and the secretion of potentially toxic xenobiotic and endobiotic substances. They are also more active in glycolytic and ketogenic reactions. Under certain conditions fat is deposited in the hepatocytes and it appears first in the more centrally disposed cells. Thus the cytosol of a given hepatocyte exhibits differences in composition at different times in relation to feeding and whether fat or glycogen has been deposited.

The canaliculus

The lumen of the canaliculus is approximately $0.75\,\mu m$ in diameter. Microvilli project from the canalicular membrane into the lumen, providing a large surface area for secretion. Membranes of adjacent hepatocytes are joined by tight junctions near the canaliculus (Fig. 6.2C). These junctions are leaky and permit paracellular exchange between the plasma and the canaliculus.

The canaliculus is involved in transport of substances into the lumen, but it is also a contractile structure. Actin filaments are present in the microvilli, and both actin and myosin fibres are present in the cytoplasm surrounding

the canaliculus. Contractions of the canaliculi can be stimulated by extracellular ATP. The contractions involve actin–myosin interaction as in smooth muscle cells. They probably pump bile towards the ducts. Atony (lack of contractile function) of the canaliculus causes cholestasis (reduced bile flow).

The junctions of the bile canaliculus with the bile ducts at the periphery of a lobule consist of an intermediate structure called the ductules or canals of Hering. Here the hepatocytes that form the canaliculus are gradually replaced by smaller cells with dark nuclei and poorly- developed organelles. These are the ductule cells. They are underlain by a distinct basal lamina. The lumen of the ductule eventually joins that of a bile duct in the portal area.

Extrahepatic ducts

The extrahepatic ducts are lined by tall columnar epithelium (Fig. 6.5) that secretes mucus. There is a layer of connective tissue beneath the epithelium, with numerous elastic fibres, mucous glands, blood vessels and nerves. In the common bile duct there is also a layer of smooth muscle cells. These cells are sparse in the upper region of the duct but form a thicker layer of oblique and transverse fibres in the regions of the sphincter of Oddi near the duodenum (see below).

Bile

Composition and functions

Bile is secreted at a rate of 250–1000 mL/day in the adult. It is isosmotic with blood plasma. It is a composite of two different secretions; one originating in the hepatocytes, and the other in the cells that line the bile ducts (Fig. 6.5). The two secretions mix together in the ducts.

Secretion of the duct cells

The secretion from the duct cells is a watery alkaline fluid that is rich in bicarbonate. It comprises approximately 25% of the total bile volume. Its function is, first, to provide an appropriate pH for the process of micelle formation (see below), which requires a neutral or slightly alkaline environment. Second, it contributes (together with pancreatic juice and intestinal secretions) to the neutralization of stomach acid in the intestinal chyme. This is important both for micelle formation and digestive enzyme action in the small intestine (see Ch. 8). In addition the neutralization of acid in the duodenum protects the mucosa from ulceration. The secretion contains Na^+, K^+, Cl^- and HCO_3^- ions. Its composition is similar to that of alkaline pancreatic juice. At basal rates of secretion the ionic composition resembles that of plasma. However as the flow increases upon stimulation (by a meal) the Cl^- concentration decreases and the HCO_3^- concentration increases. This is due to the presence of a Cl^-/HCO_3^- exchange mechanism in the duct cells. HCO_3^- ions are extracted from the bile and Cl^- is added to it, a process similar to that involved in the secretion of alkaline juice from the pancreatic duct cells (see Ch. 5). At high flow rates, the bile is not in contact with the duct cells for sufficient time to allow appreciable modification to take place and there is proportionately less bicarbonate extracted, resulting in a more alkaline bile. Thus, the secretion becomes more alkaline at flow rates higher than the basal level.

The volume of the alkaline secretion, unlike the secretion produced by the hepatocytes, is not directly determined by the concentration of bile salts in the blood. It has been termed the 'bile acid-independent' component of bile. The control of this secretion during a meal, like that of alkaline pancreatic juice and the alkaline fluid secreted from Brunner's glands in the duodenum, is via the release into the blood of the hormone secretin, from the walls of the duodenum. This occurs mainly in response to the presence of acid in the duodenum. The hormone circulates to stimulate all of these alkaline secretions. As it is released in response to acid chyme in the duodenum this mechanism provides a feedback control of the pH of the intestinal contents.

Secretion from the hepatocytes

The hepatocytes secrete a primary juice into the canaliculi. It contains a number of inorganic monovalent and divalent ions, and various organic substances (Table 6.1). The latter include lipids; bile acids, lecithin and cholesterol, all of which are sequestered together in micelles. Bile secretion is a major route whereby cholesterol is lost from the body. The bile acids are essential for the effective digestion and absorption of dietary fats. There are also some proteins in bile, including albumin, polymeric immunoglobulin A (pIgA) that protects the biliary tract and the upper intestines from infection, and some plasma-derived enzymes. Bile also contains bile pigments, chiefly bilirubin, that have been conjugated with glucuronic acid. The pigments are breakdown products

Table 6.1 Comparison of the concentrations of some substances in hepatic and gall bladder bile

Constituent electrolytes	Hepatic bile (mM)	Gall bladder bile (mM)
HCO_3^-	28	10
Cl^-	100	25
K^+	5	12
Na^+	145	130
Ca^{2+}	5	23
Organic molecules		
Bilirubin	0.7	5.1
Cholesterol	2.6	16.0
Lecithin	0.5	3.9
Bile salts	26.0	145.0

Loss of gall bladder bile via a fistula can quickly deplete K^+ reserves, unless replacement therapy is started.

of haemoglobin. Bile also contains numerous other compounds that are extracted from the blood, metabolized by the liver, and excreted. Many of these substances are potentially toxic endogenous or exogenous substances such as steroid hormones, drugs and environmental toxins that have been detoxified and conjugated in the liver. Conjugation serves to increase the polarity of a substance and therefore its solubility in water (see below). Bile remains isosmotic with plasma at different rates of flow. This implies that an increase in secretion of bile acids and metabolites by the liver is accompanied by an increase in water secretion resulting in an increase in bile volume. This is known as the choleretic effect.

Biliary lipids

The structures of the major lipids present in bile are shown in Figure 6.6. The bile acids are derivatives of cholesterol and contain the cyclopentanoperhydrophenanthrene nucleus. One, two or three alcohol groups are attached to this nucleus and there is a short hydrocarbon chain ending in a carboxyl group (Fig. 6.6). Primary bile acids (cholic acid and chenodeoxycholic acid) are synthesized by the liver hepatocytes. Secondary bile acids (deoxycholic acid and lithocholic acid) are formed by dehydroxylation of primary bile acids in the intestines, by bacteria (Fig. 6.6). The bile acids are usually conjugated in the hepatocyte, with amino acids, largely glycine or taurine. The ratio of glycocholates to taurocholates is normally approximately 3:1 but the exact proportions depend on the relative availability of the two amino acids. The conjugated primary and secondary bile acids are reabsorbed actively in the ileum (see Ch. 8). However, bile acids may be deconjugated by bacteria in the small intestine and colon. Some of the unconjugated bile acids are absorbed by passive diffusion. Bile acids synthesized

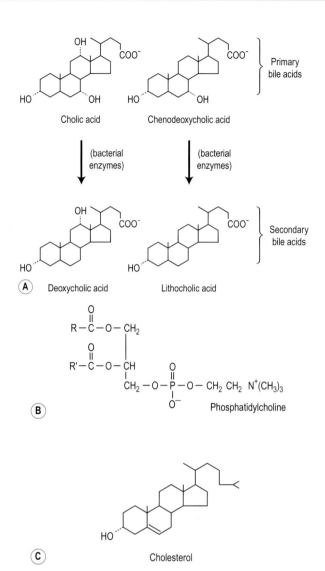

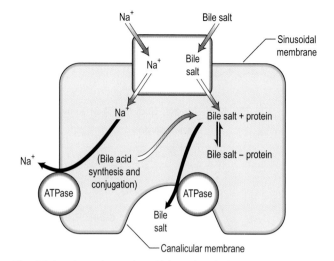

Fig. 6.7 Uptake and secretion of bile acid in the hepatocyte.

Fig. 6.6 (A) Structure of primary and secondary bile acids and their modification by intestinal bacteria. (B) Structure of phosphatidylcholine (R, palmitic acid; R', oleic or linoleic acid). (C) Structure of cholesterol.

de novo in the liver, and absorbed unconjugated bile acids, are reconjugated in the liver. In physiological fluids bile acids form salts with Na^+ and K^+ ions.

Uptake of bile salts from the blood into the hepatocyte is an active process that occurs against a concentration gradient (Fig. 6.7). It derives its energy from a Na^+/K^+-ATPase that pumps Na^+ out of the cell and involves a Na^+/bile salt cotransporter system located in the sinusoidal membrane. The process is driven by the electrochemical gradient for Na^+ set up by the pumping out of Na^+ ions. Another mechanism for bile acid transport, which involves a transporter with a wider specificity, has also been characterized. The different bile salts compete with each other indicating that they share the same transporter. Inside the hepatocyte the bile salts bind to protein, thereby keeping the intracellular concentration of free bile salts low. These proteins may be involved in transport of the bile acids through the cell.

Bile salts are secreted into the canaliculus against a considerable electrochemical gradient. The transport across the canalicular membrane is Na^+-independent. The energy may be partly derived from the membrane potential which is approximately 40 mV (negative inside the cell), but an ATPase-dependent pump that is specific for bile acids is present in the canalicular membrane and this is the major mechanism for bile salt transport across this membrane (see Fig. 6.7). It is distinct from the Na^+ gradient-driven bile acid uptake transporter in the sinusoidal membrane.

Bile acids are held in micelles in bile. They can be concentrated several-fold in hepatocyte bile as they are still held in micellar form. Bile acids are powerful detergents, and their sequestration in micelles may reduce their detergent and cytotoxic actions.

The major phospholipid in bile is a phosphatidylcholine (lecithin) with a unique fatty acid pattern: palmitic acid forms the outer ester bond and either oleic acid or linoleic acid the inner ester bond (Fig. 6.6). The immediate source of this phospholipid is a preformed pool in the liver cell membranes. The cholesterol in bile is also mainly derived from a preformed pool but an appreciable proportion is derived via *de novo* synthesis in the liver. The cholesterol in bile is not esterified to any significant extent (Fig. 6.6).

Inside the hepatocytes the phospholipid and cholesterol probably exist as components of membranes of intracellular vesicles. The membranes of these vesicles are incorporated into the plasma membrane by fusing with it. The rate of secretion of phospholipid and cholesterol appears to be linearly related to the rate of bile salt secretion. Bile salts are secreted into the canaliculus first. The detergent action of these may be responsible for removing the other lipids from the canalicular membrane. The ratio of cholesterol to phospholipid is fairly constant (approx. 0.3 in the human). Some biliary phospholipid and cholesterol is present in bile in vesicles. These vesicles can incorporate bile salts and are gradually converted to micelles.

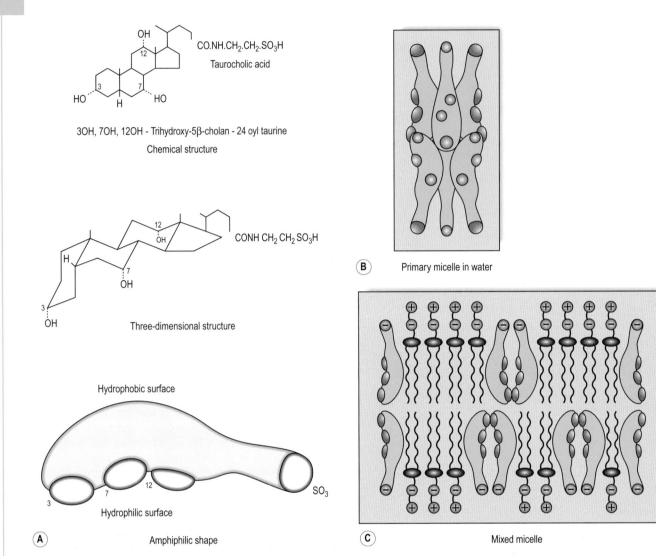

Fig. 6.8 (A) Electrical polarity of a conjugated bile acid. (B) Primary micelle, composed of bile salts, showing orientation of the amphiphilic lipid in the micelle. (C) Mixed micelle, containing bile acid and phospholipid, illustrating surface net negative charge and outer shell of cations (mainly Na^+ ions).

Micelle formation

Bile salts are essential for the formation of micelles in bile. The bile salt molecule is amphiphilic; the roughly planar ring system is hydrophobic and forms one side of the molecule. The alcohol groups, the carboxyl group, and the peptide bond of the bile acid, all project from the other side, imparting a net negative charge, and therefore a hydrophilic nature to that side of the molecule (Fig. 6.8). A micelle has a hydrophilic shell region and a hydrophobic core region. Newly formed (primary) micelles are initially composed of bile salt molecules. The bile salts orientate themselves in the micelle with the hydrophobic side in the core and the hydrophilic side in the shell (Fig. 6.8). Primary micelles can sequester very little cholesterol. However, they take up phospholipid to form mixed micelles. Phosphatidylcholine is also an amphiphilic molecule; the long chain fatty acyl chains forming the hydrophobic domain that resides in the core region of the micelle and the phosphorylcholine group the hydrophilic domain which projects into the shell region (Fig. 6.8). The mixed micelle can hold more cholesterol than the primary micelle. In the presence of phosphatidylcholine larger micelles tend to form than in its absence. It is therefore known as a 'swelling' amphiphile. Cholesterol, which is extremely insoluble in water, resides in the core of the micelle. As the net charge on all micelles is negative they repel each other, thereby preventing coalescence, and inducing the formation of a stable suspension. The negatively charged micelle collects an outer shell of cations, mainly Na^+ ions. A micelle is disc-shaped, and its thickness approximates that of a lipid bilayer.

If the concentration of bile acids is too low for micelles to form, cholesterol precipitates out and gallstones form (Case 6.1: 1–3).

Two properties of bile salts determine whether they will participate in micelle formation:

1. The Krafft point, which is the temperature below which micelles composed of the particular bile acid will not form. Most bile acids have Krafft points well below body temperature, although the secondary bile acid lithocholic acid has a high Krafft point and is incapable of forming micelles at body temperature.

Case 6.1
Gallstone disease: 1

An obese middle-aged woman explained to her general practitioner that she had suffered several attacks of severe 'gripping' pain in the upper abdomen. However, there were no abnormal physical signs at the time she was seen by the doctor. Upon questioning she said that the attacks had started after meals. The pain built up gradually to a maximum and lasted for several hours. Her description of the location of the pain indicated that it was epigastric, and in the right upper quadrant of the abdomen. She also said that during a recent severe attack her husband had remarked that the 'whites' of her eyes (the sclera) had appeared yellow. In addition the patient had noticed that her urine became dark in colour, and her stools were pale and greasy-looking and tended to float in the lavatory pan. The doctor suspected that the patient was suffering from gallstones. This was subsequently confirmed by an ultrasound scan, and the patient was referred to a surgeon for a cholecystectomy (surgical removal of the gall bladder).

Examination of the details of this case provokes the following questions:

- What would an ultrasound scan show in gallstone disease? How could the findings explain the cause of the patient's pain?
- How can the abnormal appearance of the patient's stools be explained? What abnormalities of the digestive process does it indicate?
- How can the yellowing of the sclera (a symptom of jaundice) be explained?
- How would the composition of the bile entering the duodenum differ from normal after cholecystectomy? Would cholecystectomy have deleterious consequences for the normal functioning of the body?
- What is the composition of gallstones? Why do they form?
- How can gallstone disease be treated?

These issues will be addressed later in this chapter.

Case 6.1
Gallstone disease: 2

Detection and cause of pain

Gallstones (biliary calculi) are hard masses that can be present in the gall bladder or the bile ducts (Fig. 6.9). They can be classified broadly into two types:

1. Those composed largely of cholesterol
2. Those composed largely of bile pigment.

Both types may be calcified, but usually are not. Cholesterol stones tend to be large (often in excess of 1 cm in diameter), and several may be present in one individual. The attacks of pain (biliary cholic) experienced following meals are due to transient obstruction of the cystic duct when the gall bladder contracts. The pain in this patient is due to the pressure of the bile behind the stone. However, most individuals with gallstones are asymptomatic, and require no treatment.

Gallstones that are sufficiently calcified (<20% of all gallstones) can be detected by plain abdominal radiography. These may be cholesterol stones with a calcified shell, or pigment stones composed mainly of calcium bilirubinate. Pure cholesterol stones are radiolucent and cannot be detected using this technique.

The simple rapid technique of ultrasonography is usually employed to reveal gallstones (Fig. 6.9). This provides an overall

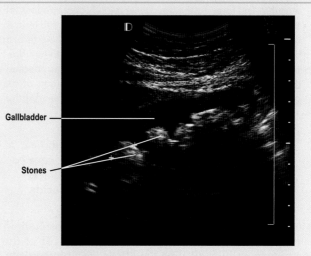

Fig. 6.9 An ultrasound scan showing a distended gall bladder and radio-opaque stones within the lumen.

gallstone detection rate of over 90%. It also allows evaluation of the thickness of the gall bladder wall; an abnormally thick wall indicates a diseased gall bladder, usually secondary to chronic inflammation, but occasionally due to a carcinoma.

Gallstones: composition, formation and occurrence

Many compounds can precipitate in bile to form stones, but approximately 80% are formed from cholesterol, with a variable Ca^{2+} content. The rest are composed largely of bile pigments and Ca^{2+} salts.

Cholesterol stones

If the concentration of bile acids or phospholipids relative to cholesterol in the bile falls, cholesterol will not be held in micelles. The bile then becomes supersaturated with cholesterol, and this tends to precipitate out as microcrystals. These microcrystals coalesce to form gallstones. Some cholesterol stones are composed purely of cholesterol. In these cases the stones tend to be large, solitary and pale yellow in colour. Smaller cholesterol stones can form and these are often of mixed composition but usually contain more than 70% cholesterol. These are also pale yellow and are usually multiple. They are of variable size and are laminated, with a dark central nucleus. The cholesterol crystals deposit around this nucleus, and then become hardened by the precipitation of organic salts.

Cholesterol gallstones tend to develop when there is a high-ratio of cholesterol to bile acids or lecithin in the bile. This can be due to high cholesterol secretion, as a consequence of a high fat diet, or to congenital hypercholesterolaemia. They may also form if there is reduced bile acid secretion, as a consequence of bile acid malabsorption in the ileum, or reduced lecithin secretion. The bile acid pool in an individual is fairly constant (see below) but in people with gallstones it tends to be smaller than average. Gallstone formation may happen at night as bile acid secretion falls (even further) and when blood concentrations are low (see below). The ratio of cholesterol to bile salts and lecithin is raised by a high-fat diet, as fats are converted to cholesterol in the liver. Interestingly, gallstones are common in South American women whose diet includes diosgenin-rich beans, because diosgenin increases cholesterol secretion. Inflammation of the gall bladder may also contribute by increasing reabsorption of bile salts or water in the gall bladder, thereby encouraging the cholesterol to precipitate out in the bile.

Women tend to have a higher cholesterol: phospholipid ratio than men which may account for the fact that four times more women than men suffer from gallstones. Genetic and racial factors also appear to be important. Cholesterol gallstones are also found in diseases of the ileum, such as Crohn's disease (see Ch. 8), which lead to reduced bile salt reabsorption.

Pigment stones

Pigment stones are usually of small diameter (a few m), and dark brown or black in colour. When they occur, they are usually multiple. They contain 40–95% pigment and less than 20% cholesterol. They constitute approximately 20% of all gallstones. They can form if there is an overload of unconjugated bilirubin resulting from haemolytic anaemia, burns or crush injury. A high incidence of pigment gallstones is seen in patients with haemolytic states (such as sickle cell anaemia). The bile becomes supersaturated with unconjugated bilirubin and it precipitates out. The free bilirubin combines with calcium in the bile to form insoluble calcium bilirubinate. This forms the nidus of a stone, and degradation products of bilirubin aggregate on this core to form pigment stones. A deficit in the conjugating ability of the liver can also result in the formation of pigment gallstones. In addition, infecting organisms that contain β-glucuronidase, an enzyme that deconjugates bilirubin glucuronide, can be responsible. Until recently a form of the disease where highly calcified pigment stones were present occurred in oriental countries (notably Japan). It was caused by infestation of the biliary duct with parasites that contain this enzyme. Its incidence has diminished as hygiene and nutrition have improved. Unfortunately, however, as the diet has become 'westernized' the incidence of cholesterol gallstones has increased. There is also a tendency for pigment stones to form in patients with cirrhosis of the liver due to stasis in the biliary tract.

---

2. The critical micellar concentration, which is the minimum concentration of a particular acid required for micelle formation. The critical concentration is usually well below the concentration of bile acids present in bile, and micelles easily form.

Micelle formation is also dependent on the phospholipid concentration, and on the ionic strength and pH of the medium: neutral or alkaline conditions are a prerequisite. The alkaline secretion from duct cells has an important role in this respect.

Micelle formation determines the volume of bile secreted. An individual micelle may be composed of 20 or so molecules of lipid but it constitutes only one osmotic particle. Thus a simple chemical analysis of the composition of bile does not indicate its osmolarity. Bile is in osmotic equilibrium with blood plasma and any increase in its content of osmotic particles is followed by increased secretion of fluid (the choleretic effect). When biliary lipids are secreted into bile however, micelle formation enables bile to be highly concentrated with respect to its lipid constituents without the enormous increase in volume that would accompany an equivalent secretion of water-soluble molecules.

Conjugation of metabolites and drugs

A number of other anions (mostly in conjugated form), in addition to bile acids, appear in bile. Their concentrations may be 10–1000 times that of their precursors in the plasma, indicating that active transport mechanisms exist for the removal of their precursors from the blood, or for their secretion into the canaliculus. Some of these anions

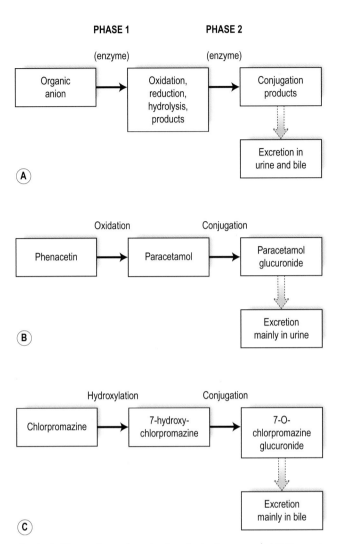

PHASE 1   **PHASE 2**

(enzyme)   (enzyme)

Organic anion → Oxidation, reduction, hydrolysis, products → Conjugation products → Excretion in urine and bile

(A)

Oxidation   Conjugation

Phenacetin → Paracetamol → Paracetamol glucuronide → Excretion mainly in urine

(B)

Hydroxylation   Conjugation

Chlorpromazine → 7-hydroxy-chlorpromazine → 7-O-chlorpromazine glucuronide → Excretion mainly in bile

(C)

Fig. 6.10 Biotransformation of anions in the hepatocyte. (A) General scheme involving two phases. (B) A drug (phenacetin) which is metabolized in the liver, secreted into the blood, and excreted in the kidney. (C) A drug (chlorpromazine) which is metabolized in the liver and excreted in the bile.

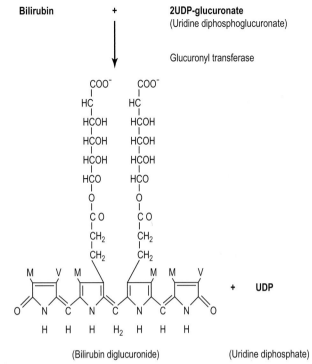

Bilirubin   +   **2UDP-glucuronate**
(Uridine diphosphoglucuronate)

Glucuronyl transferase

+   **UDP**

(Bilirubin diglucuronide)   (Uridine diphosphate)

Fig. 6.11 Conjugation of bilirubin in the hepatocyte.

are of endogenous origin, such as bile pigments or steroid hormones, and others are xenobiotics such as drugs or toxins, or their metabolites. Many of these organic anions undergo biotransformation in two phases in the liver cells. Figure 6.10 shows a general scheme for these reactions. Phase I metabolism makes the molecule more polar. It can be from oxidation, reduction or hydrolysis. The most common type of phase 1 reaction is oxidative. These oxidative reactions are catalysed by a complex enzyme system, known as the mixed function oxygenase system, present in the endoplasmic reticulum. The most important enzyme in this system is cytochrome P-450, a haem protein which is part of the electron transfer chain, that catalyses an intermediate hydroxylation step in phase 1 oxidative reactions.

Some drug oxidation reactions involve specific enzymes. Ethanol oxidation, for example, is catalysed by alcohol dehydrogenase, and monoamine oxidase inactivates many biologically active amines, including adrenaline and serotonin. Reduction reactions are less common, but one important clinical example is the inactivation of the anticoagulation drug warfarin.

Phase 2 involves conjugation of the anion with a more strongly ionizable group that introduces a negative charge, or increases the negative charge, on the molecule, making it more hydrophilic. The most common phase 2 reaction involves the production of glucuronides. These glucuronidation reactions are all catalysed by UDP-glucuronyl transferase (Fig. 6.10). Steroid hormones, thyroid hormones, bilirubin and many drugs are converted to glucuronides in the liver. The formation of bilirubin diglucuronide is described below and is illustrated in Figure 6.11. However, many compounds are conjugated to form sulphates, in the presence of glutathione. Others are conjugated to amino acids or to certain hexoses.

These transformations enable the organic anion that is generated to be handled by anion transporters (see below) in the canalicular membrane. The conjugates are usually more water soluble and less toxic than their precursors, although some (e.g. 7-O-chlorpromazine glucuronide) may be more toxic, and as a consequence may damage the biliary system, or act as carcinogens (especially in the lower part of the duct system). Furthermore, some conjugated drugs become less hydrophilic after being acted upon by bacteria in the colon. They may then be absorbed by passive absorption in the colon and recycled via the liver (the enterohepatic circulation), in which case they can be difficult to eliminate from the body. Their toxicity is thereby increased. In liver diseases such as cirrhosis, in which the hepatocytes are damaged, there may be an increase in the half-life of a drug because the capacity of the liver to metabolize and secrete it is decreased.

Determinants of preferential excretion into bile

Some organic anions are excreted preferentially via the bile and some via the urine. The processing of two important drugs to glucuronides is indicated in Figure 6.10. One of these, the analgesic drug phenacetin, is converted to paracetamol glucuronide, which is secreted by the liver into the blood to be excreted mainly by the kidney. The other, the antipsychotic drug, chlorpromazine, is converted to 7-O-chlorpromazine glucuronide, which is excreted mainly in the bile. In the human, small organic anions of molecular mass less than 500 Da are excreted exclusively by the kidney while bigger anions are preferentially excreted into bile. Conjugation with glucuronic acid or glutathione serves to increase the molecular mass of a substance by 176 Da and 306 Da, respectively and conjugation may therefore increase the likelihood of secretion of the anion into bile. The reason for this discriminatory threshold for excretion in bile is unknown but the anion transporters in the canalicular membrane (see below) may show molecular size specificity. Another possibility is 'molecular sieving' by tight junctions between the hepatocytes; according to this hypothesis, all anions are secreted into the canaliculus but the small ones leak back into the plasma across the tight junctions.

Many drugs are toxic to the liver in high doses; one of these is paracetamol. Case 6.2: 1 describes the consequences of an overdose of this drug. The reasons for its toxicity at high concentrations in the blood are described in Case 6.2: 2, and the possible treatments are described in Case 6.2: 3.

Transport of organic ions

Transport into the hepatocyte

Organic ions are transported in the blood largely by high affinity binding to albumin and consequently the concentrations in plasma of the free ions are low. However, the amount of material extracted in a single pass through the liver is often greater than that in free solution. The mechanism for this is unknown.

Uptake of 'cholephilic' anions by the hepatocyte involves membrane carrier proteins with high affinity binding sites. Competition studies indicate that the carriers are shared by several anions. Thus bilirubin, sulphonamides, salicylates and sulphobromophthalein share the same carrier. This carrier is known as the organic anion transporter (oatp). Transport of anions via this mechanism is energy requiring and can be against enormous concentration gradients. It involves a chloride antiport system.

Transport into bile

Transport of anions across the canalicular membrane into the bile can be against a 100-fold concentration gradient. The membrane potential difference, which is approximately 40 mV, intracellular negative, can only account for transport of organic anions against a threefold concentration gradient. At least three specific ATP-dependent active transport mechanisms are present in the canalicular membranes for the transport of organic ions (Fig. 6.12). The ATP-dependent transporters and the membrane potential-dependent transporter are distinct proteins. The membrane potential-dependent transporter is a glycoprotein. One of the ATP-dependent transporters is responsible for transport of bile acids and has been

---

Case 6.2	Paracetamol overdose: 1

A teenager who had just failed her examinations was discovered unconscious in her bed and rushed into hospital. An empty bottle of paracetamol tablets was found in her bedroom and it seemed likely that she had ingested a whole bottle of tablets. Her stomach was washed out as soon as she arrived in casualty. The girl's blood paracetamol levels were monitored for 12 h and from the results it was predicted that she might suffer liver damage. She was given intravenous acetylcysteine over the following 20 h. After about 48 h she seemed to have recovered, but then she became aggressive and 2 days later she started to vomit, and became delirious. At the time of her relapse, she had become jaundiced, her liver was tender, and her serum transaminase levels and prothrombin levels were found to be extremely high. These findings indicated that acute hepatic necrosis was present and it was decided that her best chance of survival would be to have a liver transplant. Luckily a suitable donor liver was available.

After the transplant operation, the patient's serum bilirubin levels, prothrombin time and serum albumen were monitored to determine the progress of her recovery.

After studying the details of the above case history we can ask the following questions:

- Why are high blood levels of paracetamol toxic to the liver?
- Why did the patient suffer a relapse after she appeared to have recovered?
- Why did the patient appear jaundiced after her relapse?
- How can the patient's aggressive behaviour be explained?
- Why were the patient's serum prothrombin and transaminase levels excessively high, and what is the significance of this finding?
- Why was the patient treated with intravenous acetylcysteine?
- Why was a liver transplant necessary?

described above. Another is known as the canalicular multiorganic anion transporter (cMOAT). It transports many organic anions including bilirubin glucuronide, and conjugates of various xenobiotics. It does not transport unconjugated bilirubin. The jaundiced mutant (Tr-) rat that exhibits hyperbilirubinaemia is deficient in this transporter. A similar defect is present in Dubin–Johnson syndrome in the human. The third transporter is actually a group of phosphoglycoproteins (Pgps), known as P-transporters, which bind ATP. They transport mainly hydrophobic, neutral compounds, and organic cations, into bile. One P-transporter, known as the multi-drug transporter 3 (mdr-3), transports many cationic drugs across the canalicular membrane including certain peptides and anti-cancer drugs such as daunomycin. Interestingly the expression of the P-transporters is temporarily increased after partial hepatectomy.

Metabolism of bilirubin

Bilirubin, which is reddish-orange in colour, is the major bile pigment produced by breakdown of either haemoglobin or myoglobin in the reticuloendothelial system. Figure 6.13 shows the formation of bilirubin from haem, the porphyrin moiety of haemoglobin. Some of the intermediate product, biliverdin, a green pigment, is also usually present in bile, and in bile that has been stored the bilirubin reoxidizes to form biliverdin, and the bile tends to turn green. (These pigments are bound to albumin in the circulation.)

Free bilirubin from the blood enters the liver cells via an anion transporter that exchanges it for Cl^-. Inside the cell, it is bound to specific cytoplasmic proteins, known as ligandins (or Y and Z proteins). It is then conjugated to glucuronic acid to form bilirubin diglucuronide, in a reaction catalysed by glucuronyl transferase (Fig. 6.11).

Case 6.2 — Paracetamol overdose: 2

Toxicity

Liver

Paracetamol has potent analgesic and antipyretic actions but its anti-inflammatory actions are weaker than those of many other non-steroidal anti-inflammatory drugs (NSAIDs). It is given orally. A therapeutic dose of paracetamol is normally metabolized in the liver by conjugation to form soluble glucuronide or sulphate derivatives that can be excreted in the urine. Its half-life in the blood is 2–4h. It may act therapeutically by inhibiting a central nervous system-specific cyclo-oxygenase isoform such as COX-3, although this has not yet been proved.

High toxic levels of paracetamol cause nausea and vomiting. A dose of approximately 10g of paracetamol is sufficient to cause toxicity. The damage to the liver is due to the conjugating enzymes becoming saturated, that results in the drug being converted by mixed function P-450 oxidases to N-acetyl-p-benzoquinone imine (NAPBQI). The latter compound causes cell death by:

- Depleting intracellular glutathione, causing oxidative stress. When glutathione is depleted, intermediate metabolites build up and these also contribute to hepatocyte cell death
- Binding to cell proteins to produce NAPBQI protein adducts
- Increasing lipid peroxidation and membrane permeability
- Oxidizing SH groups on Ca^{2+}-ATPases resulting in sustained increases in intracellular Ca^{2+} and activation of Ca^{2+} activated proteases.

Note: Alcohol ingestion should be avoided if paracetamol has been taken for a headache because alcohol is an enzyme inducer and therefore it enhances the formation of toxic metabolites of paracetamol. Thus, the combination of a normally safe dose of paracetamol and a high level of blood alcohol can lead to liver damage. This combination is particularly dangerous if there is underlying liver disease (as can be the case in an alcoholic).

The hepatotoxic effects of paracetamol metabolites take more than 24 hours to inflict significant damage to hepatocytes. That is why the patient had a relapse after she appeared to have recovered. She appeared jaundiced after her relapse because the damaged liver could not excrete bilirubin in the bile. Consequently, it accumulated in the blood. The bilirubin in the blood would be predominantly unconjugated bilirubin because of the widespread damage to the liver cells where it is normally conjugated.

The excessively high concentrations of serum transaminase in the patient's blood and prolonged prothrombin clotting time are other manifestations of liver damage because transaminases are inappropriately released from dying hepatocytes and liver cell failure results in reduced production of clotting factors such as prothrombin. Determination of these parameters enables the extent of the liver damage to be assessed, and its progress monitored.

Other tissues

The patient's aggressive behaviour was due to encephalopathy that can accompany hepatic necrosis. The encephalopathy is due to high concentrations of toxic substances in the blood as a result of the inability of the liver to detoxify and excrete them. These cross the blood–brain barrier to damage the central nervous system. An EEG (electroencephalogram) can be used to monitor the encephalopathy.

Paracetamol and other NSAID can also cause nephrotoxicity and renal failure. This occurs mainly in patients with diseases where glomerular filtration is compromised, such as heart or liver disease. This effect is due to ischaemia in the kidneys because NSAIDs such as paracetamol inhibit the synthesis of prostaglandins, which are vasodilators.

Treatment

Drugs

Intravenous acetylcysteine was administered to the patient because paracetamol can be conjugated to form sulphates, as well as glucuronides. The sulphation reaction requires glutathione. Acetylcysteine increases glutathione synthesis in the liver and this increases the conjugation of paracetamol to paracetamol sulphate, which can be excreted. Glutathione itself is not administered because it does not readily penetrate the liver. If the patient is seen soon after ingesting the paracetamol overdose (within 12h) the liver damage may be prevented by this treatment.

Note: Forced diuresis or renal dialysis would not have been useful in this patient because these procedures do not increase the excretion of paracetamol or its metabolites as the compounds bind tightly to tissues.

Transplantation

A liver transplant was necessary in this patient because, although the ability of the liver to recover function is well recognized, if over 80% of the hepatocytes have been irreversibly damaged, sufficient function will not be recovered. This degree of damage would have been present in this case.

Determination of prothrombin time, and serum albumen and bilirubin concentrations enables the function of the transplanted liver to be assessed and monitored. The production of clotting factors and albumen is seen within hours. As the new liver becomes functional, the bilirubin levels gradually fall because the liver regains its ability to sequester it from the blood and excrete it into the bile. The process of excreting the bilirubin takes several weeks. Thus, prothrombin time and albumen levels are sensitive tests for monitoring early transplant function.

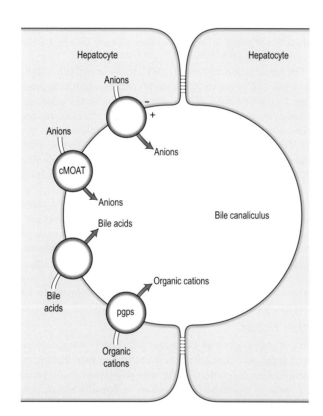

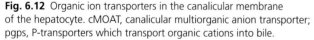

Fig. 6.12 Organic ion transporters in the canalicular membrane of the hepatocyte. cMOAT, canalicular multiorganic anion transporter; pgps, P-transporters which transport organic cations into bile.

The glucuronide is more soluble than free bilirubin. Some of the bilirubin diglucuronide escapes into the blood and may be excreted by the kidney, but most is excreted actively via the cMOAT transporter system into bile.

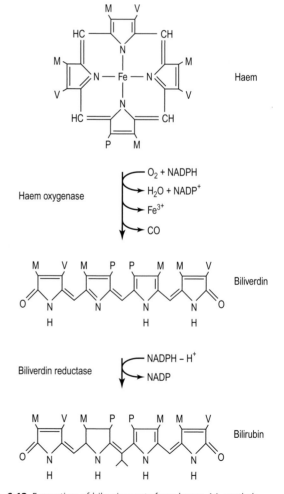

Fig. 6.13 Formation of bile pigments from haem. M, methyl; V, vinyl; P, propionyl; CO, carbon monoxide.

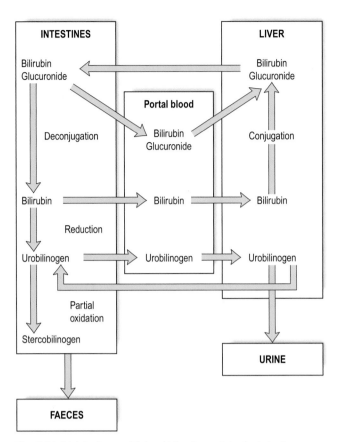

Fig. 6.14 Metabolism and fate of bile pigments in the intestines.

Box 6.2 Jaundice and its causes

Jaundice becomes obvious when the plasma bilirubin concentration exceeds 34 μmol/L. It can be classified into three types, depending on the location of the defect that causes it:

1. *Prehepatic (or haemolytic) jaundice.* Excessive haemolysis of red blood cells and haemoglobin breakdown to bilirubin can exceed the capacity of the liver to excrete it. This type of jaundice is most frequently associated with haemolytic anaemia of various types. The bilirubin present in the plasma is largely unconjugated as it has not been taken up and conjugated by the liver.

2. *Intrahepatic (or hepatocellular) jaundice.* A variety of defects in the liver itself can also give rise to hyperbilirubinaemia. These include decreased uptake of bilirubin into hepatocytes, defective intracellular protein binding or conjugation, or disturbed secretion into the bile canaliculi. This type of jaundice is most commonly seen in acute hepatitis. Although the primary failure is due to hepatocyte damage that results in accumulation of unconjugated bilirubin, there is also secondary biliary stasis that provides a mixed picture with secondary accumulation of conjugated bilirubin.

    In Crigler Najjar disease there is an inherited deficiency of glucuronyl transferase and high concentrations of unconjugated bilirubin are present in the plasma, causing jaundice. The affected individuals may develop kernicterus (deposits of pigment in the brain) that can cause nerve degeneration. Exposure to light degrades the pigment, and children born with this disease can be treated by phototherapy. Gilbert's syndrome is another condition in which unconjugated bilirubin accumulates in the blood. In this case glucuronyl transferase activity is reduced by approximately 70%. This results in mild, intermittent jaundice that normally does not require treatment. Conjugation of some drugs is also usually impaired in these conditions.

    At birth, infants have little ability to conjugate bilirubin but it develops within the first few weeks of life. Thus some babies are jaundiced soon after birth, as unconjugated bilirubin is not readily excreted. This condition is known as physiological jaundice of the newborn. Exposure to light can be employed in these infants to deplete the excess bilirubin.

3. *Post-hepatic (or obstructive) jaundice.* Blockage of the intrahepatic or extrahepatic bile ducts by, for example, gallstones, also causes jaundice as the bile is refluxed into the blood. This is commonly referred to as post-hepatic or obstructive jaundice (Case 6.1: 4). In this case the bilirubin is largely conjugated.

If bilirubin subsequently becomes deconjugated in the biliary system, pigment gallstones may form (see Case 6.1: 3).

Fate of bile pigments in the gastrointestinal tract

After delivery to the intestines most conjugated bilirubin is eliminated in the faeces. This is because the intestinal mucosa is not very permeable to the conjugated metabolite. However, some may be deconjugated by the action of bacteria in the intestines and the free bilirubin formed can be absorbed to some extent, by passive diffusion into the portal blood because it is more lipid-soluble than conjugated bilirubin. It is then returned to the liver (via the enterohepatic circulation, see below). Intestinal bacteria can also convert bilirubin to colourless derivatives known as urobilinogens, which can also be absorbed into the portal blood. These are mostly excreted in the bile but some are excreted in the urine. Urobilinogen remaining in the gut is partially reoxidized to stercobilinogen, the reddish-brown pigment responsible for the colour of the faeces. Figure 6.14 outlines the fate of excreted bile pigments.

Failure of the body to excrete bile pigments results in accumulation of the pigments in the blood plasma (hyperbilirubinaemia), causing jaundice. This is manifest as yellowing of the skin, sclera and mucous membranes. Box 6.2 describes this condition and its causes.

Proteins in bile

Most proteins in bile are plasma proteins, although some are derived from cells of the hepatobiliary system. The plasma proteins are mostly synthesized in the liver

Gallstone disease: 4

Obstructive jaundice

The yellowing of the patient's sclera was due to high concentrations of conjugated bilirubin in the blood. Bile backs up in the hepatobiliary system when there is a blockage of the bile duct and is refluxed into the blood. Thus, in this case, the plasma bilirubin has been conjugated by the liver cells. The presence in the blood of abnormally high concentrations of conjugated bilirubin or certain other constituents of bile, such as the enzyme alkaline phosphatase, indicates hepatobiliary disease. The non-clearance of bilirubin from the body may not in itself be particularly damaging. However, when jaundice is present it is likely that many other potentially toxic materials have also accumulated in the blood as a consequence of their reflux from the bile or impaired secretion from the hepatocyte. This can lead to impaired mental function and malaise.

The patient's urine was dark-coloured because the bilirubin conjugates in the blood are water-soluble, and are therefore excreted by the kidney. Unconjugated bilirubin binds tightly to albumen. Therefore, in healthy individuals, not much bilirubin is excreted in the urine. Conjugated bilirubin binds much less tightly to albumen and when the conjugate is present in high concentrations in the blood, some of it is filtered in the glomerulus of the kidney and is only partially reabsorbed in the tubules. Thus excretion of bilirubin glucuronide by the kidney (bilirubinuria) reflects the presence of bilirubin conjugates in the blood. When the bile ducts are blocked, bile pigments cannot gain entry to the gastrointestinal tract and consequently, the faeces are pale and clay-coloured (acholic).

and secreted into the blood, but some plasma proteins are normally present in bile, including unaltered active enzymes and antibodies.

Some proteins exhibit relatively low bile:plasma concentration ratios. Two non-specific pathways exist for protein transport in hepatocytes:

- Paracellular sieving. This pathway is responsible for secretion of smaller proteins
- Pinocytosis (membrane vesiculation) followed by transport of the pinocytotic vesicles and exocytosis. This pathway does not discriminate in relation to molecular size.

There are also receptor-linked pathways for the secretion of some proteins. One example is immunoglobulin A (IgA) that is transported by receptor-mediated vesicle transport in the duct cells. This protein provides immunological protection for the biliary and intestinal tracts.

Excessive secretion of these molecules across the canalicular membrane can occur when the intracellular microtubular guiding system which directs the vesicles which house them to the sinusoidal membrane is disrupted and the secretory vesicles are misdirected to the canalicular pole of the cell. The release of some plasma membrane-derived enzymes, such as alkaline phosphatase, into bile is promoted by bile salts. This enzyme has no known function in bile but raised alkaline phosphatase in plasma is used as a biochemical marker of liver disease. It is usually elevated in any form of cholestasis, including biliary cholic.

The gall bladder

Anatomy and histology

The gall bladder is a pear-shaped sac. In the human adult it is approximately 8 cm long and 4 cm wide, but it is capable of considerable distension. It is lined by a mucous membrane that is thrown into numerous folds (rugae) when the gall bladder is contracted (Fig. 6.15). As the gall bladder fills with bile the folds flatten out. The cystic duct conveys the bile to the hepatic duct (Fig. 6.1).

The wall of the gall bladder is composed of three layers, the mucous membrane, the muscularis, and the adventitia (or serosa, see Fig. 6.15). The epithelium of the mucous membrane is composed of high columnar cells with basally located nuclei. The apical (luminal) borders of the cells are provided with microvilli, consistent with their absorptive function. They resemble the absorptive cells of the small intestine. Beneath the epithelial cells is the lamina propria, which is a coat of loose connective tissue. Around the mucous membrane is a thin coat of smooth muscle, the muscularis externa. Most of the smooth muscle fibres run obliquely but some run circularly and some longitudinally. Many elastic fibres are present within the connective tissue between the muscle fibres. Outside this muscle layer is an outer coat of dense fibroconnective tissue, the adventitia (or serosa) that is covered by peritoneum.

At the neck of the gall bladder, the mucous membrane is thrown into a spiral fold that has a core of smooth muscle (Fig. 6.15). This extends into the cystic duct and is known as the spiral valve. Its function may be to prevent sudden changes in the filling and emptying of the gall bladder.

Functions

The functions of the gall bladder are to store and concentrate bile, and to deliver it into the small intestine during a meal. In the human adult, it has a capacity of 30–60 mL. Gall bladder bile is an isotonic solution but some of its components are highly concentrated (Table 6.1). The endothelial cells actively reabsorb Na^+ ions from the bile, by exchange for K^+ ions. The Na^+ ions are pumped into the lateral spaces between the epithelial cells. Anions, largely Cl^- and HCO_3^-, follow passively, down the electrochemical gradient. The extraction of HCO_3^- ions tends to make the gall bladder bile less alkaline. Thus gall bladder bile is less concentrated with respect to Na^+, Cl^- and

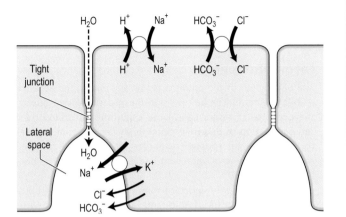

Fig. 6.16 Transport of ions in the gall bladder.

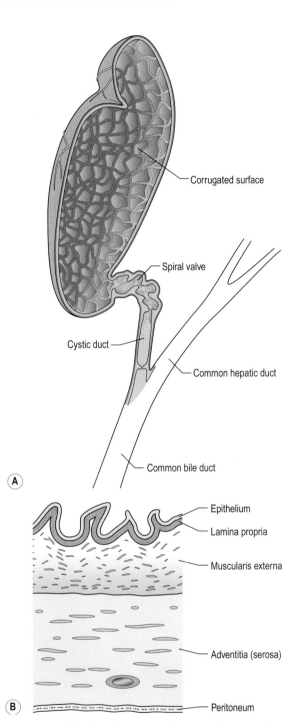

Fig. 6.15 The gall bladder. (A) Structural features. (B) Layers of the gall bladder wall.

the gall bladder. The ions and water then pass through the basement membrane into the blood capillaries (Fig. 6.16).

Table 6.1 compares the composition of gall bladder bile with hepatic bile. Ca^{2+} ions are not absorbed by the gall bladder to any appreciable extent and Ca^{2+} is therefore concentrated in gall bladder bile. K^+ ions are also concentrated. The organic constituents are highly concentrated in gall bladder bile, but it remains isosmotic with plasma. The bile pigments in hepatic bile impart a golden-brown colour to it, but gall bladder bile is almost black because the pigments are more concentrated. Bilirubin, bile acids, lecithin and cholesterol are 5–10 times more concentrated in gall bladder bile than in hepatic bile.

Bile may be lost from the body if there is a fistula between the common bile duct and the skin, as may be provided as a complication of biliary surgery. This results in impaired fat absorption in the small intestine. Loss of significant amounts of K^+ ions (present in high concentrations in gall bladder bile) can also occur, and replacement with KCl has to be instigated in the clinical management of patients with such fistulae.

Gallstones can form in the gall bladder or the ducts, causing obstruction of the passage of bile into the duodenum. As micelles are important for fat digestion and absorption, this can lead to fat malabsorption (Case 6.1: 5). (The condition can sometimes be managed by the oral administration of bile acids, see Case 6.1: 6.)

Gall bladder contraction

The gall bladder exhibits muscle tone and contractions even in the interdigestive period. It also contracts between meals to deliver bile intermittently into the duodenum. The contractions coincide with the migrating myoelectric complex of the small intestine (see Ch. 7). These fasting contractions may cause mixing of the bile, reducing the likelihood of cholesterol crystals accumulating and forming gallstones.

The major stimulus for gall bladder contraction after a meal is a high blood level of CCK, the hormone that is released in response to fat in the duodenum. It acts on

HCO_3^-, than hepatic bile. The pumping of Na^+ out of the endothelial cell at the basal surface keeps its concentration low inside the cell, and this provides the driving force for Na^+ ions to enter the cell via the apical membrane (down their concentration gradient). Transport in the apical membrane occurs partly via exchange for H^+ ions and partly by symport with Cl^- ions. As a consequence, water is transported passively, down the osmotic gradient, out of

Fat malabsorption

The pale colour of the patient's stools was due to the absence of bile pigments (see below), and the greasiness was due to the presence of abnormally large quantities of unabsorbed fat. Elimination of excessive amounts of fat is known as steatorrhoea. The fat caused the faeces to float, and to smell abnormally offensive because it had been fermented by bacteria in the colon.

Bile acids play an important role in the digestion of lipid, and in the absorption of lipid- and fat-soluble vitamins (vitamins A, D, E and K). Consequently, in severe cholestasis such as when the common bile duct is obstructed by gallstones,

bile acids are not delivered to the small intestine and as a consequence, lipids are not absorbed. Fat malabsorption causes flatulence and diarrhoea. The duration of the time period over which fat malabsorption is present in gallstone disease before it is treated is usually relatively short and for that reason, fat-soluble vitamin deficiency is unusual, except in the case of vitamin K as body stores of vitamin K are very limited. Deficiency of this vitamin leads to deranged blood coagulation.

Restriction of dietary fat reduces steatorrhoea, but then vitamin K supplements are required to prevent failure of blood clotting.

Treatment

Surgery

In gallstone disease, where stones are present in the gall bladder, surgical removal of the gall bladder is often performed using 'keyhole' surgery (Fig. 6.17). If a gallstone is present in the biliary duct, sphincterectomy can be employed. This involves passing an endoscope down through the mouth into the duodenum (Fig. 6.18). The sphincter of Oddi can then be divided to allow the stone to be removed.

The digestive processes are not seriously impaired after removal of the gall bladder because hepatic bile simply flows directly into the duodenum. A greater volume of unconcentrated bile enters the intestines, but the extra fluid is

absorbed, so dehydration does not occur. One consequence is that bile acids may enter the small intestines more rapidly, and therefore, a higher proportion may be eliminated from the body. However, this reduction in the bile acid pool is normally rectified by increased synthesis in the liver.

Lithotripsy

A non-invasive treatment for gallstones, involving the use of ultrasonic vibrations, known as lithotripsy, can be performed.

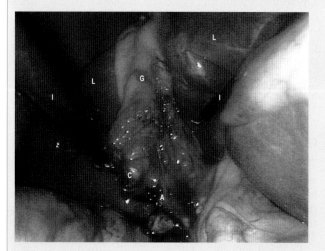

Fig. 6.17 Gall bladder surgery being performed laparoscopically. The gall bladder (G), divided cystic duct (C) and cystic artery (A) are seen, with the liver (L) lying behind. (I) Instruments for lifting and dividing the gall bladder structures.

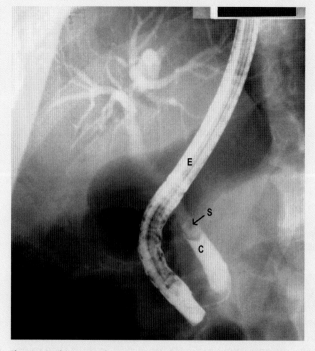

Fig. 6.18 This X-ray shows an endoscope (E), which has been passed into the duodenum. Contrast has been injected (retrograde) into a dilated common bile duct (C), which contains a calculus (S).

In this procedure, focused ultrasound waves are used to disrupt the gallstones and the fragments formed are carried in the bile into the small intestines and subsequently eliminated from the body. Lithotripsy is not widely employed because the stone fragments can get lodged in the common bile duct, resulting in obstructive jaundice. (Kidney stones are more commonly treated using this technique.)

Treatment with bile acids

Gallstones can be treated by oral administration of bile acids. Cholesterol supersaturation in bile in patients with gallstones is usually due to a diminished bile acid pool. The ingested bile acids are absorbed in the ileum and taken up by the liver and then secreted in the bile (Fig. 6.19). Thus if a bile acid is fed in substantial amounts, the bile acid pool is expanded. This enables more cholesterol to be retained in micelles, rather than precipitating in the bile. The bile acids slowly dissolve the gallstones over a period of time, usually several months. Chenodeoxycholic acid (Fig. 6.6) can be effective. Ursodeoxycholic acid (ursodiol), a derivative of chenodeoxycholic acid that is relatively abundant in polar bear bile, is even more effective. These particular bile acids are effective because they increase cholesterol sequestration in micelles and (unlike cholic acid and deoxycholic acid) they do not suppress bile acid synthesis. Ursodiol also inhibits cholesterol absorption in the intestine and decreases the synthesis of cholesterol in the liver. This causes reduced plasma cholesterol levels, and for this reason, ursodiol has also been considered for the treatment of coronary heart disease.

The main side-effect of bile acid treatment is diarrhoea, secondary to incomplete absorption of the ingested bile salts.

Small gallstones disappear relatively quickly with bile acid treatment. However, it is the large stones which are usually responsible for the symptoms of gallstone disease, and so alleviation via this means takes a long time. Moreover, most individuals with gallstones present with acute symptoms, which are often associated with a dysfunctional gall bladder. Therefore the use of bile salt therapy is limited. Furthermore, life-long therapy with bile salts would be required to prevent the stones recurring.

Thus cholecystectomy remains the primary choice for the removal of gallstones.

CCK-A receptors on the smooth muscle of the gall bladder. Gastrin, a related peptide, released by the stomach antrum in response to peptides also stimulates gall bladder contraction. In addition, distension of the stomach antrum stimulates contraction via a nervous reflex. The gastric mechanisms involved in the control of bile release are presumably preliminary to the emptying of chyme from the stomach.

Vasoactive intestinal peptide (VIP), pancreatic polypeptide (PP), and stimulation of the sympathetic nerves to the gall bladder, all cause gall bladder relaxation. Bile acids in the duodenum also inhibit gall bladder contraction (a feedback control).

The sphincter of Oddi

The hepatic bile duct penetrates the wall of the duodenum, at the same location as the pancreatic duct. Part of the way through the duodenal wall, the hepatic duct and the pancreatic duct fuse. The lumen of the fused duct is relatively wide and this region is known as the ampulla of Vater. It opens into the lumen of the duodenum, and at the opening are the duodenal papillae. Circular smooth muscle is associated with the ampulla and with the regions of the hepatic and pancreatic ducts that are associated with it (Fig. 6.1). This constitutes the sphincter of Oddi. The closure of this sphincter prevents bile from entering the intestine. As a result, the bile that is formed while it is closed is diverted into the gall bladder. In addition there are smooth muscle fibres that run in parallel with the bile and pancreatic ducts. When these fibres contract, the ducts shorten and become wider to increase the flow of the digestive juices through them. The main stimulus for relaxation of the sphincter muscle is CCK. Thus when the levels of CCK increase in the blood during a meal, the gall bladder contracts and the sphincter of Oddi relaxes, and bile enters the duodenum. These events act in concert to allow bile to enter the small intestine when a meal is being processed in the gastrointestinal tract.

The enterohepatic circulation of bile acids

Conjugated bile acids are secreted by the liver, released into the duodenum, and eventually absorbed in the ileum into the portal blood. They are then taken up by the liver and secreted again. This cycle is repeated over and over again. This is known as the enterohepatic circulation of bile acids. The secretion of the bile acid-dependent fraction of bile from the hepatocytes is not controlled to any great extent by hormones or nerve impulses originating in the gastrointestinal tract, although CCK may be a weak stimulus. The normal stimulus for increased secretion of bile salts is a high bile salt concentration in the blood (Fig. 6.19). The bile salts are secreted more or less continuously but the rate of secretion increases when the blood concentration increases. The concentration in the portal blood normally increases after a meal when the bile acids have been absorbed.

Thus, food in the gastrointestinal tract indirectly controls:

- The secretory process, as bile acids do not enter the duodenum in any appreciable amounts until the gall

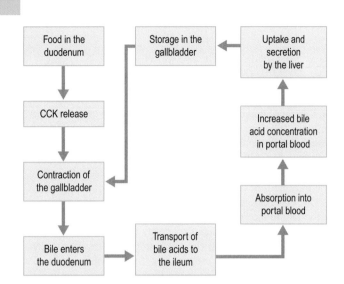

Fig. 6.19 The enterohepatic circulation of bile acids.

bladder contracts and the sphincter (of Oddi) relaxes, when they can subsequently be absorbed in the ileum into the portal blood, to stimulate secretion

- Access of bile to the chyme in the intestines, by stimulating gall bladder contraction and sphincter (of Oddi) relaxation via CCK release into the blood.

Most of the pool of bile salts may be recycled twice during a meal, and between 3 and 14 times a day depending on the number of meals taken and the fat content of the meals. Fat in the chyme elicits CCK release which stimulates gall bladder contraction and sphincter relaxation. As bile acids are important for lipid digestion and absorption (see Case 6.1: 5), this control constitutes a positive feedback mechanism. The uptake of bile acids from the intestines enables small gallstones to be successfully treated by oral administration of a bile acid, as this will be secreted by the liver to increase the concentration in the bile and dissolve the stones (see Case 6.1: 6).

The total bile acid pool (approx. 3.0 g in the adult) is kept constant. The rate of synthesis is normally very low because most of the conjugated bile acids that enter the small intestine are actively reabsorbed and returned to the liver (Fig. 6.19). Normally only a small proportion, approximately 10%, is lost in the faeces. The liver keeps the size of the pool constant by synthesizing an amount equivalent to that lost. *De novo* synthesis is a response to low levels of bile acids in the blood. If for any reason bile acids are not reabsorbed in the intestines (e.g. disease of the ileum) then *de novo* synthesis of bile acids increases. However, if the enterohepatic circulation is interrupted (e.g. after resection of the terminal ileum), the rate of synthesis is not sufficient to compensate for the loss via the faeces. The result is malabsorption of fats and fat-soluble vitamins. The commonest cause of this is Crohn's disease of the terminal ileum (see Ch. 8).

Control of the hepatobiliary system during a meal

Bile is secreted at a rate of between 250 and 1500 mL/day in the human adult. Several different functions of the hepatobiliary system are under physiological control; secretion of alkaline fluid from the ducts, the secretion of bile from the hepatocytes, contraction of the smooth muscle in the wall of the gall bladder to release the stored bile, and relaxation of the smooth muscle in the sphincter of Oddi, which allows the bile into the duodenum.

The control of alkaline bile secretion (like that of gastric juice and pancreatic juice) during a meal can be divided into three phases according to the location of the ingested material:

1. The cephalic phase, which is the response to the approach of food or the presence of food in the mouth.
2. The gastric phase, which is the response to food in the stomach.
3. The intestinal phase, which is the response to food in the duodenum.

The bile acid-dependent fraction is secreted more or less continuously, but the gall bladder usually only contracts forcefully during a meal. Thus although secretion is continuous, bile acids usually only enter the gastrointestinal tract in appreciable amounts during a meal, i.e. when they are required.

Cephalic phase

The cephalic phase is mediated via impulses in nerve fibres in the vagus nerve. It is due to the sight and smell of food, and the activation of taste and touch receptors by food in the mouth. In this phase there is an increase in the secretion of alkaline bile from the duct cells, which would presumably minimize the effects of increased acid secretion in the stomach during the cephalic phase. Weak contractions of the gall bladder and relaxation of the sphincter of Oddi also occur.

Gastric phase

Peptides, caffeine or alcohol in food in the stomach, and distension of the stomach walls cause increased release of gastrin from the pyloric antrum and activation of nerve fibres in the vagus nerve. These influences stimulate alkaline juice secretion from the bile ducts and weak contractions of the gall bladder.

Intestinal phase

The intestinal phase is the most important of the three phases for the control of both the secretion of alkaline bile and the contraction of the gall bladder. It is mediated largely via the peptide hormones secretin and CCK that are released from the walls of the duodenum into the blood. Secretin is released in response mainly to acid in the chyme. It acts on receptors on the duct cells to stimulate the release of alkaline bile. Its action is potentiated by CCK.

CCK is the most potent stimulus for gall bladder contraction. The most potent stimulus for CCK release is fat in the duodenum: when fat is not present in a meal,

contraction of the gall bladder is weak. CCK also causes relaxation of the sphincter of Oddi, thereby enabling the bile to flow freely into the duodenum. Bile acids exert a negative feedback control on gall bladder contraction and sphincter relaxation, by inhibiting the release of CCK from the duodenum.

THE SMALL INTESTINE

Chapter objectives

After studying this chapter you should be able to:

1. Describe the structure of the small intestine and the major cell types present in the mucosa.

2. Understand the processes of water and electrolyte secretion and absorption in the small intestine.

3. Understand the mechanisms of diarrhoea, its consequences and treatment.

4. Describe the motility of the small intestine, and its control.

Introduction

In the human, most digestion and absorption occurs in the small intestine. Digestion in the stomach is dispensable and it is only preparatory. Pancreatic juice and bile from the liver enter the duodenum (Fig. 7.1). Intestinal juice is secreted along the entire length of the intestine from glands in the wall. In the normal individual, digestion is substantially complete when the chyme passes into the colon. The small intestine normally also absorbs over 95% of the water which enters the gastrointestinal tract. There is considerable reserve of function, and two-thirds of the small intestine can be removed without serious impairment of the quality of life.

Absorption is the central process of the digestive system and all other physiological processes that occur in the gastrointestinal tract subserve it. In this chapter we shall deal with the absorption of water and monovalent ions. Digestion and absorption of other nutrients will be dealt with separately. We shall also consider how the contractile activity of the intestines mixes and propels the food towards the ileum.

The importance of water and electrolyte absorption in the intestines is illustrated in this chapter, by the problems encountered in cholera, a condition in which there can be a massive loss of fluid from the body (Case 7.1: 1).

Intestinal phase of digestion

When chyme enters the small intestine from the stomach, it causes the release into the blood of the hormones

secretin and CCK from endocrine (APUD) cells in the walls of the duodenum. Secretin stimulates secretion of alkaline pancreatic juice, alkaline bile, and alkaline intestinal juice. CCK stimulates secretion of enzyme-rich pancreatic juice. It also causes contraction of the gall bladder and relaxation of the sphincter of Oddi, which promotes the entry of bile and pancreatic juices into the duodenum

---

Case 7.1 Cholera: 1

An elderly man was carried by his son into a hospital, which was situated in a remote region of Bengal. The man appeared emaciated. He said he had initially been vomiting and suffering from abdominal distention. Now he was suffering from copious diarrhoea. The duty doctor noted that the man's skin lacked turgor. The man's pulse was barely detectable but his pulse rate was rapid (100 b.p.m.). The younger man was also suffering from diarrhoea, but he was less severely affected. The doctor suspected that they were both victims of the latest cholera epidemic. Such epidemics are not uncommon in the region because of contamination of food and drinking water with the bacterium *Vibrio cholerae*. The elderly man was provided with electrolyte fluid via an intravenous drip. His plasma and urine K^+ and HCO_3^- concentrations were monitored. He was also given intravenous tetracycline for 2 days. The younger man was given some packets containing a mixture of salt (NaCl) and sugar (glucose) and a supply of clean drinking water. He was told to dissolve the salt and sugar in clean water from the hospital supply and to drink large quantities of the solution over the next few days. He was given tetracycline to take by mouth. Both patients had recovered within a few days.

We shall address the following questions:

- What causes cholera?
- Why were the patients treated with tetracycline?
- Why was it necessary to monitor the patient's plasma and urine K^+ and HCO_3^- concentrations?
- How would the patients' acid–base status have changed?
- What adjustments in respiratory and renal function would be taking place in response to the changes in acid–base status?
- How does the *V. cholerae* bacterium cause diarrhoea?
- Could other treatments counteract the effect of the toxin on the crypt cells?
- What is the rationale for treating people suffering from cholera with (a) oral fluid containing NaCl and glucose and (b) intravenous fluid? What is the likely composition of the intravenous fluid?
- Why was the elderly man's pulse (a) feeble and (b) rapid?
- What adjustments in cardiovascular and renal function would take place in response to the hypovolaemia?
- Are changes in intestinal motility involved in this condition?

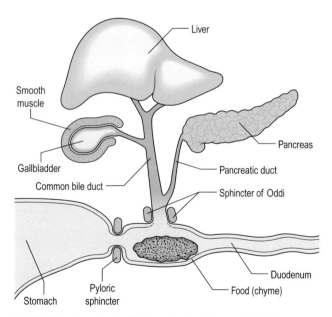

Fig. 7.1 Structures involved in the duodenal phase of digestion. Pancreatic juice and bile from the liver enter the duodenum during the intestinal phase. The entry is controlled by the pressure generated when the gall bladder contracts and by relaxation of the sphincter of Oddi. These juices, and juices from the intestinal walls, mix with the acid chyme arriving from the stomach.

(Fig. 7.1). At the same time, these hormones inhibit gastric emptying which enables processing of the contents of the small intestine to occur before the next portion of chyme enters from the stomach, and prevents the intestinal chyme from becoming too acid. The latter is important because the action of pancreatic enzymes and lipid absorption require an alkaline or neutral pH.

The chyme also stimulates contraction of the smooth muscle of the intestines, which mixes the intestinal contents and propels it towards the ileum. The intestinal phase of the control of digestion is summarized in Table 7.1.

Anatomy and structure

In the adult human, the small intestine consists of approximately 6 m of 3.5 cm diameter tubing that is coiled in the abdomen. It leads from the stomach to the colon (Fig. 7.2). The duodenum comprises the first 25 cm or so. This region differs from the rest of the small intestine in having no mesentery. The adjacent region is the jejunum that comprises approximately 40% (2.5 m) of the small intestine. The remaining distal part is the ileum. The longitudinal smooth muscle in the wall is normally partially contracted (tone). After death, when it is relaxed, the small bowel reaches a length of approximately 7.5 m.

Duodenum

The duodenum has an essential role in mixing digestive juices, derived from the liver and pancreas, and its own wall with the food. It forms an arc ending in a sharp bend, the duodeno-jejunal flexure. The head of the pancreas lies within the arc, with which it shares a blood supply via the pancreatico-duodenal artery (Fig. 7.2). At approximately two-thirds of the way down the descending part of the duodenum are two papillae. The major duodenal papilla is the location of the duct where the bile and pancreatic juice empty into the duodenum via the ampulla of Vater. The opening of the ampulla is controlled by the sphincter of Oddi (Fig. 7.1). An accessory pancreatic duct, present in most individuals, opens at the tip of the lesser papilla.

The surface of the duodenum is folded. The folds are known as plicae circularis (circular folds). Most are crescent-shaped, and do not disappear when the intestine is distended. The mucosa of the small intestine is covered with tiny projections, known as villi. These are tongue-shaped in the duodenum.

Two types of glands are present in the duodenal mucosa. At the base of the villi are tubular invaginations that reach almost to the muscularis mucosae, known as intestinal glands or crypts of Lieberkühn (Fig. 7.3). The submucosa of the duodenum contains coiled compound tubular mucous glands known as glands of Brunner that secrete an alkaline fluid rich in mucus. These glands are more numerous in the proximal region of the duodenum. They usually open at the base of the intestinal glands.

Jejunum and ileum

No anatomical feature separates the jejunum from the ileum. The structure of the jejunum and ileum is basically similar to that of the duodenum. However, there is a gradual decrease in diameter, and in the thickness of the wall, and in the number of mucosal folds, with distance from the duodenum (Fig. 7.4). The folds are absent altogether from the terminal ileum. In addition the villi gradually become less numerous, smaller, and more finger-like, with distance from the duodenum. Numerous

Table 7.1 Control of secretion and motility during the intestinal phase

	Effect	Hormone
Secretion		
Duodenal (alkaline)	Stimulation	Secretin
Bile (alkaline)	Stimulation	Secretin
Bile (hepatocyte)	None	
Pancreatic juice (alkaline)	Stimulation	Secretin
Pancreatic juice (enzyme-rich)	Stimulation	CCK
Smooth muscle		
Stomach	Relaxation	CCK, secretin
Gallbladder	Contraction	CCK
Sphincter of Oddi	Relaxation	CCK
Intestinal	Contraction	Various

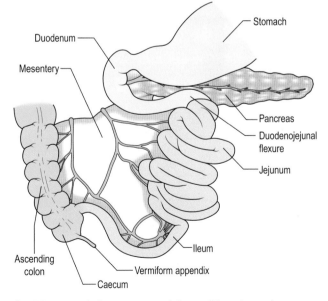

Fig. 7.2 Anatomical arrangement of the small intestine and associated structures.

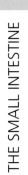

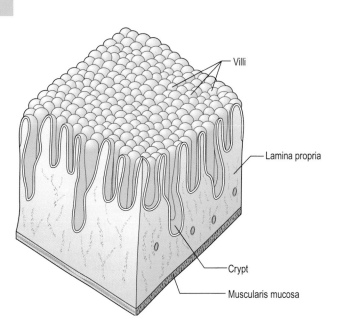

Fig. 7.3 Structure of the submucosa of the small intestine, showing the relationship of the glands to the villi.

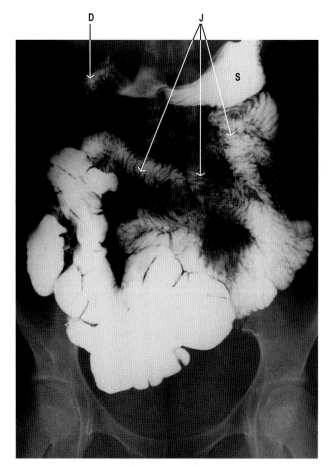

Fig. 7.4 An X-ray of the small bowel taken 2 h after ingestion of barium. The mucosal outline of the jejunum (J) is clearly seen, showing the dense mucosal folds that maximize the surface area. The stomach (S) and duodenum (D) are also visible.

lymph nodes, called Peyer's patches are present in the mucosa and submucosa of the ileum. The junction between the ileum and the large intestine is the ileocaecal junction. It consists of a ring of thickened smooth muscle, known as the ileocaecal sphincter (see Ch. 10), which reduces reflux from the colon.

The jejunum and ileum are on a mesentery. This contains the arterial blood vessels (branches of the superior mesenteric artery), and the veno-lymphatic drainage vessels, which are supported in fatty connective tissue, and is covered by mesothelium.

Blood supply

At rest, approximately 10% of the cardiac output flows to the intestine. The blood vessels in the jejunum and ileum are derived from the superior mesenteric artery. Numerous arterial branches form an extensive network in the submucosa that supplies the wall of the intestine (Fig. 7.5).

Nerves, hormones and local paracrine factors control the intestinal circulation. Stimulation of the sympathetic nerves (which follow the arteries) causes vasoconstriction and reduced blood flow, enabling a redistribution of blood away from the intestine. This is particularly important during low cardiac output states such as shock, or during exercise when extra blood is required for skeletal muscle. In the blood vessels of the villi, the vasoconstriction is relatively short-lived. This is due to vasodilator metabolites, such as adenosine, which accumulate during the vasoconstrictor response.

The splanchnic blood flow increases by 50–300% during a meal (functional hyperaemia). Distension of the walls of the intestine and substances present in the chyme stimulate the blood flow. Other stimuli include products of carbohydrate and lipid digestion in the proximal small intestine, and bile acids in the distal ileum. Gastrin, CCK, secretin, serotonin and histamine all have

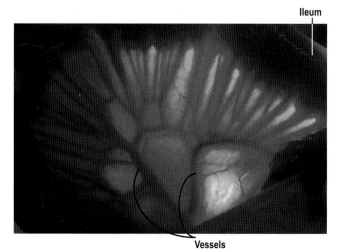

Fig. 7.5 A photograph of the vascular arcade in the ileum, showing the multiple arterial anastomoses in the mesentery.

the capacity to increase blood flow, and may be involved in this response during a meal.

The nutrients absorbed across the absorptive cells are transported to the liver in the portal veins (Ch. 6).

Countercurrent exchange in the villi

The blood vessels of the villi (Fig. 7.6) constitute a countercurrent exchange system, whereby there is net diffusion of dissolved substances across the interstitium from the venule to the arteriole, or vice versa, depending on which limb has the higher concentration. Thus oxygen tension is higher in the ascending arterial blood because it is extracted from the blood in the capillaries, and it diffuses from the ascending to the descending limb. This results in a lower oxygen tension at the tips of the villi than at their bases. The relative hypoxia at the tip has been causally implicated in the shedding of the epithelial cells from the tips of the villi. In hypovolaemic shock, a situation where hypotension is present, the reduced perfusion pressure together with increased smooth muscle relaxation that accompanies it, leads to a reduced oxygen supply. This can cause the tips of the villi to become severely hypoxic. During hypovolaemic shock this can lead to ulceration of the intestines, which can develop within hours of the onset of hypovolaemia. Such acute ulcers are seen in patients who have suffered severe burns, especially children, and after major haemorrhage, such as a leaking aortic aneurysm.

Structure of the intestinal wall

The wall of the small intestine has the same basic structure as other regions of the gastrointestinal tract (see

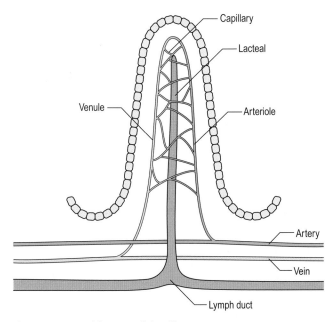

Fig. 7.6 Structural features of the villus.

Ch. 1). Beneath the serosa is the muscularis externa that consists of two layers of smooth muscle, an outer longitudinal coat and an inner circular coat. Preganglionic parasympathetic nerve fibres of the vagus nerve synapse with the cells of the terminal ganglia in the myenteric plexus. The postganglionic nerves stimulate muscle contraction and gland secretion (see Ch. 1). Postganglionic sympathetic nerve fibres arising largely from the prevertebral ganglia mostly innervate their target effector cells directly. The submucosal plexus contains a few parasympathetic ganglia of the vagal nerve, but postganglionic sympathetic fibres from the superior mesenteric plexus form the major proportion of the extrinsic nerves present.

Beneath the submucosa is the muscularis mucosae which consist of two thin layers of muscle with some elastic tissue. The inner muscle layer consists of circularly disposed fibres and the outer layer longitudinally disposed fibres. The muscularis mucosae permit localized movement of the mucous membrane. Small bundles of muscle fibres extend from it to the epithelium. Some of the fibres end on the epithelial basement membrane. Beneath the muscularis mucosa in the lamina propria is a layer of connective tissue that supports the epithelium and contains collagen, reticular fibres and some elastic fibres. It also contains blood capillaries and lymph capillaries that are situated close to the epithelial surface, especially in the villi (Fig. 7.6). It also contains numerous lymphatic nodules. Lymphocytes and plasma cells gain access to this layer across the epithelial membrane. These cells protect the tissue against bacteria that enter across the epithelial membrane. The plasma cells produce IgA immunoglobulins. The innermost layer is the epithelium which is described below.

The villus

The villus is regarded as the unit of absorption. Its length varies between 0.5 and 1.5mm, depending on its location in the small intestine. The structure of the villus is depicted in Figure 7.6. Each villus contains a blood capillary network and a blind-ended lacteal (or lymph vessel). It is covered by simple columnar epithelium. Most of these cells have numerous cytoplasmic extensions, known as microvilli at the luminal surface. The microvillous surface of the intestine is known as the brush border.

Histology

The mucosa of the small intestine is simple columnar epithelium. Four cell types are present:

1. Absorptive cells that produce digestive enzymes and absorb nutrients from the chyme

2. Goblet cells that produce mucus which lubricates the surface and protects it from mechanical damage

3. Granular cells (cells of Paneth) that produce enzymes and protect the intestinal surface from bacteria

4. APUD cells that produce peptide hormones which regulate secretion and motility in the gastrointestinal tract, liver and pancreas. The general function and structure of APUD cells are described in Chapter 1.

The four cell types arise from undifferentiated cells in the crypts of Lieberkühn. The granular and endocrine cells remain at the bottom of the crypts but the absorptive and goblet cells slowly migrate up the sides of the villi, to the tips. Figure 7.7 shows the cell types and their typical locations in the mucosa. The cells that migrate are eventually shed from the tips. The process of migration from the crypts to the tips of the villi occurs over 3–6 days in the human. Thus, most of the intestinal epithelium is renewed every few days. The columnar cells mature as they travel towards the tips of the villi, and their functions change. There is a gradual transition from base columnar cells in the crypts (Fig. 7.7) to villous columnar cells; their size increases progressively as they ascend the walls of the crypts and villi, and their content of free ribosomes decreases, while their content of rough endoplasmic reticulum increases.

Cell types

Villous epithelium

About 90% of the cells covering the villi are the absorptive columnar cylindrical cells. Most of the rest are goblet cells, but ≤0.5% are endocrine cells. The absorptive cells have abundant cytoplasm and mitochondria but few ribosomes. They have a thick striated microvillous border and convoluted lateral cell membranes. Figure 7.7 shows the structure of an absorptive cell, and the structure of microvilli. The rough endoplasmic reticulum and Golgi saccules are well-developed in columnar cells at the base of the villi but less prominent in cells at the tips of the villi. The columnar cells produce a cell coat that is composed of glycoproteins, but the cells at the base of the villi are more active in this respect than the other cells, as is consistent with their well-developed Golgi saccules. Some of the glycoproteins present are enzymes involved in the digestion of nutrients such as disaccharides (see Ch. 8). They act *in situ* but are also active after being shed into the lumen.

Crypt epithelium

The base of the crypt contains approximately equal numbers of small columnar cells and Paneth cells. The small columnar cells have sparse cytoplasm containing few mitochondria and little rough endoplasmic reticulum and a small Golgi apparatus. However, they contain numerous free ribosomes, consistent with their active protein synthesizing function. They have smooth lateral membranes and are relatively undifferentiated. These are the stem cells that give rise to the other cell types.

Paneth cells are highly differentiated, possessing abundant rough endoplasmic reticulum and a prominent Golgi apparatus. They synthesize enzymes, such as lysozyme, and sequester them in zymogen granules, from which they are released into the lumen by exocytosis.

There are also oligomucous cells that contain few mucus globules in the crypts. These are the precursors of the goblet cells. They can divide but they lose this ability when they become distended with mucus after migrating up the villus.

Endocrine cells comprise about 1% of the cells in the crypts. They have a narrow apex, and a wide basal region that is packed with dense argentaffin granules. These cells produce hormones such as secretin, CCK, somatostatin or endorphins. Others produce serotonin.

There are a few caveolated cells, characterized by invaginations of the cell membrane extending into its cytoplasm (caveolae). They have long microvilli that contain long bundles of straight filaments that extend into the cytoplasm, and filaments encircling the apical region. Their role is unknown.

Intestinal secretions

An alkaline fluid containing electrolytes, mucus and water, is secreted throughout the length of the small intestine. The precise composition of the secretion, and the mechanisms that control it, vary from one region to another. It is secreted by the immature cells in the crypts of Lieberkühn. The mechanisms involved are outlined in Figure 7.8. The key step is the active transport of Cl^- across the basolateral membrane of the cell. Cl^- is actively transported into the cell via a co-transporter protein that transports Na^+, K^+ and $2Cl^-$. The transport of Na^+ down its electrical gradient is the driving force for the operation of this transporter. The K^+ is transported back out via K^+ channels in the same membrane. This K^+ flux maintains the electrical potential difference (cytosol negative) across the cell membranes. This potential difference contributes to the driving force for the basolateral influx of Na^+ across the basolateral membrane, and also for Cl^- transport across the luminal membrane. Cl^- is transported into the lumen via the cystic fibrosis transport regulator (CFTR, see Ch. 5) which is an electrogenic Cl^- channel in the luminal membrane. Na^+ is then transported into the lumen between the cells, down the electrochemical gradient produced by the extrusion of Cl^- from the cell. The opening time of the CFTR channel is prolonged by increased cAMP. Therefore secretion by the crypt cells is stimulated by substances that elevate cAMP, such as vasoactive intestinal peptide (VIP) and prostaglandins. Ca^{2+}-mobilizing agents such as acetylcholine potentiate the actions of these substances. The mechanism of action of cholera toxin is also via increasing intracellular cAMP. In this case it causes a massive secretion of fluid (Case 7.1: 2). There is a defect in the CFTR channel in cystic fibrosis (see Ch. 5). The first manifestation of cystic fibrosis can be postnatal constipation (meconium ileus) that is directly related to absence of the CFTR channel.

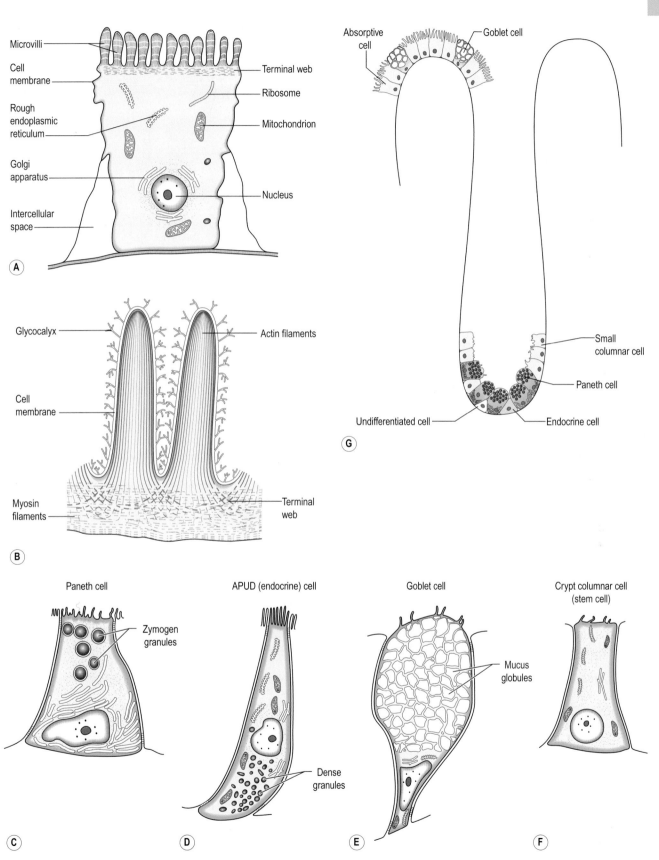

Fig. 7.7 Cell types in the intestinal epithelium. (A) Absorptive columnar cell. (B) Structure of microvilli of the absorptive cell. (C) Paneth cell. (D) Endocrine cell. (E) Goblet cell. (F) Undifferentiated columnar cell. (G) Localization of the different cell types in the epithelium of the crypts and the villi.

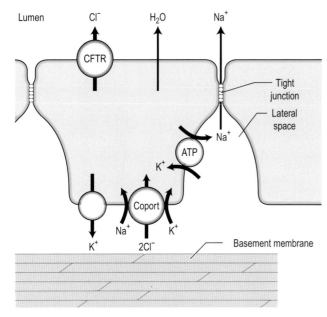

Fig. 7.8 Mechanism of secretion of electrolytes and water by the immature cells of the crypts of Lieberkühn.

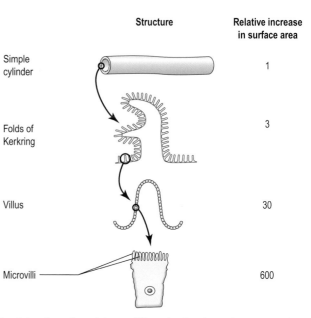

Fig. 7.9 Adaptation of the small intestine for absorption. Comparison of the surface area of a segment of the small intestine with a simple cylinder of the same length and diameter.

Control of secretion in the small intestine

Secretion in the small intestine can be controlled by hormones, paracrine factors and nervous activity. Gastrin, neurotensin, serotonin, histamine, prostaglandins, and a number of other hormone and paracrine factors stimulate the epithelial cells directly. The cells are innervated by secretomotor neurones, mainly from ganglia in the submucosal plexus but also from ganglia in the myenteric plexus. The submucosal neurones release ACh, VIP, substance P and serotonin, and probably other transmitters, to stimulate secretion. Parasympathetic nerves innervate neurones in the enteric nerve plexi. They enhance secretion via ACh release onto neurones in the plexi. Parasympathetic tone contributes to the basal secretion. Reflexes triggered by distension of the lumen of the small intestine, and the presence of various substances (glucose, acid, bile salts, ethanol, cholera toxin) in the intestinal chyme, stimulate secretion. These reflexes involve intrinsic and extrinsic (parasympathetic nerves).

Noradrenaline inhibits secretion in two ways: it acts directly on the epithelial cells (via α-adrenoreceptors), and it acts on neurones in the submucosal ganglia to inhibit secretory nerves that stimulate the epithelial cells. Somatostatin acts humorally on the crypt cells, as an inhibitory neurotransmitter. It is released from the enteric secretomotor nerves, and from the nerve fibres that innervate the crypt cells. It inhibits secretion by decreasing the levels of cAMP in the epithelial crypt cells. The effect of somatostatin to inhibit secretion has led to use of its analogues such as octreotide in the treatment of secretory diarrhoea, and to reduce fluid loss from small bowel (ileocutaneous) fistulae.

Absorption

Most substances are absorbed in the proximal small intestine and most of the contents of the small intestine have normally been absorbed by the time the chyme reaches the middle of the jejunum. However, a few substances such as vitamin B_{12} and bile salts (see Ch. 8) are actively absorbed in the ileum.

Surface area of the small intestine

The rate of transport of materials across the small intestine is proportional to its surface area. The surface area of the small intestine is vast. This organ is therefore well-adapted for absorption. Its area is approximately 600 times greater than that of a simple cylinder of the same length and diameter, by virtue of the presence of mucosal folds, villi and microvilli (Fig. 7.9). When the surface area is reduced, malabsorption of many substances ensues. In coeliac disease, for example, which is characterized by flattened villi, and therefore reduced surface area, there is malabsorption of many nutrients, including protein, resulting in malnutrition (see Ch. 8). The children who present with this condition have weight loss, diarrhoea and a failure to thrive.

Barriers to absorption

There are a number of barriers to transport from the intestinal lumen to the blood: the unstirred layer, the luminal plasma membrane, the cell's interior, the basolateral plasma membrane, the intercellular space, the basement membrane of the capillary and the cell membranes

Causes, mechanism of action and changes in electrolyte and acid–base balance

Causes

The *V. cholerae* bacterium present in contaminated water and food produces a toxin that elicits a massive secretion of fluid and electrolytes. The effect is produced mainly in the proximal small intestine. Epidemics in the Indian subcontinent usually occur in the early summer before the monsoon breaks. The bacteria are harboured in the gall bladder in asymptomatic carriers, which may comprise up to 5% of the population in this region.

Treatments with antibiotics such as tetracycline or chloramphenicol is effective but should be regarded as ancillary to rehydration therapy (see below). Thus, for example, tetracycline treatment decreases the average duration of the disease by 60%.

Anticholera vaccines have been developed, but these are of limited use during epidemics because it takes 2–3 weeks for them to become effective.

Bacteria are normally destroyed by gastric acid in the stomach, normally providing some protection. Increased susceptibility to the disease is seen in individuals with achlorhydria or those who have had a partial gastrectomy.

Mechanisms of cholera toxin action

Hypersecretion

There is an increased secretion of Cl^-, Na^+ and water into the crypts of Lieberkühn in patients with cholera. The cholera toxin is an 84000kDa protein produced by *V. cholerae*. It binds to monosialoganglioside (G_{m1}) receptor molecules in the brush border membrane of the crypt cells, mainly in the proximal intestine. This results in activation of adenyl cyclase, which causes an increase in cAMP in the cells. The increase in cAMP causes activation of the CFTR Cl^- channels in the brush border resulting in an increase in the secretion of Cl^-. Na^+ and water secretion increase as a consequence. Cholera victims sometimes produce up to 20L of watery stool per day. Treatment with somatostatin analogues such as octreotide which inhibit secretion by decreasing the levels of cAMP counteracts the effect of cholera toxin.

The intramural nerves are also involved in the mechanisms of the toxin action because substances that block nerve activity reduce the effects of the toxin. However, the precise neural mechanisms involved are unclear.

Hypermotility

Hypermotility of the small intestine can result in water and electrolytes being delivered rapidly into the colon. It can be delivered so fast that the colon may not be able to absorb it before it is lost in the faeces. This mechanism is also involved in conditions such as cholera, as distension of the intestines by the large volumes of secreted fluids stimulates peristaltic activity, which propels the fluid rapidly along the intestines.

Changes in electrolyte and acid–base balance

Secretions of the small intestines contain large amounts of HCO_3^-, Na^+ and Cl^- ions. K^+ is absorbed during a meal, down the concentration gradient set up by the absorption of water (see below). However, when the concentration of K^+ in the lumen is reduced below approximately 25mM the concentration gradient favours net secretion into the lumen. This occurs via the paracellular pathway. In diarrhoea, the luminal contents become diluted with respect to K^+ and it is therefore transported into the lumen. Considerable losses of K^+ can occur, leading to hypokalaemia.

As HCO_3^- is secreted into the lumen, H^+ is transported into the blood, which becomes transiently acid. Excessive loss of HCO_3^- in secreted intestinal fluid causes a severe acidosis. The transient acidity in the blood is normally neutralized by the alkaline tide that accompanies the secretion of acid in the stomach (see Ch. 3). If there is excessive loss of alkaline fluid from the gastrointestinal tract however, the acidity in the blood is proportionately increased and it cannot be buffered. This metabolic acidosis will be partially compensated in the short term by an increased rate and depth of breathing which results in CO_2 being blown off from the body. Longer-term adjustments are brought about by reabsorption of HCO_3^- in the tubules of the kidney, and excretion of H^+ (see the companion volumes: *The Respiratory System* and *The Renal System*).

K^+ is required for cell growth and division, enzyme action, cell excitability, muscle contraction, acid–base balance and volume regulation. Hypokalaemia (reduced serum K^+ concentration) causes hyperpolarization of cell membranes and reduces the excitability of neurones, cardiac muscle, and skeletal muscle. Severe hypokalaemia can cause paralysis, cardiac arrhythmias, decreased ability to concentrate urine, and death, which is usually due to cardiac arrest.

of the endothelial cell of the capillary or lymph vessels. The luminal border of the enterocyte is the effective barrier for the absorption of many substances but for some substances it is the basolateral border or the endothelial cell membrane. Transport across some of the plasma membranes involved, for example the membranes of the endothelial cells, is via simple passive diffusion. However, for transport across others, special mechanisms such as active transport, facilitated diffusion or pinocytosis (endocytosis) exist.

Potential difference across the small intestine

A potential difference exists across the wall of the small intestine, the serosal side being positive with respect to the mucosal side. In the case of a charged ion, transport is the net effect of the forces due to the concentration gradient and the potential difference (see Ch. 1). Thus net transport of anions from the lumen can occur passively down the electrochemical gradient.

The size of the potential difference varies along the length of the small intestine. The magnitude of the potential difference is determined by the active transport of electrolytes, in particular Na^+, which occurs against the electrical gradient (see below). The magnitude of the potential difference is increased in the presence of glucose that stimulates the active transport of Na^+. Table 7.2 compares the potential difference in different regions of the small intestine in the presence and absence of glucose in the lumen.

Routes of absorption

The rate of absorption of a substance by passive diffusion is determined by its ionization and its lipid solubility. Substances can be absorbed via two routes: water-filled pores, and the lipid membrane.

Pore route

Water-soluble substances, with low molecular diameter can diffuse through water-filled pores in the cell membrane. The pore diameter in the small intestine varies between 40 and 340 nM. Bulk fluid movement drags small solute molecules through the pores in the moving stream of fluid (solvent drag). Thus if water absorption is increased by any means (e.g. hormonal influences), then the rate of passage of the dissolved substances is increased. Examples of small soluble substances that are absorbed by this route are urea, creatinine, some monosaccharides (mannitol, xylose, fucose) and ions.

Lipid route

The rapid rate of absorption of many substances can only be explained by their passage through the lipid of the cell

membrane. The cell membrane can be regarded as a sea of lipid with proteins embedded in it. Lipid–soluble substances dissolve in the lipid and diffuse rapidly through the membrane. Examples of lipid–soluble substances transported by this route are alcohols and long–chain fatty acids.

Absorption of drugs

Lipid soluble drugs

The importance of lipid solubility is illustrated in Table 7.3, where the rates of absorption of a selection of barbiturate drugs are compared. Compounds with the highest lipid solubility are absorbed at the fastest rate. Thus hexethal, the compound with the greatest lipid solubility chloroform/water coefficient of those listed is absorbed four times as fast as barbital even though it has the greatest molecular size.

Weak electrolyte drugs

A weak electrolyte exists as the undissociated molecule in equilibrium with the dissociated ion products. The equilibrium for a weak acid can be represented by the equation:

$$HA \leftrightarrow H^+ + A^-$$

where HA represents the undissociated weak acid, and A^- the anionic component. The undissociated molecule is lipid soluble but the ions are not. Thus the undissociated molecule is transported rapidly through the lipid

Table 7.2 Potential difference in different regions of the small intestine in the presence and absence of glucose

	Potential difference (Vm)		
	Upper jejunum	**Mid-intestine**	**Lower ileum**
Glucose absent	2.9	4.7	3.8
Glucose present	7.3	11.1	7.4

The potential difference rises in the presence of glucose, thereby increasing the passive transport of anions into the cells.

Table 7.3 Effect of lipid solubility on the absorption of barbiturates

Compound	Chloroform/ water coefficient	Absorbed (%)
Barbital	0.7	12
Butethal	11.7	24
Hexethal	>100	44

membrane. Removal of the undissociated acid from the equilibrium causes more of the undissociated molecule to form. This then diffuses across the membrane. In this way the substance can be rapidly absorbed. The rate of transport will depend on the proportion present in the undissociated form, i.e. it will depend on its pK and the pH of the solution in which it is dissolved. Thus in situations where the proportion of unionized molecule is increased the rate of absorption will be high. Many drugs are weak electrolytes. For a weak acid the rate of absorption can be increased if the pH of the solution is lowered below the pK value because the equilibrium will be shifted to the left. The opposite applies to a weak base which has a high pKa. Figure 7.10 illustrates this for two drugs: 5-nitrosalicylic acid, an aspirin derivative, which is a weak acid, and quinine, which is a weak base. In the upper small intestine, the pH of the chyme tends to be slightly acid, thereby favouring the absorption of weak acids. Furthermore, some weak acids such as aspirin can be absorbed in the acid environment of the stomach (see Ch. 3).

Strong electrolyte drugs

Strong acids (pKa <3.0) and bases (pKa >10) are very poorly absorbed. Clinically important drugs such as the muscle relaxants tubocurarine and hexamethonium that are strong bases, have to be administered intravenously. However for others, such as the aminoglycoside antibiotics, their poor absorption is an advantage because they can be used to sterilize the gut before intestinal surgery, without producing systemic effects.

Factors that affect gastrointestinal absorption of drugs

In most cases, approximately 75% of a drug is absorbed within 1–3h, but the rate of absorption can be altered by local factors, including changes in intestinal motility or splanchnic blood flow.

In many diseases gastrointestinal motility is slowed and this increases the time over which absorption takes place. Excessively increased motility can reduce the proportion of a substance that is absorbed. Some drugs, for example, muscarinic antagonists, can slow motility, and others such as metoclopramide can increase it.

Particle size and formulation of a drug can be significant factors in the rate of absorption. Capsules, or tablets can be given a resistant coating, which enables them to remain intact for some hours, thereby delaying absorption. A sustained absorption can sometimes be achieved by including a mixture of slow and fast release particles in a capsule.

Chemical properties that can cause reduced absorption rate include the ability to bind strongly to Ca^{2+} in milk for example. Liquid paraffin, which is lipophilic, retards the absorption of lipid–soluble vitamins.

Absorption into the blood or lymph

Some substances are absorbed solely by passive diffusion. Others are absorbed by both passive and specialized mechanisms: at a rapid rate by a specialized mechanism, and at a slow rate by passive diffusion (see Ch. 1).

A substance that is absorbed into the blood or lymph can be transported across the luminal and basolateral membranes of the enterocyte and, if it is transported into the blood, it crosses the membranes of the endothelial cells of the capillary. In many cases a given substance is transported across each membrane by a different mechanism. A good example is the transport of Na^+ that is by carrier-mediated facilitated diffusion across the brush border, by active transport across the basolateral border (see below), and via passive diffusion across the endothelial membranes of the capillaries.

Some substances are preferentially absorbed into the blood capillaries of the villi, and some into the lacteals (Fig. 7.6). Two properties determine whether a given substance is absorbed into the blood or the lymph; its size, and its lipid solubility. Large molecules, particles, and lipid–soluble substances, are transported into the lymph. Most lipids are sequestered in chylomicrons prior to transport into the lymph, and certain intact proteins can be absorbed in trace amounts in some individuals (see Ch. 8). Most other substances, that is, small, water-soluble substances, are absorbed into the blood. Transport across the endothelial cells of blood and lymph vessels is always passive and occurs down a concentration or electrochemical gradient. Substances that are absorbed into the lymph eventually gain access to the blood via the thoracic duct. The reasons for a particular substance being preferentially absorbed into the blood or lymph are outlined below.

Absorption into the blood

Both capillaries and lymph vessels are freely permeable to low molecular weight water-soluble substances. However, there is an extensive network of capillaries in each villus but only a single lacteal and therefore there is a greater surface area available for transport into the blood than into the lymph, and a greater blood volume.

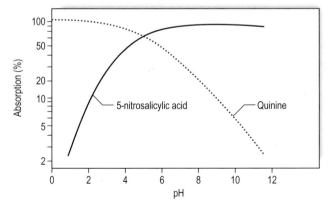

Fig. 7.10 Effect of pH on the absorption of weak electrolyte drugs in the small intestine. Absorption of a weak acid, 5-nitrosalicylic acid (pKa 2.3), and a weak base, quinine (pKa 8.4).

Furthermore, blood flow is much greater (approx. 500 times faster) than lymph flow. This ensures the rapid removal of the transported substances, which are carried away via the rapidly flowing blood and helps to maintain a favourable concentration gradient for transport. Thus, most (>95%) low molecular weight, water-soluble substances are absorbed into the blood.

Absorption into the lymph

The endothelial cells of the blood capillary contain pores (fenestrae) with diameters in the range 20–50 nM. They also have a basement membrane. The pores are large enough to admit large molecules, but they cannot cross the basement membrane, and are therefore excluded from the blood capillary. Lipids are delivered to the lateral spaces as components of large protein–bound particles (chylomicrons), which are excluded from the capillaries for the same reason.

The endothelial cells of the lacteals lack a basement membrane. They do not contain pores, but when they are viewed under the microscope the endothelial cells appear to be displaced relative to each other at their lateral borders (as though movement can occur between adjacent cells). It seems likely therefore that transient gaps form between adjacent cells. Large molecules or particles are probably transported to the lymph between the cells via these gaps. Peristalsis and the pumping action of the villi (see below) aid absorption into the lacteals, probably by promoting the formation of the gaps.

Transport of water and electrolytes in different regions of the small intestine

The cells at the tips of the villi are specialized for water and ion transport while those in the crypts produce net secretion of water and ions. However, the rate of transport varies along the length of the intestines because the villi are larger and the brush border surface is greater per unit area in the proximal region of the small intestine than the distal region (see above). Thus, the fluxes of water and nutrients tend to be greater in the jejunum than the ileum, except where localized special transport mechanisms exist. The surface area in the colon is less than in the small intestine and therefore less net transport occurs in the colon. Flux of ions and water occurs both through the cells and across the tight junctions between them. The tight junctions are leakier in the proximal small intestine than the distal regions. This also results in a greater paracellular flux per unit area in the jejunum than the ileum. The result is that most absorption occurs in the proximal small intestine.

Absorption of water

Water transport in the gastrointestinal tract is largely a function of the small intestine (see Ch. 1). The stomach is almost impermeable to water but the small intestine is highly permeable. The colon is permeable to water but less so than the small intestine.

The transport of water in the small intestine can occur either from the lumen to the blood or from the blood to the lumen. Net transport is down the osmotic gradient and it will occur in whichever direction the osmotic forces determine. It will be secreted into the lumen if the chyme is hypertonic to plasma and absorbed into the blood if it is hypotonic. The chyme entering the duodenum from the stomach is usually initially hypertonic. Rapid gastric emptying, as may occur after surgery, results in the contents of the small intestine being abnormally hypertonic. This causes an influx of water into the small intestine. If excessive, this can cause severe diarrhoea.

The digestion of complex nutrients in the duodenal chyme results in a further increase in osmolarity. The prevailing osmotic forces result in the secretion of water in this region, and the intestinal contents normally become isotonic with plasma in the duodenum.

In the jejunum and ileum, water is absorbed from the lumen into the blood down the osmotic gradient produced as a result of the absorption of nutrients in these regions. More water absorption occurs in the jejunum than the ileum. The chyme remains isotonic throughout the jejunum and ileum where water is absorbed as a consequence of the absorption of other substances.

A major determinant of the osmotic gradient in the small intestine is the active transport of Na^+ ions (see below). Cl^- ions are absorbed passively down the electrochemical gradient as a consequence of Na^+ absorption. In addition the absorption of other ions, for example K^+, by passive diffusion, depends on the concentration gradients set up as a consequence of water absorption. Moreover, some sugars and amino acids are absorbed by symport mechanisms with Na^+. Thus, all of these processes are interdependent and they will therefore be considered together. Figure 7.11 shows the consequences of failure of membrane transport in the small intestine.

Absorption of sodium, chloride and potassium

Na^+ transport occurs throughout the length of the small intestine. The transport of sodium across the epithelial cells of the small intestine is by both passive diffusion and active special mechanisms. The mucosal surface of the small intestine is electronegative with respect to the serosal surface, favouring the passive transport of Na^+ into the lumen. The electrochemical gradient is largely due to the secretion of Cl^- into the lumen (Fig. 7.8). The passive flux of Na^+ is via the paracellular pathway. However, the permeability for Na^+ decreases along the small intestine, being highest in the duodenum and lowest in the ileum, due to the gradual decrease in both the brush border surface area and in the leakiness of the tight junctions from jejunum to ileum.

Most Na^+ is transported from the lumen of the small intestine into the blood by active mechanisms. This involves the transcellular route. It is usually transported in the absence of a chemical gradient as the chyme in the

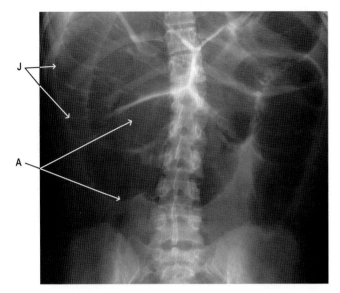

Fig. 7.11 A plain abdominal X-ray showing obstruction to the small bowel. The jejunum (J) has become grossly dilated and filled with air (A) and fluid, due to failure of membrane transport.

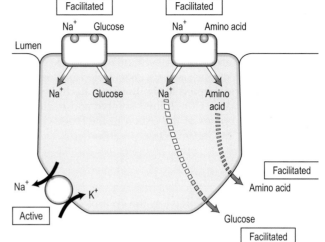

Fig. 7.12 The secondary active transport of Na$^+$ via the Na$^+$/glucose and Na$^+$/amino acid co-port systems in the absorptive cells of the proximal small intestine.

small intestine is normally isotonic with plasma, but it is obviously transported against the small electrochemical gradient present. The processes involved are illustrated in Figure 7.12. The key process is the active transport of Na$^+$ out of the cell, across the lateral border via a Na$^+$/K$^+$ ATPase pump, which simultaneously pumps K$^+$ into the cell. This maintains the low concentration of Na$^+$ within the cell. The Na$^+$ concentration gradient set up by this pump is the driving force for the transport of Na$^+$ from the lumen of the intestine into the cell. This diffusion across the luminal brush border of the cell is therefore down the concentration gradient. However, transport across this membrane occurs at a faster rate than it would by simple passive diffusion. This is because the Na$^+$ ions are transported on carrier proteins in the brush border membrane. One of these carriers is the Na$^+$ dependent/glucose transporter (SGLT 1, see Ch. 8). It only functions if glucose, or galactose (which competes with glucose), is present in the lumen. The transporter has a binding site for glucose and a binding site for Na$^+$. Both binding sites must be occupied for the transport process to take place, and then both Na$^+$ and the hexose are transported into the cell via this co-port system (see Fig. 7.12 and Ch. 8). The transport of Na$^+$ and glucose by this means is inhibited by the presence of high concentrations of K$^+$ in the lumen. This is because K$^+$ occupies the Na$^+$ binding site to inhibit the transport process. Inside the cell, where there is a high concentration of K$^+$, the displacement of Na$^+$ from the carrier by K$^+$, may be responsible for Na$^+$ being released into the cell's cytoplasm. The transport of hexoses, including glucose, is described in more detail in Chapter 8.

Neutral amino acids also stimulate Na$^+$ absorption via a co-port system involving transporter molecules. This mechanism also depends on the Na$^+$ concentration gradient set-up by the operation of the Na$^+$/K$^+$ ATPase pump in the lateral border of the cell (see Fig. 7.12 and Ch. 8).

The net rate of absorption of Na$^+$ is highest in the jejunum because the glucose and neutral amino acid transporters are situated mainly in this region. Sugars and amino acids produce a lesser stimulation of Na$^+$ absorption in the ileum where the transporters are less numerous.

The active transport of Na$^+$ out of the cell across the lateral border increases its concentration in the lateral spaces. Cl$^-$ and other monovalent anions are transported down the electrical gradient created, mainly via the paracellular pathway, through the tight junctions, into the lateral spaces. This occurs in the duodenum, jejunum and ileum, although the proportion transported via this route is greater in the duodenum, where the tight junctions are leakiest.

The accumulation of ions within the lateral spaces creates an osmotic gradient, and water is transported down this osmotic gradient, via the paracellular pathway, into the spaces. The spaces expand during a meal because of this increase in osmolarity. The transport of water out of the lumen results in concentration of the chyme. This increases the concentration, and therefore the concentration gradient for ions such as K$^+$. These are then transported passively between the cells into the lateral spaces. Thus, the transport of many substances ultimately depends on the active transport of Na$^+$ out of the epithelial cells.

Na$^+$ can also be actively absorbed in exchange for H$^+$ that is secreted into the lumen, i.e. via a N$^+$/H$^+$ exchange mechanism. This anion exchange operates in the lower small intestine and the colon. It is the major route for active Na$^+$ transport in the ileum, where the glucose and amino acid transporters are less numerous than in the jejunum, and in the colon. However, the ileum and colon can absorb Na$^+$ against a higher potential difference than can the jejunum. The anion exchange mechanism is illustrated in Figure 7.13. The H^+ secreted into the lumen reacts with HCO_3^- to form carbonic acid. The HCO_3^- arises via transport out of the cells because of the operation of a Cl^-/HCO_3^- exchange mechanism whereby Cl^- is absorbed in exchange for HCO_3^-. Thus active transport of Na^+ and Cl^- is coupled in this way. The carbonic acid formed in the lumen is hydrolysed to give CO_2 and water. CO_2 is lipid soluble and it diffuses across the membranes of the cells into the blood. In this way H^+ and HCO_3^- are effectively reabsorbed.

Control of absorption

Various factors are involved in the control of water and electrolyte absorption by the cells near the tips of the villi. These include endocrine, paracrine and nervous influences. Glucocorticoids stimulate electrolyte and water absorption in both the small and large intestines, probably by causing an increase in the expression of the Na^+/K^+-ATPase pumps in the basolateral membrane of the epithelial cell. Opioids (acting on δ-opioid receptors) also stimulate water and electrolyte absorption. Somatostatin stimulates electrolyte and water absorption in the ileum and colon. Noradrenaline also increases Na^+ absorption, probably following its release from sympathetic nerves on to enteric nerves that innervate the absorptive cells. Absorption can be inhibited by inflammatory mediators such as histamine and prostaglandins that are released from cells of the gastrointestinal immune system.

Diarrhoea

Diarrhoea is defined clinically as a loss of fluid and solutes from the gastrointestinal tract in excess of 500 mL/day. The causes are infectious agents, toxins, drugs, food, or anxiety. The mechanisms responsible for loss of fluid can operate in the small intestine or the colon.

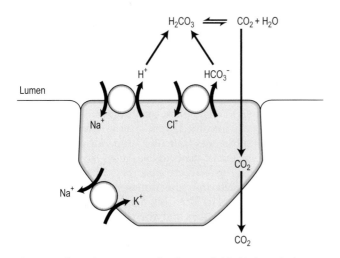

Fig. 7.13 The active transport of sodium and chloride ions via the Na^+/H^+ exchange and Cl^-/HCO_3^- exchange systems, respectively, in the small intestine.

Diarrhoea can be classified as four types, according to the mechanism responsible: secretory diarrhoea, diarrhoea due to defective ion transport, osmotic diarrhoea and diarrhoea due to increased intestinal motility. However, several or all of these mechanisms may co-exist.

Secretory diarrhoea

In secretory diarrhoea, the secretions of the small intestine are so copious that the capacity of the colon to reabsorb the excessive water is overwhelmed. Food poisoning caused by bacteria (e.g. *V. cholera* or *Escherichia coli*) causes this type of diarrhoea. The bacteria produce toxins that bind to receptors in the membranes of the secreting crypt cells to increase intracellular cAMP, which stimulates a massive secretion (see Case 7.1: 2). The treatment of this condition by rehydration therapy is described in Case 7.1: 3. The massive secretion of fluid in cholera can cause hypovolaemia (Case 7.1: 4).

Case 7.1 Cholera: 3

Rehydration therapy

Individuals suffering from cholera are treated with (1) intravenous fluid and electrolytes, or with (2) oral fluid, salt and sugar, depending on the severity of their symptoms.

Intravenous rehydration

The intravenous fluid would consist of water containing electrolytes in concentrations that are isotonic with plasma. The massive fluid loss can lead to dehydration, hypovolaemia, renal failure and death. Particular attention is paid to K^+ and HCO_3^- replacement as excessive losses of these ions can have rapid and dangerous consequences.

Oral rehydration therapy

The discovery of the co-port mechanisms for Na^+ transport in the small intestine revolutionized the treatment of food poisoning due to *V. cholerae* or *E. coli*, where excessive fluid loss and dehydration can occur. Prior to the discovery of the co-port mechanisms, approximately 50% of individuals suffering from cholera died, due to collapse of the extracellular fluid volume (ECF). Treatment was by administration of large quantities of salt solution, a regimen that was only partially effective. Oral rehydration therapy with a solution of glucose and common salt has dramatically reduced the death rate. The solution used should be isotonic or hypotonic, as a hypertonic load will create an osmotic gradient for the transport of more water into the lumen. Inflammation and damage to the mucosa are not normally present and the digestion and absorptive mechanisms are not affected. Therefore glucose can be replaced with table sugar (sucrose) as it is digested to glucose (and fructose). Replacement of glucose with starch can also be effective because digestion of each starch molecule results in numerous glucose digestion products, and it can therefore be ingested as a dilute solution that does not constitute a great osmotic load.

Excessive activation of intrinsic neurons in pathological conditions may also cause secretory diarrhoea. Some of these neurons release VIP that increases intracellular cAMP. Others release transmitters such as acetylcholine or substance P that cause increased intracellular Ca^{2+}, which can also mediate excessive secretion from the crypt cells.

Defective ion transport

As active transport of Na^+ is a major determinant of the osmotic transport of water from the lumen into the blood, the presence of inhibitors of Na^+ transport will inhibit water transport to cause diarrhoea. Bile acids inhibit Na^+ absorption in the colon, if they are not absorbed in the terminal ileum. Furthermore, fat malabsorption results in fermentation of lipids in the colon to produce toxins that inhibit Na^+ absorption. Inflammatory mediators such as histamine and prostaglandins released from cells of the gastroimmune system that inhibit Na^+ absorption may be involved in the secretory diarrhoea of inflammatory bowel disease and Crohn's disease. However, noradrenaline can increase absorption, and in diabetes when sympathetic neurodegeneration is present, diarrhoea can be a problem.

A defect in ion transport can also result in failure to absorb water. In congenital chloridorrhoea, for example, the Cl^-/HCO_3^- exchanger is absent from the brush border membrane (see Case 7.2: 1 and 2). A congenital defect in the Na^+/H^+ exchanger has also been described. In these conditions the defective exchanger protein is lacking in the jejunum, ileum and colon. In the duodenum and jejunum, the glucose and amino acid co-port mechanisms promote Na^+ and water absorption, but these transporters are not present in the ileum or colon. Therefore it is impairment of Cl^- transport in distal regions of the gastrointestinal tract that results in diarrhoea in these congenital transporter deficiencies.

Osmotic diarrhoea

The presence of hypertonic fluid in the intestinal lumen can cause osmotic diarrhoea. High concentrations of salts such as SO_4^{2-}, Mg^{2+} and PO_4^{3-}, which are only slowly absorbed in the intestine can be responsible. Magnesium sulphate solution is commonly used as a laxative. The osmotic gradient set-up favours water transport into the lumen. Absorption disorders can also give rise to osmotic diarrhoea. If nutrients that are normally absorbed in the

---

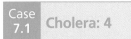

Cholera: 4

Hypovolaemia: cardiovascular and renal adjustments

Cause of feeble rapid pulse rate

In hypovolaemic conditions the blood volume is reduced, and the cutaneous veins collapse, leading to reduced venous return. This results in a reduced end-diastolic volume in the left ventricle, leading to a reduced cardiac output (see the companion volume *The Cardiovascular System*). This is manifest clinically as a low pulse, and collapsed peripheral veins. Reduced baroreceptor stimulation leads to reduced vagal tone and increased sympathetic tone, and this causes an increase in heart rate, and an increase in contractility of the myocardium. The increased sympathetic activation also leads to general venoconstriction leading to increased venous return. The reduced blood flow to the intestinal mucosa can be so severe as to lead to necrosis of the tissue, due to a decreased oxygen supply.

Adjustments in function to correct the reduced ECF

The major adjustments however, are those brought about by changes in renal function. The kidneys respond to the decrease in ECF volume by decreasing the urine output. The mechanism involves sympathetic vasoconstriction in the kidney, and retention of Na^+ ions and water, as a result of increased release of aldosterone and antidiuretic hormone (ADH), respectively.

Congenital chloridorrhoea: 1

A premature infant who was born with a distended abdomen, developed diarrhoea soon after birth. The chloride content of the fluid on the infant's napkin was extremely high (95 mmol/L). The child appeared dehydrated and during the first week of life, blood analyses showed that she was hyponatraemic, hypochloraemic and hypokalaemic. Later, she developed a metabolic alkalosis, and her faeces were acid. Fortunately she was quickly diagnosed as having congenital chloridorrhoea. In this rare condition the Cl^-/HCO_3^- exchanger is absent from the luminal membranes of the jejunum, ileum and colon. Initially intravenous electrolyte replacement therapy was instituted, but after a few weeks, electrolyte replacement therapy (a solution of KCl and NaCl) could be given orally.

Perusal of this case history could provoke the following questions about this condition:

- Why are abnormally high amounts of Cl^- lost in the faeces?
- How does this defect result in diarrhoea?
- Is the fluid loss likely to be due to the absence of the exchanger in the small intestine or the large intestine, or both?
- Why did alkalosis develop in the child and why were the child's faeces acid?
- What is the basis of oral replacement therapy with KCl and NaCl?
- Why was it not necessary to include glucose in the oral replacement fluid?

Case
7.2   Congenital chloridorrhoea: 2

Defect and consequences

In this condition, the inherited defect is an absence of the Cl^-/HCO_3^- exchanger in the brush border membrane in the small intestine and in the colon. The exchanger transports Cl^- out of the lumen, in exchange for HCO_3^- (Fig. 7.13). The Na^+/H^+ exchanger is normal in this condition, but eventually the acidity of the luminal contents inhibits the Na^+/H^+ exchange mechanism as well.

Diarrhoea

If the exchanger protein is absent, Cl^- transported across the gut wall is reduced, and Cl^+ is lost in the faeces. The high concentrations of electrolytes present in the lumen cause water to be transported into the lumen by osmosis (osmotic diarrhoea). The absence of the exchanger in the jejunum is less important than its absence in the ileum and colon, because water is transported as a consequence of $Na^+/glucose$ and $Na^+/amino$ acid co-port mechanisms in the jejunum. These co-port systems are not numerous in the ileum and not present in the colon. So the osmotic forces in the ileum and colon cause water malabsorption.

Treatment

The child was treated by administration of NaCl and KCl solution for the following reasons: the child's plasma Cl^- concentration was low because of the absence of the Cl^-/HCO_3^- exchanger, and the Na^+ concentration was low because of the consequent inhibition of the Na^+/H^+ exchanger which transports Na^+ into the blood in exchange for H^+. The K^+ was low because K^+ is transported into the lumen down its concentration gradient. If water accumulates in the lumen, as in diarrhoea, this gradient will favour transport into the lumen, as the contents become more dilute.

Thus the oral replacement therapy given will correct the hyponatraemia (low blood Na^+ concentration), the hypokalaemia (low blood K^+ concentration) and the hypochloraemia (low blood Cl^- concentration).

The transport of water as a consequence of the $Na^+/glucose$ co-port mechanism in the upper small intestine is not affected in this condition, and it is probably operating optimally. As the mechanisms that are defective are the Cl^-/HCO_3^- exchanger and the Na^+/H^+ exchanger that operate mainly in the distal small intestine and colon, the presence of glucose in the solution administered would serve no purpose.

Metabolic alkalosis

The exchanger protein that is absent in congenital chloridorrhoea transports Cl^- into the blood in exchange for HCO_3^- that is transported into the lumen. If the exchanger is absent, HCO_3^- accumulates in the blood and causes alkalosis. The Na^+/H^+ exchange system transports Na^+ into the blood in exchange for H^+, which is transported into the lumen. This is normally neutralized by the HCO_3^- transported into the lumen in exchange for Cl^-, but in this case the HCO_3^-/Cl^- exchanger is absent in the membranes and H^+ would be lost in the faeces.

---

small intestine cannot be absorbed for any reason, the osmotic pressure in the lumen is increased. Furthermore, when these nutrients enter the large intestine they may be fermented by colonic bacteria so that each molecule is degraded to a number of products, thereby increasing the osmolarity even further. The volume of water transported into the lumen as a consequence may be too great for the colon to reabsorb it, and diarrhoea results. An example of such a condition is lactase deficiency in which lactose (milk sugar) cannot be digested. This sugar enters the colon unchanged, but it is fermented by colonic bacteria to smaller products. This causes an increased osmotic potential (see Ch. 8).

Hypermotility of the intestines

Where hypermotility of the intestines is present, water and electrolytes may be delivered to the colon at a rate that is too fast for the water to be absorbed in the colon. The causes of intestinal hypermotility are not clear, but in cases of malabsorption, colonic bacteria may ferment unabsorbed nutrients to produce toxins that increase motility. One example is lipid malabsorption, where lipids are fermented to produce hydroxylated fatty acids that increase motility in the colon (as well as inhibiting Na^+ transport, see above).

The treatment of diarrhoea is outlined in Box 7.1.

Motility in the small intestine

The smooth muscle of the small intestine performs two major functions. First, it is responsible for a thorough mixing of the digestive juices arriving from the liver and pancreas with the chyme received from the stomach. Second, it is responsible for moving the contents, usually slowly, but sometimes rapidly, along the 5 m separating the stomach from the colon. This enables one meal to make way for the next. However, it is important that the food is retained in each location for sufficient time to allow mixing, digestion and absorption of food substances.

Smooth muscle contracts spontaneously, even during fasting, although the contractions increase in strength and frequency after food has been ingested. The fine local and temporal control of intestinal motility in the different segments of the intestine is integrated by nervous and hormonal mechanisms.

Box 7.1 Treatment of diarrhoea

Oral rehydration therapy

Severe acute diarrhoea requires maintenance of fluid and electrolyte balance, with occasional use of antibiotics. Maintenance of fluid and electrolyte balance is of paramount importance. The use of oral rehydration therapy (fluid containing NaCl and glucose) is described in Case 7.1: 3. This treatment is particularly important in small children with diarrhoea, in whom the fluid and electrolyte loss can rapidly become life-threatening.

Antibiotics

Antibiotics can be useful in the treatment of diarrhoea in enteritic conditions such as amoebic dysentery, typhoid and cholera, which are caused by bacteria and protozoa. Milder types of bacterial and viral enteritis generally resolve without being treated. *Campylobacter* is a common infection that causes diarrhoea (in developed countries) and this can be treated with erythromycin. However, in many underdeveloped regions of the world enteritis is usually caused by viruses.

Antimotility drugs

Antimotility drugs, including opiates, codeine and loperamide, can be used to treat diarrhoea. These increase the tone and rhythmic activity of the intestine, but decrease its propulsive activity. They also inhibit secretion in the intestine. They are not usually used in infective diarrhoea.

Absorbents

Absorbents such as kaolin, chalk and charcoal are also used to decrease diarrhoea, but their mechanism of action is not entirely clear. They may act by adsorbing microorganisms and toxins, by altering the intestinal flora in some way, or by coating and protecting the intestinal mucosa.

Non-steroidal anti-inflammatory drugs

Agents that reduce secretion or increase absorption can also reduce diarrhoea. Non-steroidal anti-inflammatory drugs such as aspirin and indometacin are effective. The mechanism is probably due to inhibition of prostaglandin synthesis.

Types of motility

Spontaneous contractions

The smooth muscle of small intestine displays spontaneous activity even when a meal is not present in the gastrointestinal tract. This activity is tonus. Spontaneous contractions of smooth muscle occur in the absence of stretch, hormones or nervous activity due to the uneven amplitude of the oscillating membrane potential (see Ch. 1). The inherent mechanisms of tone and rhythmicity may be augmented by a background of transmitters such as acetylcholine released from nerves in the vicinity. This slow wave activity of the smooth muscle in the duodenum is influenced by that in the stomach. Some longitudinal muscle fibres from the stomach cross the pyloric sphincter region to the duodenum (see Ch. 4). The frequency of contractions in the duodenum (approx. 12/min) is higher than in the stomach. Every fifth contraction of the muscle in the duodenal bulb is augmented by a contraction of the antrum due to the transmission of the slow waves via the fibres crossing the sphincter. This acts to prevent the duodenal contents flowing back into the stomach.

There is also a regular type of spontaneous contraction, known as the moving myoelectric complex (MMC, see below), which moves distally down the intestine. Transmitters released during the progression of the MMC (see below) may be responsible for augmenting other types of spontaneous muscle activity. In addition catecholamines such as noradrenaline released from sympathetic nerves, and adrenaline released into the blood, during fasting and in times of stress, can reduce the tone of the smooth muscle.

The migrating myoelectric complex (MMC)

In fasting individuals there are cycles of smooth muscle contractions with an average frequency of approximately 1.5h. These are the MMCs. Each cycle involves contraction of several adjacent segments of the small intestine, and it lasts approximately 10min. The contractions occur sequentially in adjacent groups of segments. They actually begin in the stomach and migrate via the proximal small intestine 'aborally' towards the colon (Figure 7.14). In the fasting state, the periodic sweeping of the contents towards the colon may clean the intestine of residual food and secretions. It may also prevent the migration of colonic bacteria into the ileum. As one sweep reaches the terminal ileum, another starts in the duodenum. MMCs also occur when a meal is being processed, but then they are more frequent, and less ordered. Presumably they then assist in sweeping the digested contents of the lumen towards the colon.

Mixing and propulsion during a meal

Segmentation mixes the contents of the lumen when a meal is being processed, while peristalsis is responsible for propelling the chyme along towards the colon.

Segmentation

Segmentation involves contraction of rings of circular muscle situated at intervals along a region of the small intestine (Fig. 7.15A). The contractions remain stationary. These rings of muscle then relax, and then adjacent segments contract. The overall effect is a continuous rhythmic division and subdivision of the intestinal contents that results in a thorough mixing of the chyme in the lumen. Segmentation increases in frequency and strength when chyme enters the duodenum. It occurs more frequently in the duodenum (approx. 12 contractions/min) than

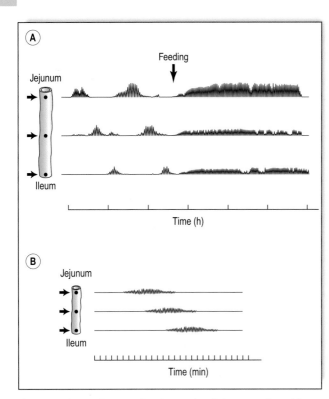

Fig. 7.14 The moving myoelectric complex. (A) Contractile activity. (B) Electrical activity.

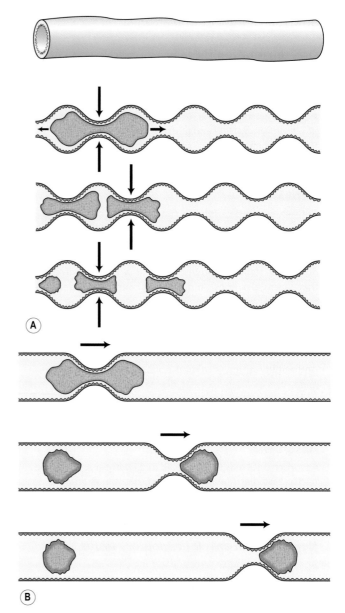

Fig. 7.15 Motility in the small intestine. (A) Segmentation. (B) Peristalsis.

in the jejunum or ileum (approx. 8 contractions/min). This is appropriate because the need for mixing is greatest in the duodenum, where the alkaline pancreatic juice and bile mix with acid chyme from the stomach to provide the appropriate neutral or slightly alkaline conditions necessary for digestion and micelle formation. Rhythmic (concertina-like) back and forth movements also occur, but may simply be as a result of segmentation. At any one time, a group of segments contract and this is followed by a period of rest. In the jejunum segmentation occurs as bursts of contractions that last approximately 1 min, followed by an interval when the contractions are weak or absent. This pattern is known as the minute rhythm.

Contraction of a ring of smooth muscle forces the chyme forwards and backwards, but because segmentation is more frequent in the proximal regions, the chances of the material being pushed towards the colon are greater than it being pushed towards the stomach. Thus although segmentation is responsible for mixing the chyme, it also aids propulsion of the chyme towards the colon.

Peristalsis

Peristalsis involves the sequential contraction of adjacent rings of smooth muscle in the aboral direction,

followed by relaxation of these rings of muscle, causing a wave of contraction that propels the chyme towards the colon (Fig. 7.15B). In the human, after a meal has been eaten, peristaltic activity in the small intestine is infrequent and of low strength. Furthermore, each wave of contraction travels only about 10 cm. It is for this reason that resection of segments of the intestine do not interfere with propulsion. However, there are occasional waves of intense contraction, known as peristaltic rushes, which travel the entire length of the small intestine. Both the short and the long waves are responsible for moving the chyme along the intestine towards the colon.

Contraction of the muscularis mucosae

In addition to the above types of motility due to contractions in the circular and longitudinal layers of muscle, sections of the muscularis mucosae undergo irregular contractions. These contractions assist in the mixing of the chyme. In addition the villi contract in an irregular fashion. Contractions of the villi are most frequent in the proximal small intestine. They squeeze the lacteals in the centre of the villi, thereby emptying them of lymph and enhancing intestinal lymph flow.

Control of motility

Certain basic patterns of contractile activity may be programmed into the neural circuitry of the intrinsic nerve plexi. However, motility in the small intestine is under physiological control by various factors, including stretch, intrinsic nerves of the intramural plexi, extrinsic autonomic nerves, paracrine factors and circulating hormones.

An intrinsic property of smooth muscle is reflex contraction in response to stretch of the muscle, without the involvement of nerves or hormones (see Ch. 1). This is known as the myenteric reflex. However, reflex contractile activity due to activation of pressure receptors and chemoreceptors in the walls of the intestine is probably more important when a meal is being processed by the small intestine.

Nervous control

Activation of the intrinsic nerves in the intramural plexi can control segmentation and short peristaltic waves by influencing the basal electrical rhythm, in the absence of extrinsic nerves and hormones. However, extrinsic parasympathetic and sympathetic nerves synapse with intrinsic nerves in the nerve plexi. The extrinsic nerves mediate long-range reflexes and both extrinsic nerves and hormones modulate the activity in intrinsic nerves. Segmentation and peristalsis are increased by activation of parasympathetic nerves, and inhibited by stimulation of sympathetic nerves. Activation of the sympathetic nervous system, during stress for example, results in release of adrenaline into the circulation and this also inhibits motility. Sympathetic activation also causes marked vasoconstriction of the gastrointestinal blood vessels (see Ch. 1).

Many transmitters, in addition to acetylcholine and the catecholamines, can influence intestinal motility. These include peptides, amines and nucleotides. The peptides include VIP, somatostatin, VIP, substance P and opioids. Peptides may be released from nerves and APUD cells to influence the gastrointestinal contractility.

The initiation and propagation of the MMC depends largely on enteric neural activity. If the enteric neurones are blocked at a particular level the MMC does not propagate past the block.

Hormonal control

Many peptide hormones are secreted by the stomach and small intestine in response to activation of pressure receptors and chemoreceptors to control motility. Gastrin, which is released into the blood in response to peptides in the stomach, and secretin and CCK, released in response to acid and fat respectively in the intestinal chyme, all increase intestinal motility if injected.

Motilin, a peptide that is released from the walls of the duodenum and jejunum into the blood when the intestinal chyme becomes alkaline, increases peristalsis if injected into the blood. It seems likely that when the acid in the chyme has been neutralized and the nutrients in the chyme have been digested that chyme becomes more alkaline, because alkaline juices are still being produced. A resulting increase in blood concentration of motilin would then cause the chyme to be moved on. Interestingly the plasma levels of motilin oscillate in phase with the MMCs, indicating that this hormone may be involved in initiating the MMC. This possibility is supported by the fact that intravenous injections of motilin initiate MMCs that strongly resemble those that occur naturally. Another view is that motilin is released as a result of the MMC but then helps to coordinate the events involved in it.

Another peptide hormone released from the small intestine when food material is present is enteroglucagon. It is released in response to glucose and fat in the chyme. This hormone inhibits peristalsis, and its role may be to allow time for the absorption of glucose and fat before the chyme is moved on towards the colon. Endogenous opioids may inhibit intestinal motility and as a consequence constipation is one of the most common side effects of opiate therapy used for pain relief.

Reflex control

Activation of pressure receptors by distension of the walls is involved in the reflex control of intestinal motility. A bolus of food placed in the small intestine will cause the smooth muscle behind it (in the orad direction) to contract, and that in front of it, to relax. Furthermore, over-distension of the walls of one part of the intestine by food results in relaxation of the rest of the intestine (the intestino-intestine reflex). The pressure receptors are probably near the longitudinal muscle layer. The afferent and efferent limbs of this reflex involve activation of extrinsic autonomic nerves, and would therefore be absent in a patient with a bowel transplant.

Trauma of other organs outside the gastrointestinal tract, such as the kidneys and gonads, leads to inhibition of intestinal motility (atonic bowel, or paralytic ileus).

This inhibition ultimately involves activity in the sympathetic splanchnic nerve. Various regions of the central nervous system have been implicated in the control of intestinal motility in such conditions. These include the cerebellum and pituitary. However, the precise role of the central nervous system and the pathways involved are still largely unknown.

Gastroileal reflex

When food is present in the stomach, motility increases in the ileum, and the ileocaecal sphincter relaxes. This is known as the gastroileal reflex. Conversely, distension of the ileum decreases gastric motility (emptying) in the stomach (the ileogastric reflex). The gastroileal reflex appears to be mainly under the control of external nerves to the intestinal mucosa, but gastrin, released into the blood in response to food in the stomach, may augment the response.

Ileocaecal sphincter

The last portion of the ileum is separated from the colon by a ring of smooth muscle known as the ileocaecal sphincter (Ch. 10). It is approximately 4 cm long in the adult human. Relaxation and contraction of the sphincter controls the rate of entry of material into the colon. It may have a role in preventing the movement of bacteria from the colon to the ileum. This sphincter is normally closed, but when peristalsis occurs in the last portion of the ileum in response to food in the stomach (the ileogastric reflex), distension of the ileum causes reflex relaxation of the sphincter muscle. This allows a small amount of chyme to enter the large intestine. The rate of entry is appropriately slow as it enables salt and water absorption from the chyme in the colon to take place before the next portion of chyme enters. Relaxation of the smooth muscle of the sphincter is coordinated by activity in the nerves in the intramural plexi.

Drugs that affect intestinal motility

Drugs that increase intestinal motility include purgatives, which accelerate the movement of chyme through the gastrointestinal tract, and drugs that increase segmentation but not peristalsis. Purgatives can be used to treat constipation. The treatment of constipation is discussed in Box 7.2.

Box 7.2 Treatment of constipation

Purgatives (laxatives) can be used to treat constipation. These can be substances that stimulate secretion and motility, substances that cause a relative osmotic diarrhoea, emollients, which alter the consistency of the faeces, or bulk-forming agents.

Secretory laxatives

Secretory laxatives cause an increased secretion of fluid and electrolytes by the mucosa into the lumen of the intestines. This results in fluid accumulation and watery chyme that flows rapidly through the intestines. They include castor oil, the active ingredient of which is ricinoleic acid. Others are cascara, aloe, senna and fig syrup, all of which are naturally occurring anthraquinone derivatives, and phenolphthalein, bisacodyl and danthron, which are synthetic agents. Senna and cascara contain derivatives of anthracene (such as emodin) bound to sugars to form glycosides. Hydrolysis of these glycosides by bacteria in the colon releases the active anthracene derivatives. These are absorbed to act on the myenteric plexus. This results in stimulation of secretion and motility. These agents can cause abdominal cramps due to excessive stimulation of smooth muscle. Prolonged usage can result in dependence, loss of normal intestinal function, and even an atonic colon.

Osmotic laxatives

Osmotic laxatives are poorly absorbed solutes that cause the volume of chyme to increase by transport of water down the osmotic gradient into the lumen. Salts such as Epsom's salts ($MgSO_4$) or $Mg(OH)_2$, which act in this way can be used to treat constipation. They have a rapid onset laxative effect, within a few hours of administration.

The concept of osmotic diarrhoea consequent to carbohydrate malabsorption in brush border diseases, such as lactase deficiency, has been exploited by the pharmaceutical industry in the development of lactulose that is now commonly used to treat constipation. Lactulose, a disaccharide composed of fructose and galactose, is not digested in the small intestine. It is digested to its component monosaccharides, by bacteria in the colon. These are then fermented to lactic and acetic acid that act as osmotic laxatives.

Emollients

Emollients are non-absorbable substances that coat and lubricate the faeces. This accelerates their movement through the intestines, and softens the rectal contents. Examples of emollients are didactyl sodium sulphosuccinate and liquid paraffin. Liquid paraffin can interfere with the absorption of fat-soluble vitamins, and for this reason it is now seldom used.

Bulk-forming agents

Bulk-forming agents, such as bran and methylcellulose, are generally the preferred treatment for constipation as they are free from side-effects, inexpensive, and probably the most acceptable and natural of the alternatives. They consist of nondigestible cellulose fibres that become hydrated in the intestines. This decreases the viscosity of the luminal contents to increase their flow through the intestines. Hydration causes them to swell, providing bulk, with consequent activation of the defaecation reflex (see Ch. 10).

Drugs that increase motility

Drugs that increase intestinal motility include muscarinic receptor agonists such as bethanechol, and anticholinesterases such as neostigmine. Such drugs that increase segmentation without increasing propulsive activity can be used for disorders of motility in the gastrointestinal tract, such as paralytic ileus (paralysis of the ileum) that can occur following intestinal surgery. They can also be used as antiemetics (via their actions on the central nervous system, see Ch. 3) prior to procedures such as diagnostic radiography or duodenal intubation. Domperidone, a dopamine D_2 receptor antagonist can also be used to increase intestinal motility. It probably enhances motility by blocking $\alpha_1$adrenoreceptors, rather than dopamine receptors, thereby decreasing the relaxant effect of sympathetic activation of these receptors.

DIGESTION AND ABSORPTION

8

Chapter objectives

After studying this chapter you should be able to:

1. Explain the mechanisms of digestion and absorption of complex nutrients, vitamins and minerals.

2. Understand the consequences of malabsorption in intestinal diseases.

Introduction

Most digestion and absorption occurs in the small intestine. The transport of water, monovalent ions and drugs was discussed in Chapter 7. In this chapter, the digestion of complex nutrients, and the absorption of the products of digestion, as well as the absorption of vitamins and minerals will be considered.

The consequences for nutrition, of disease of the small intestine will also be addressed in this chapter. As absorption of different nutrients can occur in different regions of the gastrointestinal tract, the regions affected by the disease process determine which nutrients will be poorly absorbed. Coeliac disease (Case 8.1: 1, 2 and 3), which usually affects the proximal small intestine, and Crohn's ileitis (Case 8.2: 1, 2 and 3), which usually affects the terminal ileum, will be used to illustrate some of the general principles of absorption, as well as the specific problems encountered as a consequence of malabsorption of the nutrients that are normally absorbed in the affected regions.

Absorption

Most nutrients are absorbed at a slow rate by passive diffusion throughout the small intestine. However, many important nutrients are absorbed at a faster rate by processes which involve saturatable mechanisms (see Ch. 1). The proximal small intestine, i.e. the duodenum and jejunum, is the location of most of these special mechanisms, as most substances are absorbed predominantly in those regions. Figure 8.1 shows the approximate sites of absorption of many important nutrients. The important divalent cations, Ca^{2+} and Fe^{2+}, are absorbed mainly in the duodenum and jejunum. Hexoses, including glucose, galactose and fructose, are also absorbed in the duodenum and jejunum, as are amino acids, small (di- and tri-) peptides and some water-soluble vitamins. Fatty acids, monoacylglycerols and fat-soluble vitamins are also absorbed in the duodenum and jejunum. Cholesterol is absorbed throughout the small intestine. Vitamin C is absorbed in the proximal ileum. Vitamin B_{12} and bile salts are absorbed predominantly in the terminal ileum. Water and monovalent ions are absorbed throughout the small and large intestines. The defects in absorption seen in coeliac disease and Crohn's disease which affect different regions of the small intestine, are described in Case 8.1: 2 and Case 8.2: 2.

Absorption of important nutrients

Carbohydrates

The average daily intake of carbohydrate in the human adult is probably between 250g and 800g/day. The useful carbohydrate in the food is largely vegetable starch in potatoes, bread, pasta and rice, and to a lesser extent glycogen

Case 8.1

Coeliac disease: 1

A 25-year-old woman visited her doctor and complained of diarrhoea and flatulence. She also said she had recently lost a considerable amount of weight, and she felt weak and exhausted most of the time. She also suffered from back pain. Upon questioning she said her faeces were bulky, greasy and foul-smelling.

She recalled that she had had persistent diarrhoea throughout childhood but the symptoms had disappeared during adolescence. She was referred to a gastroenterologist. The consultant arranged for blood and faecal analyses. The faecal tests confirmed the presence of steatorrhoea. The blood tests indicated that she had iron-deficiency anaemia, folate-deficiency and Ca^{2+} deficiency. Her blood electrolyte concentrations and prothrombin clotting time were within the normal range. The consultant suspected coeliac disease and arranged for an endoscopy (telescopic visualization of the duodenum) to be performed. A biopsy of the mucosa, taken at the examination, showed flattening of the villi and excessive plasma cells in the submucosa. A further blood test, to measure the concentrations of transglutaminase antibodies was performed and this showed a high titre of the antibodies. In view of these findings the consultant told the patient to exclude wheat, rye and barley flours (but not oat flour) from her diet, and to try to ensure that it was nutritionally balanced. She was prescribed iron, folate and vitamin D supplements. This diet was not easy to follow as so many food products contain the flours, but after a few weeks the patient had vastly improved. She had gained weight and was no longer feeling constantly tired.

After reading this case history we can address the following questions:

- What is the basic defect in this condition?
- If the duodenum and proximal jejunum were the regions of the small intestine involved, which nutrients are likely to be malabsorbed? Why was iron-deficiency anaemia present? Why was the patient's clotting time measured? Is milk intolerance likely to be a complication in this condition? Why was her blood investigated for transglutaminase antibodies?
- Why was steatorrhoea present in this patient?
- What problems result from deficiencies of these nutrients?
- How would a defect in CCK and secretin release from the duodenum affect the functioning of the digestive system?
- What are the likely causes of diarrhoea in coeliac disease?
- Why were the patient's blood electrolyte concentrations measured?

(animal starch), in meat and liver. These polysaccharides are composed entirely of D-glucose subunits linked together mainly by α-1,4 glycosidic linkages. In the human, over 90% of the starch in the diet is digested and absorbed. The

Case 8.2 Crohn's disease: 1

A 17-year-old young man complained to his general practitioner that he had been suffering from abdominal pain, diarrhoea, weight loss and feelings of lassitude. The doctor examined him and found that his abdomen was distended. He ascertained that the pain was in the central and right lower quadrant. He suspected acute appendicitis, and the patient was admitted to hospital. An abdominal operation was arranged. The surgeon observed that the appendix appeared normal. However, a short length of the terminal ileum was reddened, thickened and oedematous. These features indicate Crohn's disease of the terminal ileum. No further surgery was performed. Following the operation, blood and faecal samples were obtained for analyses. The patient was allowed a few days to recuperate and was then sent home. He was prescribed codeine for the pain, and diphenoxylate (Lomotil) for the diarrhoea, and he was started on oral steroids to reduce the inflammation. He was advised to keep to a nutritious diet. The acute symptoms gradually settled, but he suffered several relapses over the next few years. He required iron supplements and intramuscular injections of vitamin B_{12}. He developed steatorrhoea.

The patient eventually suffered an intestinal obstruction. He was maintained on intravenous parenteral nutrition for 2 weeks and during this time the symptoms diminished, but they returned when he resumed normal nutrition. An emergency operation was then performed to remove the affected part of the ileum (which was causing the obstruction). Following the operation he made a good recovery. He resumed a normal diet and regained the weight he had lost. Later in life he developed symptomatic gallstone disease that required the removal of his gall bladder (cholecystectomy).

Upon consideration of the details of this case we can address the following questions:

- What is the basic defect in Crohn's disease and what causes it? Which parts of the gastrointestinal tract can be affected in this disease?
- How is the condition diagnosed? Which blood and faecal analyses would have assisted the diagnosis?
- What could account for the symptoms of weight loss and lassitude? Which nutrients are poorly absorbed in Crohn's disease? Why were diarrhoea and steatorrhoea present? Why was the patient started on iron supplements? Why was he given intramuscular vitamin B_{12}?
- Why was the patient maintained on parenteral nutrition for a while? What was the likely composition of the intravenous fluid used?
- What are the likely causes of the intestinal obstruction?
- What could be the cause of the gallstone disease that developed later in life in this patient?

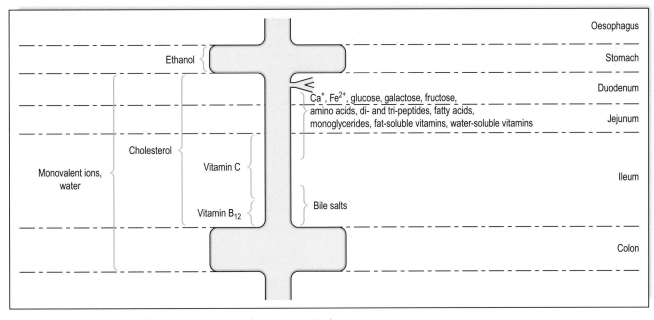

Fig. 8.1 Sites of absorption of important nutrients in the gastrointestinal tract.

remainder passes into the colon where it may be utilized by colonic bacteria.

Cellulose is another polysaccharide, which is composed of glucose subunits, present in the diet. However, it is not digestible in humans and other non-ruminants because the subunits are linked by β-1,4 glycosidic bonds that cannot be hydrolysed by the enzymes in the digestive tract. Therefore it passes into the colon. Nevertheless,

Defect and treatment

Coeliac disease is common in Northern Europe with an incidence of possibly 1 in 250. (It is rare in Africa.) Genetic and environmental factors are involved.

Defect

The disease is due to an abnormal reaction to gluten, a constituent of wheat flour. Gluten damages the enterocytes, causing atrophy of the villi, and malabsorption. The duodenum and proximal jejunum are usually more severely affected than the ileum. The damage is due to an abnormal immune response to gliadins (especially α-gliadin), components of gluten. It is a T-cell-mediated disease. Antibodies to the enzyme transglutaminase, which is released in tissues during inflammation, are present in 98% of affected individuals. The mechanisms involved in the damage have not yet been fully characterized but there is evidence that deamidation of gliadin by transglutaminase generates a recognition site for CD4$^+$ T lymphocytes; the locally activated lymphocytes trigger production of cytokines which then cause the damage. In addition transglutaminase antibodies have been shown to affect the differentiation of epithelial cells, possibly by interfering with the action of the enzyme.

Diagnosis

Determination of the serum concentration of transglutaminase antibodies is a useful tool in the diagnosis of coeliac disease. The diagnosis of coeliac disease also requires a biopsy, usually of the duodenum, which would show flattened villi, crypt hyperplasia, infiltration with lymphocytes and plasma cells and reduced cell differentiation. Figure 8.2 shows a section through the jejunal mucosa in a patient with coeliac disease. The cells cannot be replaced quickly enough by stem cell division in the crypts, and many of the cells present are immature and therefore do not absorb nutrients effectively.

Treatment

Treatment of coeliac disease involves the individual following a gluten-free nutritious diet. The gliadin peptides that cause the abnormal reactions are present in wheat, rye and barley but not oats. The latter is therefore safe for individuals with coeliac disease.

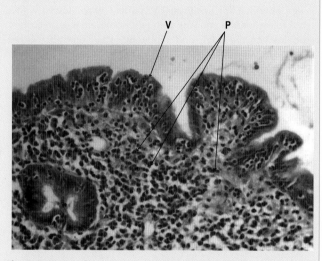

Fig. 8.2 Section through the jejunal mucosa in a patient with coeliac disease, showing flattened villi (V), and plasma cell infiltrates (P).

cellulose is an important source of dietary fibre, providing bulk that stimulates intestinal motility, and prevents constipation (see Ch. 10). In ruminants, cellulose is degraded by bacterial cellulases that hydrolyse the β-1,4 glycosidic linkages to produce D-glucose, which is absorbed.

There are appreciable amounts of disaccharides, including sucrose (table sugar), lactose (milk sugar) and maltose (malt sugar), in Western diets. The only free monosaccharide likely to be present in the diet is glucose, which is added to 'high energy' drinks and foods.

Dietary carbohydrate is utilized to provide energy for muscular and secretory activity and other metabolic functions. It is not 'essential' as a source of energy as calories can also be provided by fat and protein. However, a few carbohydrate substances, such as inositol, are 'essential' vitamin components of the diet, as they either cannot be synthesized in the body, or cannot be synthesized at a rate which is rapid enough to meet the body's requirements.

Structure of starch and glycogen

The molecular weight of vegetable starch ranges from a few thousand to 500 000. It consists of two components:

1. Amylose in which the glucose subunits are linked together in straight unbranched chains via α-1,4 glycosidic linkages (Fig. 8.4A).

2. Amylopectin which consists of branched chains, with the branches occurring at approximately every 30th glucose residue. α-1,4 linkages are present within the chains and α-1,6 linkages occur at the branch points (Fig. 8.4B).

Glycogen has a structure similar to amylopectin but the molecular weight is usually greater, between 270 000 and 100 000 000, and it has a more branched structure, the branches occurring every 8–10 glucose residues.

Crohn's disease: 2

Defect, diagnosis and treatment

Crohn's disease is most commonly diagnosed in young adults. The highest frequency is seen in Caucasians, and in the Western world. In the UK, it affects approximately 50/100 000 of the population. The cause is unknown, but it is probably multifactorial. As it is an inflammatory disease, infectious organisms, including the measles virus and *Mycobacterium pseudotuberculosis*, have been variously implicated. Autoimmunity has also been suspected because there is an association with known autoimmune conditions such as arthritis and eczema. Inherited factors are also implicated because of the high concordance in monozygotic twins, and in families. Crohn's disease in children can lead to growth retardation and delayed sexual development, probably because of poor nutrition.

Defect

Crohn's disease is an inflammatory disorder that can affect any region of the gastrointestinal tract, from the mouth to the anus. However, the terminal ileum is the commonest site to be affected (Crohn's ileitis, Fig. 8.3). In the mouth, aphthous ulcers of the buccal mucosa and tongue are seen. At the anus, skin tags, fissures and fistulae may be present. The disease is characterized by remissions and relapses. Macroscopically, the intestines appear red and swollen. Normal areas of tissue are usually present between the damaged areas. Because the inflammatory process involves all layers of the intestinal wall,

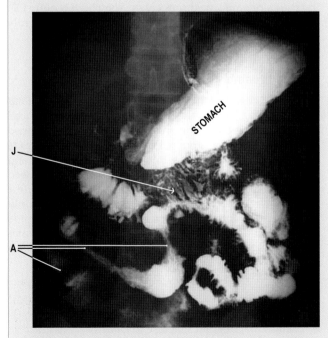

Fig. 8.3 An X-ray of the ileum, taken 15 min after ingestion of barium in a patient with Crohn's ileitis. Three narrowed segments of ileum are visible (strictures A). The normal mucosal folds of the proximal jejunum are also seen (J).

diseased segments become grossly thickened. This can give rise to obstruction. As the inflammation resolves, areas of secondary scarring (fibrosis) in the wall of the bowel also constitute obstructive regions. The mucous membrane appears 'cobble-stoned' due to longitudinal fissures and transverse oedematous folds. Aggregations of inflammatory cell infiltrates may be present, and the mesenteric lymph nodes may be enlarged due to reactive hyperplasia. Granulomas (aggregates of epithelial macrophages surrounded by a cuff of lymphocytes) may be present in the lymph nodes and the bowel wall.

The formation of enteric fistulae is a further feature of the disease. Fistulae may extend between different loops of the bowel (enteroenteric fistulae), or between the bowel and the skin (enterocutaneous fistulae, especially in the perianal areas). Gastrointestinal bleeding can also occur. This is usually mild but, because it is chronic, it can lead to iron-deficiency anaemia. There is also an increased incidence of malignant neoplasms in patients with Crohn's disease, especially in the small and large bowel. This may be related to the long-term damage to the bowel mucosa.

Diagnosis

The diagnosis of Crohn's disease is difficult because all the salient features are seen in other disorders. A combination of histology, endoscopy and radiology is usually employed. Evidence from blood analyses, including leukocytosis, elevated sedimentation rate, and thrombocytosis, is indicative of an active inflammatory process. Radiological evidence of the sites of involvement, and the chronic remitting course of the patient's illness, also assist the diagnosis. However, a definitive diagnosis requires histological assessment of the bowel and identification of granulomata.

Treatment

The management of patients with this disease includes:

- Treatment of the symptoms (diarrhoea, pain)
- Treatment with anti-inflammatory and immunosuppressive agents
- Surgical treatment where there are complications such as luminal obstruction
- Management of the patient's nutritional status, including supplementation of the diet
- Parenteral nutrition when necessary.

Total parenteral nutrition

Intravenous feeding can be used in extreme cases to rest the bowel and allow healing. The fluid administered would contain amino acids, glucose and lipid in amounts sufficient to meet the protein and energy needs of the individual, and electrolytes, vitamins and minerals in amounts sufficient to meet the estimated daily requirements. In patients with Crohn's disease total parenteral nutrition can lead to positive nitrogen balance, weight gain and temporary remission of symptoms.

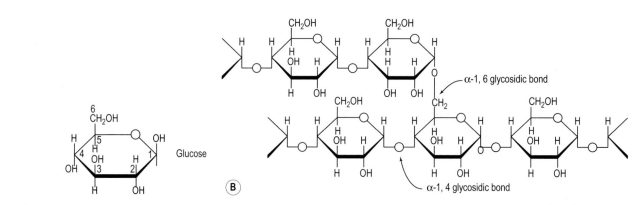

Fig. 8.4 (A) Structure of glucose showing the conventional numbering system for the carbon atoms. (B) Portion of an amylopectin molecule showing α-1,4 and α-1,6 glycosidic linkages.

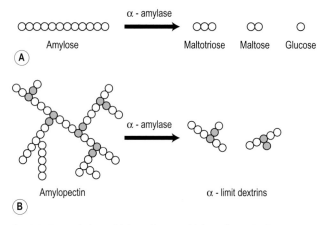

Fig. 8.5 Degradation of (A) amylose, and (B) amylopectin, by α-amylases. The filled circles indicate glucose subunits with α-1,6, glycosidic linkages.

Digestion of carbohydrate

In the gastrointestinal tract there are several enzymes that degrade starch and glycogen. These include the α-amylases secreted by the salivary glands and the pancreas, and isomaltase and glucoamylase, which are integral components of the intestinal absorptive cell membranes. Maltose, sucrose and lactose can also be degraded to their component monosaccharides by enzymes situated in the brush border of the upper small intestine (see below).

α-Amylases

α-Amylases split the α-1,4 glycosidic linkages in amylose to yield maltose and glucose, but they do not act on maltose, a disaccharide composed of two glucose subunits linked by an α-1,4 linkage. In theory α-amylase will ultimately degrade a solution of amylose to maltose, and glucose which can be released from the ends of the chains (Fig. 8.5). Intermediate oligosaccharides (dextrins) are formed in the process. α-Amylases also attack amylopectin and glycogen at their α-1,4 linkages. Intermediate

unbranched oligosaccharides and branched oligosaccharides (α-limit dextrins) are formed. Thus a mixture of products is produced (Fig. 8.5).

Salivary amylase starts the digestion of starch. It continues to act for up to half an hour in the interior of the food bolus after it has arrived in the stomach. It is eventually inactivated at the low pH produced by the gastric acid when it penetrates the food bolus. It can digest up to 50% of the starch present in food. Pancreatic juice that contains a second α-amylase is released into the duodenum when a meal is present in the digestive tract. Pancreatic amylase continues the digestion of starch and glycogen in the small intestine. It is produced in larger amounts than salivary amylase. The α-amylases from the two sources have similar catalytic properties, despite having different amino acid sequences. They both require Cl^- for optimum activity and both act at neutral or slightly alkaline pH values.

Role of brush border enzymes

Intestinal isomaltase (α-1,6 glycosidase) splits α-1,6 linkages in the branched poly- and oligosaccharides produced by amylase action in the small intestine. The combined action of α-amylase and α-1,6 glycosidase can degrade amylopectin and glycogen to a mixture of maltose and glucose, but other enzymes in the brush border speed up and complete the process of starch digestion. These are glucoamylase, which degrades small unbranched oligosaccharides, and maltase and isomaltase, which degrade maltose and isomaltose, respectively. All of these enzymes have access to the mixture of polysaccharides, oligosaccharides and disaccharides in the chyme during a meal.

The enzymes available to digest disaccharides are:

- Maltase that degrades maltose to glucose
- Sucrase that degrades sucrose to glucose and fructose
- Lactase that degrades lactose to galactose and glucose (Fig. 8.6).

Sucrase and isomaltase are synthesized as a single polypeptide chain inside the cell, and this is inserted intact into the plasma membrane. Pancreatic protease

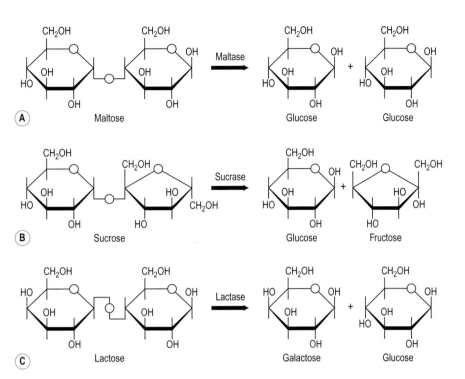

Fig. 8.6 Degradation of disaccharides by brush border disaccharidases. (A) Maltose, (B) sucrose, (C) lactose.

cleaves the polypeptide chain at a site between the active centres of the two enzyme moieties, but they remain non-covalently associated in the membrane. When sucrase is incorporated into artificial membranes, it binds sucrose at one face and releases glucose and fructose on the other side of the membrane. This has led to speculation that it is both a hydrolytic enzyme and a transport molecule. The other brush border enzymes do not appear to behave in this way. These disaccharidases are all present in the brush border of the enterocyte, and it seems that the digestion of disaccharides and small oligosaccharides actually occurs in the membrane itself. This has been inferred from the fact that after administration of a solution of a disaccharide to an animal, very little free glucose can be detected in the lumen, yet the disaccharide molecules are too large to diffuse through the pores in the membrane, and disaccharide molecules cannot be detected in the blood. It seems likely that the brush border enzymes occupy positions in the membrane that are adjacent to the hexose carriers. The release of monosaccharides occurs on the surface of the membrane and these are then transferred to the adjacent carrier molecule for transport into the cell (Fig. 8.7). Inherited disorders of brush border enzymes are described in Box 8.1. These defects result in carbohydrate malabsorption and diarrhoea.

Monosaccharide absorption

The most abundant monosaccharides in dietary carbohydrate are the hexoses, D-glucose, D-galactose, and

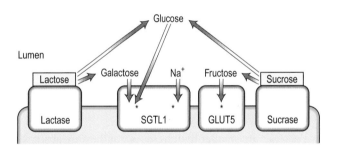

Fig. 8.7 Disaccharidases and hexose transporters in the brush border membrane. The enzymes reside in the brush border in close proximity to the hexose transporters. Disaccharides and oligosaccharides are degraded in the membrane by the enzymes, and the products are either transferred to other enzymes for further degradation or, in the case of monosaccharides, to the appropriate transporter.

D-fructose, the products of digestion of starch, sucrose and lactose. Both L-hexoses and D-hexoses are absorbed slowly by passive diffusion in the gastrointestinal tract. However, the plasma membrane of cells is relatively impermeable to polar molecules such as monosaccharides and the transport of these sugars into the enterocyte by passive diffusion is therefore slow. Glucose, galactose and fructose are absorbed by saturable mechanisms, mainly in the duodenum and jejunum. This is accomplished by membrane-associated transporters located in the brush border and basolateral membranes of the mature enterocytes. These bind the sugars and transfer them across the cell membranes and deliver them to the interstitial fluid in the lateral spaces, from where they are taken up into the adjacent capillaries to enter the portal blood.

Box 8.1 Carbohydrate malabsorption syndromes: brush border diseases

Brush border membrane disease is a collective term for conditions in which there is an absence of, or a marked decrease in the activity of a functional brush border membrane protein. These diseases are usually genetic. Sufferers may also exhibit disorders of reabsorption in the kidney proximal tubules. Several brush border diseases exist where the defect results in malabsorption of a specific carbohydrate. Intolerance of that carbohydrate in the diet develops. The unabsorbed sugar passes into the colon where some of it is fermented by bacteria. The remaining unaltered sugar and its bacterial fermentation products cause osmotic diarrhoea (see Ch. 7). The clinical symptoms of carbohydrate malabsorption are abdominal distension, gassiness, borborygmi, nausea, cramping, pain and diarrhoea. In some of these conditions, there is also a high incidence of ulceration of the mouth. Carbohydrate malabsorption is diagnosed by an oral tolerance test that involves administration of the suspected sugar by mouth, and measurement of the sugar in the blood and faeces. If the individual is intolerant of the sugar, it appears in the faeces, but it (or its normal digestion products) cannot be detected in the blood. Confirmation is by examination of a jejunal biopsy to see if the appropriate enzyme or carrier protein is absent from the mucosa.

Brush border diseases that have been characterized include:

- *Lactase deficiency*. This is a common brush border disorder that is usually expressed in adolescence or early adulthood. The enzyme, lactase, is induced by its substrate, lactose, in individuals who consume milk. There is generally a high incidence of lactase deficiency

in populations such as Mediterranean and Oriental races that do not normally consume milk after childhood, with the result that the enzyme is not present in their intestines. If milk is ingested in these individuals they experience the symptoms of lactose intolerance. A rare congenital form of lactase deficiency exists; feeding infants with this condition with normal milk causes diarrhoea. The problem can be overcome by feeding artificial milk in which lactose has been replaced by sucrose or fructose. There is a rise in H_2 elimination in the breath of affected individuals: the result of the metabolism of the unabsorbed lactose by bacteria in the colon.

- *Sucrase–isomaltase deficiency*. Individuals with this inherited brush border enzyme disease are intolerant of sucrose and isomaltose.

- *Glucose/galactose malabsorption*. In this condition, there is a genetic defect in the Na^+-dependent glucose/galactose transporter, SGLT1. Ingestion of glucose or galactose produces the symptoms of brush-border disease. Treatment involves omitting these sugars, as well as lactose (which is degraded to glucose and galactose) from the diet. Fructose is absorbed normally via the GLUT5 transporter.

Certain amino acid malabsorption diseases are also brush border diseases. These are described in Box 8.2. A congenital disease where the Cl/HCO_3^- exchanger is absent from the membranes of the jejunum, ileum and colon (congenital chloridorrhoea) is described in Chapter 7.

Pentoses are smaller than hexoses but they are absorbed at a slower rate than glucose, galactose and fructose, indicating that they are probably absorbed by passive diffusion.

Hexose transporters

There are two types of hexose transporter in mammalian cells; Na^+/glucose co-transporters which are involved in the secondary active transport of glucose, and Na^+-independent facilitative hexose transporters. Two forms of the Na^+-dependent transporter have been identified. These are SGLT1 and SGLT2, but only SGLT1 is present in the small intestine. There are at least five functional isoforms of facilitative transporter (GLUT1, GLUT2, GLUT3, GLUT4 and GLUT5). All mammalian cells express at least one of these transporters. The most studied is GLUT4, an insulin-sensitive glucose transporter present in muscle and adipose tissue (see Ch. 9). GLUT1, GLUT2 and GLUT5 are all present in the enterocyte. Figure 8.8 shows the structures of the SGLT1 and GLUT1 transporters, and their conformations in the membrane. The two molecules exhibit many similar features. The specificity of the transporters is shown in Table 8.1. An

inherited disorder where the SGLT1 is absent from the brush border has been described (see Box 8.1).

Hexose transport

The uptake of glucose across the enterocyte plasma membrane involves the binding of glucose to the Na^+/glucose cotransporter SGLT1, as described in Chapter 7. SGLT1 is present only in mature enterocytes in the upper regions of the villi. Galactose also binds to this carrier, but fructose does not. Glucose and galactose transport into the epithelial cell is via secondary active transport. The energy required is derived from the coupling of sugar transport to the transport of Na^+ down the concentration and electrical gradients from the lumen into the cell. Both Na^+ ions and the sugar are transported into the cell on the SGLT1 transporter. This represents a major route for the uptake of both the sugar and Na^+ into the enterocyte. Thus the uptake of glucose is stimulated by the presence of Na^+ in the intestinal chyme. The affinity of the carrier for glucose increases as the luminal Na^+ concentration increases. The Km of SGLT1 in the presence of Na^+ is less than 0.5 mM, but in its absence it is greater than 10 mM. The absorption of glucose is illustrated schematically

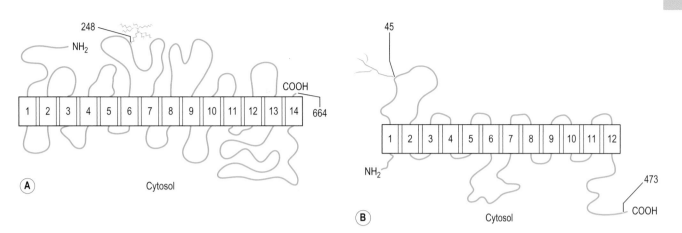

Fig. 8.8 Structure of SGLT1 and GLUT1 hexose transporters. (A) A model of the human Na$^+$/glucose transporter, SGLT1. The transporter has 664 amino acid residues. There are 12 membrane-spanning hydrophobic domains each composed of 21 residues arranged in an α-helix. N-linked glycosylation is present at residue 248 (asparagine) in a hydrophilic loop on the exoplasmic face between membrane spans 5 and 6. This may be the site which binds the hexose molecules. There is another large hydrophilic exoplasmic loop between the 11th and 12th membrane domains. The –NH$_2$ and –COOH termini are on the cytoplasmic side of the membrane. (B) A model of the GLUT 1 transporter. The model depicted represents GLUT1 that has 473 amino acid residues. A total of 12 hydrophobic membrane-spanning domains are connected by hydrophilic segments. A large exoplasmic loop present between the 1st and 2nd membrane domains contains a potential N-glycosylation site at residue 45 (asparagine), where glucose might bind. A large cytoplasmic loop is located between the 6th and 7th transmembrane domains. The –NH$_2^-$ and the –COOH termini are both on the cytoplasmic side of the membrane. The facilitative transporters GLUT1, GLUT2, GLUT3, GLUT4 and GLUT5 are structurally related to this protein.

Table 8.1 Specificity of transporters for hexoses in the enterocyte

Transporter	Glucose	Galactose	Fructose
SGLT1	+	+	−
GLUT1	+	+	−
GLUT2	+	+	+
GLUT5	−	−	+

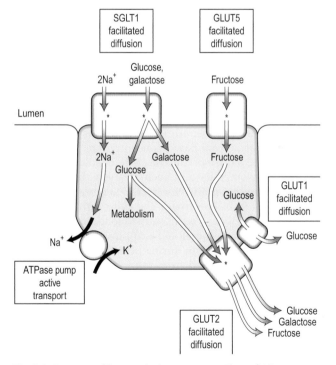

Fig. 8.9 Transport of hexoses in the enterocyte. The Na$^+$/glucose cotransporter (SGLT1) and the facilitative GLUT5 fructose membrane transporter reside in the brush border membrane, and GLUT1, GLUT2, and the ATPase pump in the basolateral membrane.

in Figure 8.9. Each carrier molecule binds two Na$^+$ ions and one glucose molecule. The glucose concentration in the cell may be higher than that in the lumen but the coupling of the transport of glucose with that of Na$^+$, enables glucose to be transported into the cell against a concentration gradient.

Fructose does not bind to SGLT1 in the brush border. It is transported into the enterocyte, down its concentration gradient by GLUT5 (which does not transport glucose, Fig. 8.9). The separate pathways for glucose and fructose transport into the enterocyte can be inferred from the fact that normal fructose absorption is present in patients with inherited glucose-galactose malabsorption (see Box 8.1), and this provides the rationale for the treatment of this condition with fructose. GLUT5 is present only in mature enterocytes on the tips and sides of the villi in the jejunum.

Some glucose is utilized by the cell for its energy requirements. The transport of the remaining glucose, galactose and fructose across the basolateral membrane is accomplished by the GLUT2 transporter, which has a low-affinity for glucose (Km 23 mM). The presence of

this low-affinity transporter allows the rate of glucose transport through the basolateral membrane to increase in proportion to the glucose concentration, which varies from 5 mM (the normal value) to 20 mM. GLUT1 is

Malabsorption and its consequences

Malabsorption

In coeliac disease, the damaged villi and loss of enterocytes leads to a reduced surface area for absorption of fat and other nutrients that are normally absorbed in the proximal small intestine. Malabsorption is exacerbated if damage to APUD cells in the duodenum results in deficiency of CCK and secretin, as these control secretion of pancreatic juice and bile, the major digestive juices in the gastrointestinal tract. Steatorrhoea (loss of fat in the faeces) was present in the patient due to fat malabsorption. Iron-deficiency anaemia was present due to iron malabsorption as iron is absorbed in the proximal small intestine.

The absorption of hexoses, amino acids, fat, fat-soluble vitamins, folate and Ca^{2+} ions could also be impaired as they are all absorbed in the proximal small intestine.

Consequences

The consequences of malabsorption in this condition, if it is left untreated, are:

- Weight loss and fatigue due to malabsorption of fuels such as carbohydrates and fat, and malabsorption of amino acids required for synthetic reactions

- Anaemia and fatigue due to iron and folate malabsorption
- Osteomalacia as a result of vitamin D and Ca^{2+} malabsorption, and the formation of Ca^{2+} soaps from fatty acids (which prevents their absorption)
- Bleeding from nose, gastrointestinal tract, vagina and ureters, as a result of increased clotting time, due to vitamin K deficiency. The blood loss would exacerbate the iron-deficiency anaemia.

Diarrhoea

The patient's blood electrolyte concentrations were measured because there can be a severe loss of electrolytes in diarrhoea (see Ch. 7).

Diarrhoea in this condition is due to:

- High concentrations of unabsorbed nutrients in the chyme which cause osmotic diarrhoea
- The delivery of large amounts of fat into the colon which results in the production of hydroxylated fatty acids by colonic bacteria. These can act as cathartics
- Milk-intolerance, due to lactase deficiency, as this enzyme is present in the enterocyte of the brush border in the proximal small intestine (see Box 8.1).

also present in enterocytes but its function is unclear. It is a high-affinity transporter that functions close to the Vmax even at normal blood concentrations. It may participate in the release of glucose at the basolateral border. However, in other tissues, such as the kidney tubules, where it is present in the basolateral membranes its function appears to be to provide the cells with a source of metabolic energy derived from the blood. Its function in the enterocyte may therefore be to provide glucose from the blood for metabolism during periods of fasting when it is not being absorbed from the intestinal lumen. The locations of the different transporters in the enterocyte are illustrated in Figure 8.9.

Malabsorption of carbohydrate is a feature of coeliac disease that involves damage to the mucosa of the proximal small intestine (see Case 8.1: 3).

Physiological regulation of hexose absorption

The transport of hexoses by the enterocyte can be regulated by diet. Thus a diet high in glucose or fructose results in upregulation of the GLUT2 transporter in the basolateral membrane, and increased transport of hexoses into the blood. Thus blood glucose levels are regulated in part by alterations in the absorptive capacity of the enterocyte.

Glucose transport into the blood can also be regulated by blood glucose concentrations. Transport of glucose across the brush border membrane, but not the basolateral membrane, is stimulated by low blood sugar (hypoglycaemia). The mechanism may involve an increase in the concentration of circulating glucagon, a hormone which stimulates cAMP formation in the cell. This hormone is released into the blood during starvation (see Ch. 9).

Paradoxically, in diabetes, chronic hyperglycaemia (high blood sugar) also stimulates intestinal glucose transport. This is partly due to an increased surface area for absorption, resulting from an increase in the number of enterocytes. However, glucagon levels are also high in diabetes and this may stimulate glucose transport by the same mechanism as during starvation. In addition there is also an upregulation of the GLUT2 transporter in the basolateral membrane in diabetic hyperglycaemia.

Protein

In the Western hemisphere, the amount of protein in the average diet exceeds that required for nutritional balance. The dietary requirement for protein in the human adult is between 30 and 50 g/day. Protein is required to supply the eight 'essential amino acids' which the body cannot

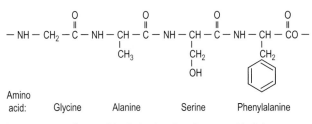

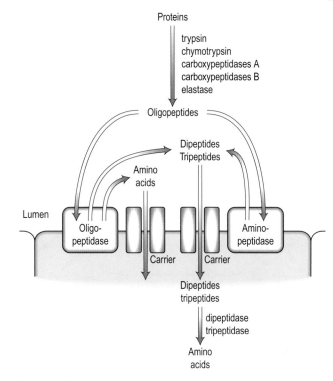

Fig. 8.10 Part of a peptide chain showing three peptide linkages.

synthesize, or cannot synthesize rapidly enough, and to replace nitrogen lost in the urine. In addition to that which is ingested, 10–30 g of protein (enzymes, mucins, etc.) is secreted into the digestive tract each day. An additional 25 g or so is derived from epithelial cells that have been shed into the lumen. Most of this protein is digested and absorbed. Approximately 10–20 g, derived from cell debris and colonic microorganisms, is eliminated in the faeces each day.

Digestion

Proteins are high molecular weight substances composed of up to 20 different amino acids, joined together in peptide linkages (see Fig. 8.10). In the adult, most protein is degraded in the digestive tract to small peptides and amino acids. This is accomplished by a variety of proteolytic enzymes. These can be divided into two categories, endopeptidases and exopeptidases. Endopeptidases cleave peptide bonds in the centre of the peptide chains, the initial products being mostly large peptides, which are subsequently degraded to oligopeptides. Exopeptidases cleave bonds at the ends of the peptide chain, splitting off amino acids one by one, in a stepwise manner: carboxypeptidases act at the C-terminal, and aminopeptidases at the N-terminal. Enzymes that specifically attack dipeptides and tripeptides are also present. The combined actions of these enzymes digest proteins to small peptides and amino acids.

Digestion in the stomach

Pepsin is an endopeptidase which is secreted by the stomach as an inactive precursor, pepsinogen, which is activated by gastric juice (see Ch. 3). It favours peptide linkages where aromatic amino acids are present. It is responsible for the digestion of only approximately 15% of dietary protein. Protein digestion is not impaired in the absence of pepsin because other proteases are available.

Digestion in the small intestine

Pancreatic juice contains three endopeptidases (Fig. 8.11):

1. Trypsin, which prefers peptide linkages where the carboxylic acid group is provided by a basic amino acid.

Fig. 8.11 Digestion of proteins and peptides, and absorption of di- and tri-peptides and amino acids in the enterocyte.

2. Chymotrypsin, which prefers linkages where the carboxylic group is provided by an aromatic amino acid.
3. Elastase, which degrades elastin.

Pancreatic juice also contains two carboxypeptidases (A and B). Carboxypeptidase A has the highest specificity for bonds where the C terminal amino acid is basic, such as lysine or arginine. The pancreatic enzymes are secreted as inactive precursors that are converted to the active enzymes in the duodenum (see Ch. 5). They all have slightly alkaline pH optima. At least 50% of the protein ingested is normally degraded in the duodenum.

A number of peptidases reside in the brush border or the cytosol of the enterocyte. They are most abundant in the cells in the jejunum. The active sites of these enzymes face the intestinal lumen and they act *in situ*, upon contact with the protein in the chyme. Enterocyte peptidases also act in the lumen where they are present as components of disintegrating cells that have been shed from the tips of the villi. One of the brush border enzymes is leucine aminopeptidase. Others are oligopeptidases, which degrade small peptides, such as tetrapeptides. There is also a dipeptidyl aminopeptidase that removes dipeptides from the N-terminal of proteins.

The products of proteolytic digestion are tetrapeptides, tripeptides and dipeptides, and some amino acids. Tripeptides, dipeptides and amino acids are transported into the epithelial cells. The dipeptides and tripeptides are degraded to amino acids by cytosolic tripeptidases

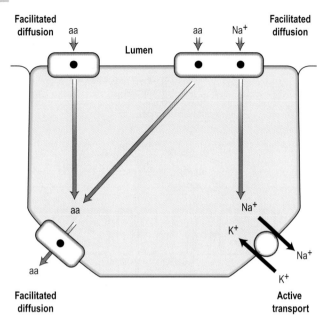

Fig. 8.12 Amino acid carrier mechanisms in the brush border and basolateral border of the enterocyte. aa, amino acid.

Table 8.2 Carriers involved in amino acid absorption in the enterocyte

Location	Carrier	Na^+-dependence	Amino acid specificity
Brush border	B	Yes	Neutral
Brush border	$B^{0,+}$	Yes	Neutral, basic and cystine
Brush border	Imino	Yes	Imino (proline, hydroxyproline)
Brush border	X_{AG}	Yes	Acidic
Brush border	β	Yes	β, mainly taurine
Brush border	$b^{0,+}$	No	Neutral, basic and cystine
Brush border	y^+	No	Basic
Basolateral border	asc	No	Small neutral
Basolateral border	y^+	No	Basic
Basolateral border	L	No	Large, hydrophobic neutral

and dipeptidases in the endothelial cells. These relationships are represented in Figure 8.11.

Absorption of protein products

Mechanisms exist in the digestive tract for the absorption of both small peptides and amino acids. In addition traces of intact protein are absorbed in some human adults.

Amino acids

The transport of amino acids across the membranes of the enterocytes into the blood can occur via passive diffusion, facilitated diffusion or active transport (Fig. 8.12). Relatively hydrophobic amino acids, such as tryptophan, are transported to an appreciable extent by passive diffusion. Only the L-isomers of amino acids are absorbed by facilitated diffusion and active transport. They are absorbed in the jejunum and the upper ileum. Carrier systems for amino acids exist in the brush border and the basolateral border (Table 8.2). At least seven specific transport systems are present in the brush border membrane, and at least three are present in the basolateral membrane. The transport of most amino acids occurs against a concentration gradient, and therefore depends on active mechanisms. Each carrier is shared by a group of amino acids. Those that share the same transport mechanism compete with each other for a binding site on the carrier protein. Table 8.2 shows the membrane locations of the transporters that have been characterized. The relationships were first discovered as a result of studies of patients with amino acid carrier deficiencies. These diseases are described in Box 8.2.

Five of the known amino acid transport systems in the brush border are Na^+-dependent co-porters, which operate in a manner resembling that of the SGLT1 glucose transporter (see above and Ch. 7). The pumping of Na^+ ions across the basolateral membrane produces concentration and electrical gradients that favour Na^+ transport into the cell. This provides the driving force for the operation of the co-transporters in the brush border. These are therefore secondary active transport mechanisms. The other two brush border transporters do not require the presence of Na^+ ions in the lumen. The specificities of the transporters are shown in Table 8.2.

Three transporters in the basolateral border are collectively responsible for the facilitated diffusion of neutral and basic amino acids into the lateral spaces (see Fig. 8.12). These transporters are present in many different types of cell. Acidic amino acids such as glutamate and aspartate are utilized by the enterocyte as energy substrates, and do not appear to be transported out of the cell by specific carrier mechanisms. The basolateral membrane also expresses carriers that transport amino acids from the fluid in the lateral spaces into the enterocyte, where they are used for protein synthesis. These systems require the presence of Na^+ ions in the intercellular fluid. Malabsorption of amino acids is a feature of coeliac disease due to damaged mucosa and the consequent loss of transporters from the epithelial cells (see Case 8.1: 3).

Absorption of small peptides

The dipeptide and tripeptide products of protein digestion are transported into the enterocyte by secondary

Box 8.2 Amino acid malabsorption diseases

The existence of different transport systems for amino acids was first deduced from the study of rare amino acid malabsorption diseases. In these autosomal recessive diseases, a group of amino acids are either poorly absorbed or not absorbed at all, while amino acids that are not in that group are well absorbed. In these conditions, there is an absence or deficiency of a specific amino acid transporter. The defect is usually present in both the small intestine and the proximal tubules of the kidney, and the amino acids that cannot be transported can appear in the urine.

These diseases include:

- *Hartnup's disease.* In this condition, the transport of neutral amino acids is defective, and neutral amino acids appear in the urine. In this case the defect is in the Na^+-dependent neutral amino acid B transporter. Children with this condition exhibit skin changes, cerebellar ataxia and mental disturbances
- *Cystinuria.* In this condition, the defect can be in either the Na^+-dependent transporter or the Na^+-independent transporter, both of which transport basic amino acids (arginine, lysine, ornithine) and cystine (see Table 8.2). In cystinuria, these amino acids appear in the urine. There is a tendency for kidney stones to develop in this condition, probably because the dipeptide cystine is poorly soluble
- *Familial iminoglycinuria.* In this condition, there is a defect in the IMINO transport system leading to impaired absorption of the imino acids, proline and hydroxyproline.

In the above diseases, amino acids that are not absorbed via the amino acid transporters can still be absorbed as components of small peptides. Therefore supplements of dipeptides and tripeptides that contain the essential amino acids that cannot be absorbed as the free amino acids can be provided in the diet. This also explains why the amino acids can appear in the urine (as a result of similar defects in the kidney tubules), even although they cannot be absorbed as the free molecules.

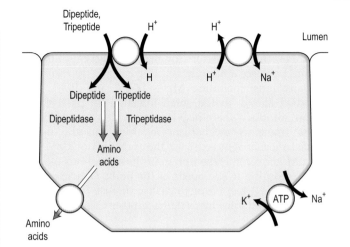

Fig. 8.13 Transport and metabolism of small peptides in the enterocyte.

Absorption of protein

Traces of intact protein can be absorbed in some adults. A foreign protein antigen that enters the circulation may provoke the formation of antibodies and the subsequent entry of that same protein may cause allergic symptoms. Intact protein can be absorbed in neonatal rodents, but it is not clear whether it can also be absorbed to any appreciable extent in the human infant. However, the absorption of antibodies present in the maternal colostrum or milk may contribute to the passive immunity of neonates. Inhibitors of proteolytic enzymes (which prevent protein degradation in the digestive tract) may be present in milk or colostrum, and so facilitate the absorption of whole proteins.

Minerals and trace elements

Chemical analysis of the human body has revealed the presence of over 20 elements. Some, such as oxygen, carbon, hydrogen and nitrogen, are abundant as constituents of organic molecules, or, in the case of oxygen and hydrogen, as components of water. Some elements are present in only trace amounts. Many enzymatic reactions will only take place if minute quantities of a particular ion are present. Therefore these substances are required in the diet.

The cations required by the body are sodium, potassium, calcium, iron, magnesium, manganese, copper, molybdenum and zinc, and the anions are chloride, iodide, fluoride, phosphates and selenate.

The body requires Ca^{2+} for a number of physiological processes, including bone and teeth formation, synaptic transmission in the nervous system and glandular secretion. PO_4^{3-} is required for bone and teeth formation, acid–base balance and many other functions. Iron is required for the synthesis of respiratory pigments such as haemoglobin, the respiratory pigment of red blood cells

active transport. The driving force for this system is the electrochemical gradient set up by the active pumping of H^+ ions across the brush border into the intestinal lumen. The small peptides are transported across the brush border via a H^+-dependent co-porter (Fig. 8.13). This transporter is specific for peptides that contain L-amino acids, and has a very low affinity for peptides that consist of more than three amino acids. Most of the small peptides transported into the cell are hydrolysed by intracellular dipeptidases and tripeptidases (Fig. 8.13). Dipeptides and tripeptides are absorbed at a more rapid rate than amino acids. Thus, an amino acid can be absorbed at a faster rate from the intestinal chyme if it is a component of a dipeptide or a tripeptide than if it is present as the free amino acid.

that transports oxygen to the tissues of the body. Mg^{2+} is required for nerve function, and as a co-factor for many enzyme reactions. Copper and zinc ions and many others are essential co-factors for enzyme reactions, and are required in trace amounts.

Many ions, including Mg^{2+}, SO_4^{2-} and PO_4^{3-}, are absorbed slowly in the small intestine by passive diffusion, although there also appears to be an additional active transport mechanism for Mg^{2+} in the ileum. Special mechanisms exist for the transport of Ca^{2+} and Fe^{2+}. Moreover, the absorption of these two ions is regulated according to the needs of the body. Deficiencies of Ca^{2+} and Fe^{2+} can occur in coeliac disease in which the proximal small intestine is damaged (see Case 8.1: 3).

Calcium

The average adult diet probably contains 1–6 g of Ca^{2+}. In addition, approximately 0.6 g enters the tract as a component of secretions. Of this 2.2 g total, only 0.7 g is absorbed. Thus after subtraction of the amount entering the tract from non-dietary sources, the net amount entering the body per day is only approximately 100 mg.

Ca^{2+} ions can be absorbed along the entire length of the small intestine. Its absorption is via both passive and active mechanisms. When its concentration in the chyme is low (<5 mM) most absorption of Ca^{2+} ions is via active transport, but when its concentration is high, an appreciable proportion is absorbed by passive diffusion. This is a consequence of the rate-limiting property of active transport. Ca^{2+} can be absorbed against a 10-fold concentration gradient, but the rate of absorption is still 50 times slower than that of Na^+.

The mechanism for the secondary active transport of Ca^{2+} ions in the enterocyte is illustrated in Figure 8.14. They are pumped out of the cell across the basolateral border by primary active transport involving a Ca^{2+}-ATPase. This pump is phosphorylated by a protein kinase, which is stimulated by a complex of Ca^{2+} and calmodulin in the cell. The phosphorylation of the pump increases both its enzymatic and its transport activities. In addition, there is a Na^+/Ca^{2+}-exchanger present in the basolateral border. Na^+ is transported down its concentration gradient into the cell in exchange for Ca^{2+}. These two mechanisms keep the concentration of free Ca^{2+} in the cell cytosol very low. The exchanger mechanism is the more effective mechanism at high levels of extracellular Ca^{2+}, and the Ca^{2+}-ATPase mechanism at low levels. The concentration gradient set up as a consequence of the extrusion of Ca^{2+} at the basolateral border provides the driving force for Ca^{2+} transport into the cell across the brush border (secondary active transport). Ca^{2+} in the chyme binds to a carrier protein in the brush border membrane that transports it into the cell by facilitated diffusion, down its concentration and electrical gradients. The carrier protein is known as the intestinal membrane calcium-binding protein (IMcal). Inside the cell Ca^{2+} is bound to another protein, known as calbindin or calcium binding protein

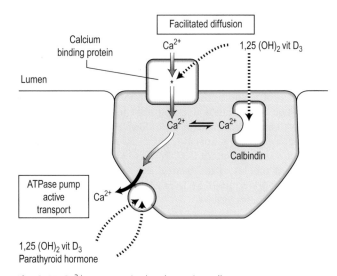

Fig. 8.14 Ca^{2+} transport in the absorptive cell.

(CaBP). This protein binds two Ca^{2+} ions per molecule. In the cell free Ca^{2+} is in dynamic equilibrium with protein bound calcium. The binding of Ca^{2+} to protein enables high amounts of Ca^{2+} to be transported into the cell without insoluble Ca^{2+} salts being formed inside the cell.

The process of calcium absorption in the small intestine is stimulated by a derivative of vitamin D_3. This vitamin can be ingested in the food (see below), or it can be formed in the skin from 7-dehydrocholesterol, under the influence of sunlight. Vitamin D_3 is converted to 1,25-dihydroxy vitamin D_3 via reactions that occur in the liver and kidneys. This vitamin behaves as a hormone in the body, and it circulates via the blood to control Ca^{2+} metabolism and homeostasis in various tissues. It is a steroid molecule that binds to nuclear receptors in the enterocytes of the small intestine to stimulate the synthesis of the brush border and cytosolic binding proteins. It also stimulates the synthesis of the basolateral Ca^{2+}-ATPase pump. Vitamin D deficiency leads to calcium malabsorption that can cause rickets in children and osteomalacia in adults (see Box 8.3).

Absorption of Ca^{2+} ions is also stimulated by parathyroid hormone, another hormone that is intricately involved with Ca^{2+} homeostasis in the body. The mechanism of action of parathyroid hormone in the small intestine is not clearly understood, although one effect is to stimulate the formation of 1,25-dihydroxy vitamin D_3. These control mechanisms enable the body to maintain a balance between the absorption and utilization of Ca^{2+}. Excess absorption results in increased Ca^{2+} excretion in the urine, which can lead to precipitation of insoluble salts such as calcium oxalate, which can lead to the formation of urinary tract stones.

Bile salts indirectly facilitate the absorption of Ca^{2+} ions by promoting the formation of micelles in the lumen of the small intestine (see Ch. 6, and below). This is partly because vitamin D is fat soluble and its absorption depends on micelle formation, and partly because bile

Box 8.3 Rickets and osteomalacia

Calcium deficiency is usually due to vitamin D deficiency, either through dietary deficiency or lack of exposure to sunlight. It can also be due to a diet low in calcium. In addition, it can be a consequence of anticonvulsant therapy (phenytoin and phenobarbital) that affects vitamin D metabolism. Malabsorption of vitamin D occurs in Crohn's disease (see Box 8.7) and coeliac disease (see Case 8.1: 3). The deficiency leads to rickets in children and osteomalacia in adults. The main defect is inadequate mineralization of bone matrix (see the companion volume *The Endocrine System*). In affected individuals there is a tendency to fractures, muscle and bone tenderness, and occasionally tetany. In children with rickets, lower limb deformities may occur.

It has been shown in animals with rickets caused by vitamin D deficiency, that their brush border membranes are deficient in IMCal transporter molecules. The transporter is induced by the vitamin, and if vitamin D_3 is administered to these animals, the binding protein appears in the brush border within 90 min of the vitamin being ingested. Treatment of the diseases is via supplementation of the diet with vitamin D and increased exposure to sunlight (which increases the synthesis of the active form of the vitamin, 1,25-dihydroxy vitamin D_3).

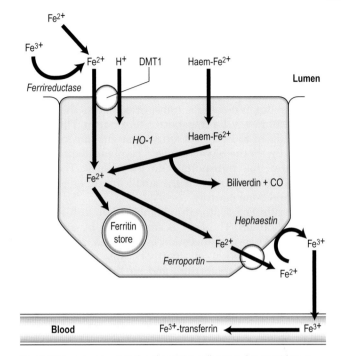

Fig. 8.15 Iron transport in the absorptive cell. *HO-1*, haemoxidase-1.

salts help to hold fatty acids in the micelles, thereby preventing them from forming insoluble Ca^{2+} soaps which cannot be absorbed. Thus, bile salt deficiency can result in negative Ca^{2+} balance. Another consequence of calcium soap formation is that Ca^{2+} is not then available to precipitate oxalic acid, a constituent of certain foods such as rhubarb. As a consequence, in bile salt deficiency where calcium soaps are formed, oxalic acid can be absorbed up to five times more rapidly than normal. Calcium oxalate kidney stones can also develop as a consequence because of the high levels of oxalate in the blood.

Calcium absorption is facultatively regulated to meet the needs of the body. The ability to absorb Ca^{2+} ions, via secondary active transport is increased by calcium deprivation. Young and growing people absorb Ca^{2+} more rapidly than do mature and elderly people. Lactating women require Ca^{2+} for milk production, and they absorb Ca^{2+} avidly.

Iron

Iron is required by the body as a component of haemoglobin and myoglobin and as a co-factor in various enzyme-catalysed reactions. Approximately two-thirds of the body iron is present in haemoglobin. Iron is ingested in several forms. The major component in normal meat-eating individuals is haem, the product of proteolytic degradation of haemoglobin and myoglobin in the intestines. Ferrous (Fe^{2+}) and ferric (Fe^{3+}) salts are usually present in the food.

Some 30–50% of the iron present in haem is released in the stomach lumen. Iron tends to form insoluble complexes with anions such as hydroxide, phosphate, oxalate and bicarbonate that are only slowly absorbed. It also forms insoluble complexes with tannins, phytins and fibre in the food. These complexes are more soluble at low pH and their absorption is stimulated by the presence of gastric acid. Furthermore, various components of food such as ascorbate (vitamin C) form soluble complexes with iron, thereby facilitating its absorption. Fe^{2+} has a lower tendency than Fe^{3+} to form insoluble complexes and is better absorbed. Fe^{3+} is only poorly absorbed. Ascorbate and gastric acid also reduce Fe^{3+} to Fe^{2+}. Removal of the stomach can lead to the development of iron deficiency anaemia as a consequence of the absence of gastric acid (see Ch. 3). Approximately half of the total amount of iron absorbed is present in haem. Figure 8.15 illustrates these processes. Absorption of iron occurs mainly in the proximal small intestine.

Haem absorption

The haem molecule consists of a porphyrin moiety containing bound iron. It is absorbed intact into the enterocyte, probably via a membrane carrier. Once inside the cell the Fe^{2+} ions are liberated from the molecule in a reaction catalysed by haem oxygenase (HO-1). Carbon monoxide (CO) and the green bile pigment biliverdin are the other products of this reaction. The free Fe^{2+} produced is thereafter processed in the same way as inorganic Fe^{2+} absorbed from the lumen. Some intact haem may be transported into the circulation but the mechanism involved is unknown.

Non-haem iron absorption

An enzyme, ferrireductase, on the extracellular surface of the enterocyte reduces Fe^{3+} to Fe^{2+} (Fig. 8.15). The Fe^{2+} is absorbed by combination with the divalent metal transporter, DMT1, which co-transports H^+ into the cell. In the cell a large proportion of the liberated Fe^{2+} enters a store, ferritin, but some is transported across the basolateral membrane via a transporter, ferroportin. The Fe^{2+} is then oxidized to Fe^{3+} by a ferroxidase enzyme known as hephaestin. In the blood, the Fe^{3+} combines with plasma transferrin that transports it to the tissues. The major stores of iron, apart from the small intestines are liver, spleen and bone marrow.

In ferritin Fe^{2+} is stored in combination with apoferritin, a β-globulin. The Fe^{2+} is surrounded by apoferritin subunits. When iron ingestion is increased, more iron is stored in the mucosal cells, partly because iron stimulates the synthesis of apoferritin, and so absorption into the blood is minimized. The Fe^{2+} in ferritin is a storage pool that is not usually absorbed. It is lost when the cells are shed from the villi. The cells disintegrate in the intestinal lumen and the liberated iron is eliminated in the faeces. Ferritin is the principal storage form of iron in tissues. It contains approximately 27% of the body's iron.

Regulation of iron absorption

The recommended dietary intake of iron in the adult is 10 mg/day for males and 15 mg/day for females of menstrual age. Normally, less than 10% of dietary iron is absorbed. In the normal adult very little iron is required because most of the iron released from erythrocytes at the end of their lifetime is recycled. The adult male or post-menopausal female loses approximately 0.6 mg/day and women of menstrual age approximately 1.2 mg/day (averaged over the monthly cycle). However, the proportion that is absorbed is tightly regulated to meet the body's needs. The amount of iron absorbed in the small intestine is approximately equal to the amount lost. Thus its rate of absorption is increased when more iron is required, for example after a haemorrhage (see below).

In iron-deficient conditions (in which haemoglobin synthesis is impaired, see Box 8.4), there is an increased expression of the transporter proteins DMT1 and ferroportin, and hephaestin, in the enterocyte (see Fig. 8.15). However, the rate of iron export from the enterocyte appears to be the main (rate-limiting) regulatory step indicating the primary role played by the rate of expression of ferroportin.

Conversely, mucosal cells that are loaded with iron have a reduced ability to take up iron. This prevents the absorption of excessive amounts, which can be toxic. In hereditary haemochromatosis, the gene mutation leads to prolonged and excessive absorption of iron (see Box 8.5).

The amount of iron absorbed in the small intestine increases following a haemorrhage, but not until 3 days after the haemorrhage has taken place. This delay was until recently believed to be due to the time taken for the absorptive cells to migrate from the crypts to the tips of

Box 8.4 Iron-deficiency anaemia

Chronic iron deficiency results in iron-deficiency anaemia, a condition in which the synthesis of the respiratory pigment haemoglobin is reduced.

In iron-deficiency anaemia the red blood cells are characteristically small (microcytes) and contain a low concentration of haemoglobin (hypochromia). In iron-deficiency anaemia the haemoglobin concentration is below 130 g/L in men and below 115 g/L in women. The prevalence is 2–5% in adult men and postmenopausal women in the developed world. Tiredness is a prominent symptom of the condition because the reduced capacity of the red cells to carry oxygen results in the body's requirement for oxygen not being met. Treatment is by oral administration of iron salts such as ferrous sulphate.

In iron-deficiency anaemia, the expression of ferroportin in the enterocyte is increased. This causes an increase in the capacity of the cell to absorb iron. There is a reduced expression of hepcidin in the liver in iron deficiency. Hepcidin circulates in the blood and signals the requirement for an increase in iron absorption in the intestine.

Iron-deficiency anaemia may be of dietary origin, due to menstrual blood loss, or malabsorption of iron in conditions such as coeliac disease (see Case 8.1: 3), chronic blood loss (as in Crohn's Disease (see Case 8.2: 3). 'Silent' chronic bleeding from the gastrointestinal tract is also a feature of all gastrointestinal cancers, and for this reason any adult with unexplained iron deficiency should be investigated for tumours of the large bowel, stomach and oesophagus.

the villi where they become mature, which takes approximately three days. The message to increase the rate of iron absorption would therefore be given to the dividing cells in the crypts, which cannot absorb iron until they are mature. However there is recent evidence to indicate that the message is given directly to the mature enterocytes. Thus the lag phase between blood loss and increased absorption of iron remains to be fully explained, but it may be due to the time taken for the events that regulate the expression of the humoral factor, hepcidin, a peptide molecule that is synthesized in the liver. Circulating hepcidin appears to signal the iron requirements of the body to the intestine by influencing the expression of ferroportin in the basolateral membrane of the enterocyte. In iron deficiency the expression of ferroportin is increased and in conditions of iron overload it is decreased. The expression of hepcidin itself (in the liver) may be partly regulated via the concentration of transferrin-bound iron in the bloodstream.

Water-soluble vitamins

The water-soluble vitamins required by the body are vitamin C (ascorbate), which prevents scurvy, and is present largely in fresh fruit, and components of the vitamin B 'complex', including thiamine, riboflavin, biotin,

Box 8.5 Haemochromatosis

Mucosal cells that are loaded with iron normally have a reduced ability to take up iron. This prevents the absorption of excessive amounts, which would be toxic. Haemochromatosis is a relatively common disorder that develops when there is prolonged excessive absorption of iron. It may also be due to excessive dietary intake. It is characterized by excessive deposits of ferritin and haemosiderin (iron binding proteins) in tissues. It can result in pigmentation of the skin (bronze diabetes), pancreatic damage (causing diabetes mellitus), cirrhosis of the liver, and (as a consequence) a high incidence of hepatic carcinoma. Hereditary haemochromatosis is an autosomal recessive congenital disorder in which the mutant gene is HFE, on the short arm of chromosome 6. It is characterized by a high rate of iron absorption in the presence of elevated, rather than depleted, body stores. The total body stores are usually between 20–40 g as opposed to 3–4 g in healthy individuals. In this condition, the mucosal regulatory mechanism is impaired, but the mechanisms involved are unclear. HFE, the protein product of the gene, is involved in the regulation of iron absorption, possibly via the regulation of the expression of hepcidin, the molecule that normally regulates iron absorption in the enterocyte. Expression of the hepcidin gene is decreased in hereditary haemochromatosis, and this facilitates iron overloading.

Treatment of haemochromatosis is by phlebotomy; removal of blood is done as often as is required to maintain low iron stores, as assessed by the concentrations of iron and iron-binding proteins in the blood, and transferrin saturation levels. A potential treatment for haemochromatosis is administration of a proton pump inhibitor that reduces acid secretion in the stomach, thereby inhibiting the reduction of Fe^{3+} to Fe^{2+}.

pantothenic acid, niacin, pyridoxine, inositol, choline, folic acid and cobalamins (vitamin B_{12}). In the main, members of the B complex are found together in nature. Furthermore, the overt manifestations of deficiency of members of this group, such as muscle weakness, fatigue and growth retardation, dermatitis and neuropathy, overlap. Water-soluble vitamins are required as cofactors in many metabolic reactions.

Most water-soluble vitamins are absorbed to an appreciable extent by simple passive diffusion, but for many, specific mechanisms are also available, although these are not all clearly understood.

Pyridoxine (vitamin B_6) appears to be transported solely via passive diffusion and then metabolized within the epithelial cell. Biotin, inositol, choline and riboflavin are absorbed by facilitated diffusion in the proximal small intestine, whilst pantothenic acid, thiamin, inositol and nicotinic acid are absorbed by active Na^+-dependent mechanisms in the proximal small intestine.

Ascorbate is absorbed mainly in the proximal ileum using a secondary active transport mechanism involving co-port with Na^+ ions, in the brush border. The operation

of the Na^+/K^+ ATPase in the basolateral border provides the gradient for Na^+ transport into the cell.

Folic acid

Folic acid (pteroylmonoglutamic acid) is formed by deconjugation of polyglutamate that is the form of the vitamin present in food. The deconjugation takes place in the brush border. It is catalysed by a zinc-activated enzyme, folate conjugase, which is maximally active at pH 5.0. Pterylmonoglutamate is transported across the apical membranes by a folate/OH^--exchange mechanism but its transport out of the enterocyte is by an unknown mechanism. Pteroylglutamate is converted to the active derivative tetrahydrofolate by folate reductase. It is then converted to 5,10-methylene-tetrahydrofolate that is required for DNA synthesis. Folate deficiency leads to macrocytic anaemia because DNA synthesis in the bone marrow is impaired.

Vitamin B_{12}

Vitamin B_{12} exists as four metabolically important forms in food: cyanocobalamin, hydroxocobalamin, deoxyadenosylcobalamin and methylcobalamin, which are mostly bound to protein. This vitamin is required for red cell maturation. For this reason pernicious anaemia develops in vitamin B_{12} deficiency. The dietary requirement for vitamin B_{12} is close to the maximum absorptive capacity, but large quantities of the vitamin are stored in the liver and these stores would normally be sufficient for at least three years if the vitamin ceased to be absorbed (as after gastrectomy, see Ch. 3). Some is lost in the bile secreted by the liver, although most of this is reabsorbed.

The cobalamins are released from their protein complexes, in the stomach, by the action of pepsin and acid. They are then rapidly bound to cobalamin-binding glycoproteins known as R proteins (haptocorrin) that are secreted in saliva and gastric juice. These complexes are degraded by pancreatic proteases in the duodenum. In pancreatic insufficiency when proteolytic enzymes are deficient, the complexes with R proteins are not degraded and the vitamin is not absorbed. The free Vitamin B_{12} (cobalamin) then combines with another glycoprotein, intrinsic factor, which is secreted by the stomach (see Ch. 3). This complex is resistant to proteolytic degradation. The formation of the vitamin B_{12}–intrinsic factor complex is necessary for the vitamin to be absorbed via active transport in the terminal ileum. The complex is a dimer of intrinsic factor that binds two vitamin B_{12} molecules. The brush border membrane of the ileal epithelial cells contains receptors for the vitamin B_{12}-intrinsic factor dimer complex. Binding of the complex to the receptor is Ca^{2+}-dependent. It seems likely that the complex is internalized by an active transport process. It dissociates within the cell, and the free vitamin B_{12} binds to another protein, transcobalamin II. This complex is then transported out of the cell, by an unknown mechanism, and

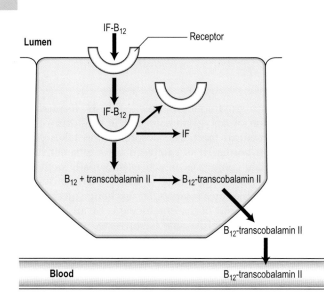

Fig. 8.16 Possible scheme for vitamin B_{12} (cobalamin) absorption. IF, intrinsic factor; B_{12}, cobalamin.

taken up into the portal blood. A scheme for its absorption is shown in Figure 8.16. The vitamin does not appear in the blood until 4 hours after it has been ingested. The vitamin B_{12}–transcobalamin II complex is taken up by receptor-mediated endocytosis in the liver for storage. In Crohn's ileitis the absorption of vitamin B_{12} is impaired because the mucosa of the ileum is damaged and the transporters are lost from the epithelial cells (Case 8.2: 3).

Vitamin B_{12} is also absorbed passively to some extent throughout the small intestine. Probably only 1–2% of the ingested vitamin is absorbed in this way, but if massive doses are eaten, enough can be absorbed to prevent pernicious anaemia. There is a shorter lag time involved in absorption by the passive mechanism than via the receptor-mediated mechanism. The causes and consequences of vitamin B_{12} deficiency are described in Box 8.6.

Lipids

Dietary lipids

The range of fat ingested by an individual varies enormously. In Western countries, it is probably between 25 and 160 g/day. Most ingested fat is neutral lipid (triacylglycerol) present in butter, margarine, cooking oil, meat, etc. In addition, some phospholipid and some cholesterol ester, components of plant and animal cell membranes are present in food, together with small amounts of other lipids.

Fat-soluble vitamins and essential fatty acids

Certain lipid molecules are 'essential' in the diet, as they are required in the body, but cannot be synthesized.

These include the fat-soluble vitamins A, D, E and K, and the essential fatty acids.

Deficiency of vitamin A results in hyperkeratosis of the skin, and xerophthalmia, a disturbance of epithelial tissues. In the human an early symptom of this condition is night blindness due to abnormal responses of the retinal rods.

Vitamin D is required for Ca^{2+} absorption (see below) and for normal calcium and phosphate metabolism. Deficiency of vitamin D and the resultant Ca^{2+} deficiency lead to abnormalities in bones and teeth, paraesthesia (due to impaired nerve conduction), skeletal pain and tetany (due to impaired muscle function).

Vitamin E is an important antioxidant. Deficiency in rodents causes sterility and muscle weakness, but its role in the human is not entirely clear.

Vitamin K deficiency causes bleeding diathesis, due to defective blood coagulation as a result of failure to synthesize prothrombin that is required for blood clotting. Part of the vitamin K requirement of an organism is supplied by bacteria that colonize the intestines.

The essential polyunsaturated fatty acids linoleic acid (C18:2) and γ-linoleic acid (present in evening primrose oil), linolenic acid (C18:3) and arachidonic acid (C20:4) are required for the proper functioning of the nervous system.

Under normal circumstances, less than 6 g of fat is eliminated in the faeces per day and most of this arises from bacterial cells and cell debris. If larger amounts of fat are eliminated the condition is known as steatorrhoea, and indicates a deficiency in fat absorption (see Case 8.1: 3 and Case 8.2: 3).

Lipid solubility

Some lipids, for example short-chain fatty acids (with a carbon chain <10), and some polyunsaturated complex lipids containing short-chain fatty acids or polyunsaturated fatty acids, are soluble in water. These are absorbed by passive diffusion. They dissolve in the membrane and are transported down their concentration gradients into the cell, and then into the portal blood. The transport of water-soluble lipids into the blood is a rapid process.

The digestion and absorption of most lipids are achieved by a variety of highly complex processes which enable the body to overcome the problem that although most lipid is insoluble in water, it has to be transferred from the gut lumen to the lymph, and eventually the blood, via aqueous media:

- The chyme in the lumen
- The cell's interior
- The interstitial fluid
- The lymph
- The blood.

A further problem is that the enzymes that catalyse the breakdown of the complex lipids, i.e. lipases,

Malabsorption in Crohn's Ileitis

If the terminal ileum is the main site involved, the absorption of bile acids and vitamin B_{12}, which are absorbed in the terminal ileum, will be the primary processes affected. If other regions are also severely affected, the absorption of many other nutrients can be impaired.

Bile acids

Bile acids are absorbed in the ileum and recycled via the enterohepatic circulation (see Ch. 6). In Crohn's ileitis, reduced bile acid absorption results in a reduced bile acid pool. This is due to the reduced surface area available for absorption and loss of bile acid transporters. If excessive bile acids are lost in the faeces, the liver cannot replace them rapidly enough (by *de novo* synthesis) to maintain the bile acid pool. Furthermore, if bacterial overgrowth is present, enzymes in the bacteria can deconjugate the bile acids, and unconjugated bile acids are not as rapidly absorbed as the conjugated derivatives.

Fats

In Crohn's disease of the ileum, fat absorption is usually impaired, leading to steatorrhoea. This is largely a consequence of defective bile acid absorption as these are important for emulsification and micelle formation. The intestinal and mesenteric lymphatics may also be extensively involved in the disease, and this can also contribute to impaired fat absorption. Malabsorption of complex lipids leads to a reduced calorie intake, but this may not be important if carbohydrate absorption is unaffected. Medium-chain triacylglycerols that contain fatty acids, which can be absorbed directly into the blood, can be substituted for long-chain triacylglycerols in the diet. This reduces the steatorrhoea.

Fat-soluble vitamins

In Crohn's disease, severe malabsorption of fat-soluble vitamins can occur. The problems associated with such deficiencies are outlined above.

Gall stone disease

A reduced bile acid pool can result in cholesterol not being held in micellar suspension and it precipitates out to form gall stones (cholelithiasis, see Ch. 6). Disruption of the enterohepatic circulation of bile acids is probably the reason why there is an increased incidence of gall stone disease in individuals with Crohn's disease.

Anaemia and vitamin B_{12}

Anaemia is common in individuals with Crohn's disease, and contributes to the patient's lassitude, and feelings of tiredness. There are a number of reasons for the development of anaemia in Crohn's disease:

- *Pernicious anaemia* due to vitamin B_{12} deficiency (see Box 8.1). If a large part of the ileum is diseased or resected, vitamin B_{12} deficiency will eventually develop, unless measures are taken to prevent it. *Note:* Folate deficiency, which also leads to macrocytic anaemia, can also occur if the jejunum is affected
- *Iron-deficiency anaemia.* Small but prolonged blood loss often leads to iron-deficiency anaemia in Crohn's disease
- *Poor nutrition.* The abdominal pain and gastrointestinal colic experienced in Crohn's disease can inhibit food intake. The resultant dietary deficiencies can also contribute to the development of anaemia (especially iron-deficiency anaemia).

Other deficiencies

- Lactase deficiency may be present due to loss of mature enterocytes (if the proximal small intestine is involved)
- Deficiencies of B complex vitamins may be present, leading to a red tongue, cracked lips, dermatitis and peripheral neuropathy. Vitamin supplements can be given when there is evidence of deficiencies.

Protein loss

In Crohn's disease, severe loss of protein, including albumen, may occur across the region of ulcerated mucosa in the intestine. This can result in hypoalbuminaemia and ascites (a fluid transudation into the peritoneum).

Diarrhoea

The diarrhoea present in Crohn's disease is partly 'osmotic' (see Ch. 7), due to quantities of unabsorbed nutrients and bile acids creating an osmotic gradient for water transport into the lumen. However, the diarrhoea is also due to the stimulation of propulsive motility by bile salts entering the colon. In addition, unabsorbed fats can be hydroxylated by bacteria in the colon, and the hydroxylated fats can stimulate colonic motility.

---

phospholipases and cholesterol esterases, are all water-soluble and insoluble in lipid, but obviously have to gain access to the lipid molecules before they can hydrolyse them. The mechanisms that enable these problems to be overcome will be described after the reactions involved in the digestion of lipids have been outlined.

Digestion

The digestion of triacylglycerol is catalysed by lipases (glycerol ester hydrolases). The major lipase in the digestive tract is secreted by the pancreas. Minor lipases are present in saliva (lingual lipase) and gastric juice,

Box 8.6 Pernicious anaemia

Deficiency of intrinsic factor, due to atrophy of the gastric mucosa, is the most common cause of pernicious anaemia. Atrophy of the gastric mucosa also leads to the inability of the stomach to secrete HCl (achlorhydria) and pepsinogen. However, it is only the lack of intrinsic factor that is serious, because pepsinogen and acid are not essential to life (see Ch. 3). Historically, intrinsic factor extracted from hog stomach was administered in this condition, and the vitamin could then be absorbed normally. Many patients developed antibodies to the intrinsic factor in their blood and it was once believed that these could be due to the presence of the foreign intrinsic factor protein in the blood. This led to the belief that the vitamin B_{12}–intrinsic factor complex was absorbed intact. However, it is now known that pernicious anaemia can be an autoimmune disease and so patients can have high antibody titres in their blood even when foreign intrinsic factor has not been ingested. Today, the vitamin is injected intramuscularly, but this is usually only necessary once every 3 months, as it is stored in the liver.

The absorption of vitamin B_{12} is impaired in pancreatic disease where proteases are deficient because it is not released from haptocorrin to which it binds in the stomach, and so cannot bind to intrinsic factor.

The complexity of vitamin B_{12} absorption is illustrated by the existence of three types of pernicious anaemia seen in childhood:

1. An autoimmune condition resulting in gastric atrophy, similar to that described above
2. A congenital deficiency of intrinsic factor with normal secretion of pepsinogen and acid
3. Congenital vitamin B_{12} malabsorption syndrome. In this condition, gastric function and release of intrinsic factor are normal but the absorption of vitamin B_{12} (in the ileum) is impaired, due to a defect in the receptors that bind the vitamin B_{12}–intrinsic factor complex.

Vitamin B_{12} is important for maturation of the red blood cells. Pernicious anaemia is characterized by a low red cell count, and high mean red cell volume (as the immature red cells present are larger than normal mature cells, i.e. they are 'macrocytic'). The symptoms that develop, if the condition is left untreated, include polyneuropathy, paraesthesia of fingers and toes, progressive weakness and ataxia, and dementia and other psychiatric problems.

but these are probably only important when the pancreatic enzyme is absent or inactive. The pancreatic enzyme cleaves the ester bonds at positions 1 and 3 in the triacylglycerol molecule, in a stepwise manner, with the formation of 1,2 diacylglycerol and 2,3 diacylglycerol intermediates. The ultimate products are 2-monoacylglycerol, which is absorbed without further degradation, and fatty acids. The overall reaction is given in Figure 8.17.

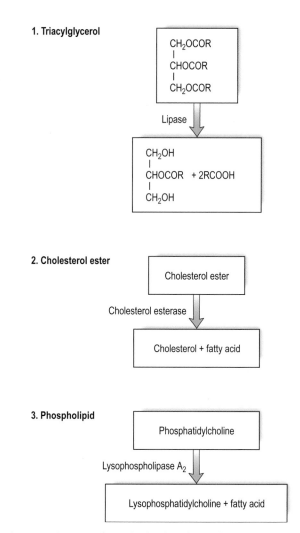

Fig. 8.17 Digestion of complex lipids in the small intestine.

Cholesterol esterase is secreted in pancreatic juice. In intestinal chyme, it forms dimers that are resistant to proteolytic digestion. It cleaves the ester bond in cholesterol ester with the formation of free cholesterol and fatty acid (Fig. 8.17). It also acts more slowly to hydrolyse triacylglycerol, lysophospholipids, monoacylglycerols and esters of fat-soluble vitamins.

Phospholipase A_2 is secreted in pancreatic juice as an inactive precursor. It is activated in the small intestine (see Ch. 5). It cleaves the ester bond at the 2 position in many phospholipids, including phosphatidylcholine (lecithin), phosphatidylserine and phosphatidylethanolamine, to give fatty acid and lysophospholipid. The hydrolysis of phosphatidylcholine is shown in Figure 8.17.

Emulsification

The process of emulsification is essential for the efficient digestion of lipids. It enables the enzymes involved to gain access to their lipid substrates. If oil is added to water it forms a layer on top of the water because it is insoluble, and is less dense than water. If some lipase is added it dissolves in the water layer and will only attack the lipid at the lipid–water interface. Therefore the rate of lipid hydrolysis is proportional to the surface area of the lipid–water interface. In the small intestine, the surface area of the lipid–water interface is increased by the process of emulsification, whereby the large droplets of lipid are broken down into tiny droplets that can be held in a stable suspension. The lipid–water interface is consequently increased enormously, enabling lipid digestion to proceed at a rapid rate.

The process of emulsification requires conjugated bile acids, which coat the lipid droplets and prevent them coalescing together. These substances are secreted in bile. Within 20 min of the beginning of a meal the gall bladder contracts and empties concentrated bile into the duodenum. The structure and release of the bile acids is discussed in Chapter 6. The emulsified droplets are 0.5–1.0 mm in diameter. A neutral or slightly alkaline environment is required for emulsification. This is normally provided by the intestinal chyme in which the alkaline secretions mix with the acid from the stomach and neutralize it.

Lipase is essentially inactive in the presence of bile acids, but colipase, a small protein (MW 10 000) present in pancreatic juice, forms a complex with lipase and bile acid, and this enables the colipase–lipase complex to spread over the surface of the minute droplets, and hydrolyse the triacylglycerol present. Triacylglycerol is hydrolysed on the surface of the emulsion droplets and the products of digestion, monoacylglycerol and fatty acids, are liberated from the droplets into the aqueous medium. The hydrolysis of triacylglycerol under these circumstances is more rapid than the absorption of its products. A small proportion of the fatty acids released from the droplets is water-soluble, and this can be absorbed directly into the blood. However, most free fatty acids and monoacylglycerols are insoluble in water. They would soon saturate the chyme and separate out into large droplets again, if it were not for the process of micelle formation.

Micelle formation

A micelle is a lipid particle of 4–6 nm diameter, which consists of an aggregate of approximately 20 lipid molecules. Bile acids are required for micelle formation. Bile itself contains micelles composed of bile salts, cholesterol and phosphatidylcholine (see Ch. 6) but in the small intestine the micelles have a more heterogeneous composition. The process of micelle formation is discussed in Chapter 6. In the small intestine, the initial constituents of the micelles in the duodenum are bile salts and 2-monoacylglycerols. These micelles then sequester other fat-soluble substances, such as long-chain fatty acids, cholesterol, fat-soluble vitamins, and phospholipids. An individual micelle may contain several or all of these molecules, although fatty acids are quantitatively the most important. Cholesterol, long-chain fatty acids

and fat-soluble vitamins, which are highly insoluble in water, are maintained in the core region of the micelle. Monoacylglycerol and lysophospholipids orientate themselves so that their acyl chains are in the core region, and their more polar regions project towards the aqueous phase (i.e. in the shell region). Bile salts are present in the shell region. The polar groups on the bile salt impart a negative charge to the surface of the micelles. This causes mutual repulsion between different micelles, keeping them in stable suspension in the chyme. The negatively charged shell collects cations such as Na^+ that form an outer shell around the micelle. When the bile acid concentration is at or above, its critical micellar concentration, the bile acid and insoluble lipids such as monoacylglycerol aggregate as micelles. With increasing bile acid concentration more monoacylglycerol molecules are carried as micelles. In the normal human the critical micellar concentration is usually well below the concentration actually present, and micelles easily form. There are certain disease states however, such as obstructive jaundice (see Ch. 6), where the concentration is too low. The critical micellar concentration (see Ch. 6) is higher for unconjugated bile acids than for conjugated bile acids. Consequently, if a considerable fraction of the bile acids is deconjugated in the intestinal lumen by bacterial action, micelle formation may be impaired.

Most fatty acids and monoacylglycerol are absorbed in the duodenum and upper jejunum, while the bile acids are absorbed more distally in the ileum. Cholesterol can be absorbed throughout the length of the small intestine, although a considerable proportion of it escapes into the colon. Thus, the composition of the micelles changes as they move down the small intestine; their content of fatty acids and monoacylglycerol diminishes while their proportional content of bile acids increases.

The constituent lipid molecules of micelles move back and forth between the micelles and the aqueous solution with great rapidity. The aqueous chyme is kept saturated with lipid molecules by the movement of fatty acids and monoacylglycerol from the micelles into the solution. Thus the micelles serve as a reservoir of these products so that the aqueous phase in contact with the enterocyte brush border is always saturated with lipid molecules, and a dynamic equilibrium between the micelle and the solution is established. The dissolved fatty acids can be absorbed. However, the micelles first have to diffuse across the 'unstirred layer' to the enterocyte cell membrane.

The unstirred layer

The unstirred layer is a layer of fluid in contact with the epithelial surface, which does not readily mix with the bulk of the chyme. It is 200–500 mm thick. Micelles and nutrients have to diffuse through this layer to the surface membrane of the enterocyte. Thus, there is a concentration gradient of nutrients across the unstirred layer with the lowest concentration at the epithelial surface. A pH gradient also exists across the unstirred layer, with the fluid in contact with the brush border being slightly more acid than the bulk of the chyme. This promotes the absorption of fatty acids as they tend to be less ionized, and therefore more easily absorbed across the lipid membrane (see Ch. 7).

Fate of lipid in the epithelial cell

Lipids can dissolve in the lipid of the brush border membrane and easily diffuse across it. The transported lipids are metabolized within the cell and used in the resynthesis of complex lipids (Fig. 8.18). The free fatty acids react with coenzyme A to form acetyl-CoA (Fig. 8.19A). Triacylglycerol is synthesized via both the α-glycerolphosphate pathway (that also operates in liver and other tissues) and via the monoacylglycerol pathway, which involves direct esterification of monoacylglycerol by fatty acyl-S-CoA, a pathway which is restricted to the mucosal cell (Fig. 8.19B,C). Phospholipid is synthesized by esterification of lysophospholipid with fatty acyl-S-CoA (Fig. 8.19D) and cholesterol ester by esterification of free cholesterol with fatty acyl-S-CoA (Fig. 8.19E).

The complex lipids are formed in the smooth endoplasmic reticulum of the enterocyte. The complex lipid molecules aggregate together to form droplets within the

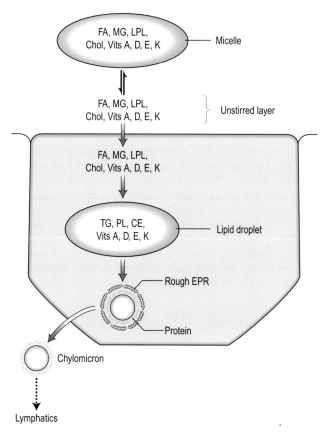

Fig. 8.18 Transport of lipids in the enterocyte. MG, monoacylglycerol; LPL, lysophospholipid; TG, triacylglycerol; PL, phospholipid; FA, fatty acids; Chol, cholesterol; Vits, vitamins.

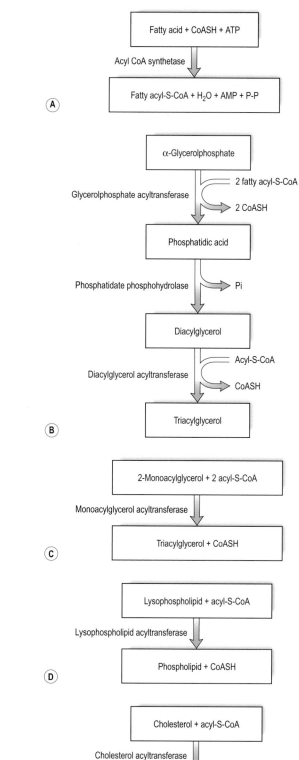

Fig. 8.19 Synthesis of complex lipids in the small intestine. (A) Formation of acetyl-S-CoA. (B) Synthesis of triacylglycerol via the α-glycerol phosphate pathway. (C) Synthesis of triacylglycerol via the monoacylglycerol pathway. (D) Synthesis of phospholipid from lysophospholipid. (E) Synthesis of cholesterol ester from cholesterol.

cell. The phospholipids form at the surface of the droplets, with their polar heads oriented towards the exterior of the droplets. The droplets become surrounded with rough endoplasmic reticulum and the ribosomes synthesize a β-lipoprotein, which, together with the phospholipid, forms a coat around the droplets (see Fig. 8.18). The droplet with its protein and phospholipid coat is known as a chylomicron. Chylomicrons vary in size from a fewnm to 750nm in diameter. The different lipids, including the fat-soluble vitamins, are sequestered together in the same chylomicrons.

The chylomicrons are extruded from the lateral surface of the cell and taken up into the lymph in the lacteals. After a meal, the intestinal lymph becomes milky due to the presence of chylomicrons. The uptake of chylomicrons into the lymph is stimulated by adrenocorticoid hormones. Defects in the process of fat digestion and absorption are described in Box 8.7. Furthermore, fat malabsorption and steatorrhoea are features of both coeliac disease and Crohn's disease (see Case 8.1: 3 and Case 8.2: 3).

Bile acids

Modification of bile acids in the small intestine

Bile acids are modified by intestinal bacteria. Primary bile acids are converted to secondary bile acids by dehydroxylation (see Ch. 6). Therefore excessive bacterial action can lead to a greater proportion of secondary bile acids in the bile acid pool. In addition, a portion of the bile acids can be deconjugated by bacterial enzymes with the release of the amino acid moieties. Conjugated bile acids have lower pKa values than the unconjugated acids, and are therefore more ionized and more water soluble at the slightly alkaline pH of the intestinal chyme. As they are ionized they exist as salts with Na^+ and other cations.

Absorption

Bile acids are absorbed from the ileum into the portal blood and transported to the liver (see Ch. 6). The absorption in the small intestine is by both active and passive mechanisms. The active transport occurs only in the terminal ileum, and only ionized conjugated bile acids are absorbed by this active process. It is very efficient so that normally only approximately 5% of conjugated bile acids reach the colon. The active transport is via a co-port carrier molecule in the brush border membrane, which also transports Na^+, in a manner similar to that in the hepatocyte (see Ch. 6). The driving force for the transport across the brush border is the electrochemical gradient created by the pumping of Na^+ out of the cell. The process whereby bile acids are transported out of the enterocyte has not yet been characterized. In Crohn's disease, bile acid absorption via the active transport mechanism is usually impaired because the terminal ileum is damaged. This leads to fat malabsorption and steatorrhoea (see Case 8.2: 3).

Box 8.7 Defects in fat digestion and absorption

Disease of various organs can lead to fat malabsorption and steatorrhoea. This a reflection of the complexity of fat digestion and absorption. Some of these diseases are described below:

- *Liver or biliary tract disease* (such as gallstone disease, cirrhosis, see Ch. 6) can result in a deficiency of conjugated bile acids and HCO_3^- resulting in impaired emulsification of lipids and impaired micelle formation. *Note*: Some drugs, for example cholestyramine, a resin used to treat diarrhoea caused by bile acids, bind bile salts thereby preventing them from forming micelles
- *Pancreatic disease* (such as chronic pancreatitis, see Ch. 5) can result in deficiency of enzymes such as lipase, which digest fats, and reduced HCO_3^-, leading to malabsorption of lipids. Other pancreatic enzymes are also deficient so malabsorption of other nutrients also occurs
- *Intestinal disease*. In coeliac disease (see Case 8.1: 1 and 2), where the villi are flattened, there is a reduced surface area available for absorption of nutrients such as fats in the affected regions. In Crohn's disease that commonly affects the ileum, the absorption of bile acids is defective and the bile acid pool is reduced. This leads to reduced emulsification and micelle formation and therefore reduced fat digestion and absorption (see Case 8.2: 3)
- *β-Lipoproteinaemia* is an inherited disorder where β-lipoprotein synthesis in the enterocytes, and elsewhere, is defective. Thus, in this condition the synthesis of the protein coat of chylomicrons is inadequate and only large chylomicrons, if any, are formed, and so fat absorption is impaired
- *Lymphatic disease* (obstruction by, e.g. a tumour) can lead to impaired transport of lipids from the lymph to the blood
- *Adrenal disease*, where there is a deficiency of adrenocorticoid hormones, can lead to impaired transport of lipids to the lymph as these hormones stimulate the uptake of chylomicrons into the lymph. (Fat absorption is depressed in adrenalectomized animals.)

Unionized conjugated bile acids are more fat-soluble than the ionized (conjugated) molecules. Glycine is a weak acid and a fraction of the glycoconjugates is unionized and therefore fat-soluble. A small amount of it is absorbed passively through the lipid membrane. Taurine conjugates are almost completely ionized at the pH of the small intestine and are therefore not absorbed in this way. Excessive deconjugation of conjugated bile acids by intestinal bacteria leads to decreased absorption and a greater loss to the colon with a resulting decrease in the size of the bile acid pool. However, unconjugated bile acids are more fat-soluble than conjugated bile acids and a proportion is absorbed by passive transport in the intestines.

Bile pigments

Bile pigments are lipid substances with limited solubility in aqueous solution. Unconjugated bilirubin is more lipid soluble than conjugated bilirubin, and it can be absorbed by diffusion across the lipid membrane of the enterocyte. Bacterial action in the intestines deconjugates some of the conjugated bile pigments, with the result that some bile pigment is reabsorbed into the portal blood. The metabolism of bile pigments by bacteria and their absorption via the enterohepatic circulation is described in Chapter 6.

Fat malabsorption

Fat digestion and absorption is a very complicated process necessitating the proper functioning of many organs including the liver, the pancreas and the small intestine. For this reason many different defects of digestion and absorption can result in malabsorption of fats and steatorrhoea. Some of these defects and the diseases responsible are described in Box 8.7. Diseases where fat malabsorption is a prominent feature include coeliac disease (see Case 8.1: 3) and Crohn's disease (see Case 8.2: 3).

THE ABSORPTIVE AND POST-ABSORPTIVE STATES

9

Chapter objectives

After studying this chapter you should be able to:

1. Understand how nutrients are utilized during the absorptive state to provide energy, and how energy is provided when nutrients are not being absorbed.

2. Consider how the absorptive and post-absorptive patterns of metabolism are controlled by hormones, and how this control is impaired in diabetes mellitus.

Introduction

The nutrient state of the blood depends on whether or not a meal is being processed in the gastrointestinal tract. When nutrients such as glucose and lipid are being absorbed, and their concentrations in the blood are high, the pattern of energy metabolism is known as the absorptive state. In this state, a fraction of the blood glucose is used by various tissues to meet their immediate energy needs. The excess glucose and the absorbed lipid are stored as glycogen and lipid that can be used to provide energy between meals or during fasting: a pattern of energy metabolism known as the post-absorptive state. The change from the absorptive state pattern to the post-absorptive state pattern is brought about by changes in the blood concentrations of insulin and other hormones. The importance of maintaining the appropriate patterns of metabolism can be illustrated by considering the metabolic defects present in insulin-dependent diabetes mellitus (IDDM, or type I diabetes), in which the secretion of insulin is severely impaired. In this chapter we shall consider the metabolic abnormalities present in this condition, and the consequences of these defects (Case 9.1: 1 and 2).

Case 9.1 — Insulin-dependent diabetes mellitus: 1

A 12-year-old girl was taken to see her doctor. Her parents were worried because she seemed listless and was losing weight. They said she also seemed to be drinking a lot and was frequently having to pass urine. The doctor noticed that her breathing was rapid and shallow (Kussmaul breathing), and that it smelled of acetone. The patient provided a sample of urine. Clinistix tests on the urine sample indicated the presence of glucose and ketones. An appointment was made for her to attend a diabetes clinic. She was told to fast from the evening before the appointment. A blood sample was taken and the blood glucose concentration was found to be (11.1 mmol/L). This is above the normal range (3.5–7.0 mmol/L), indicating the presence of hyperglycaemia (high blood glucose). Hypoinsulinaemia (low plasma insulin) and ketoacidosis (high levels of ketone bodies in the blood) were also noted. The results confirmed that the patient was diabetic. She was later taught how to inject herself with insulin, which had to be done three times a day, before meals.

After considering the details of this case we can address the following questions:

- Why is this patient likely to be suffering from insulin-dependent diabetes mellitus (IDDM) rather than non-insulin-dependent diabetes mellitus (NIDDM)? What are the basic defects in each condition? Would the concentration of plasma insulin be low in both conditions? What is the explanation for the listlessness in this patient?
- How is the control of blood glucose changed in diabetes mellitus?
- Why did the patient's breath smell of acetone? Why was her acid–base status changed? Why was her breathing abnormal (rapid and shallow)? How would the body normally compensate for the acidosis?
- What are the mechanisms responsible for the high urine output (polyuria), glucosuria and ketonuria, in this patient?
- Are hormones other than insulin also affected in diabetes mellitus?

Case 9.1 — Insulin-dependent diabetes mellitus: 2

Defect and cause

The patient was likely to be suffering from IDDM. This condition affects mostly young people, the commonest age of onset being between 10 and 14 years, whereas NIDDM usually affects people in middle or later life. Hyperglycaemia is a characteristic of both conditions. In IDDM, it is due to reduced secretion of insulin as a result of necrosis of the pancreatic β-cells. In NIDDM, destruction of many β-cells eventually occurs, but plasma insulin concentrations are not usually low until later in the disease (see Box 9.2). It is sometimes referred to as 'insulin-resistant diabetes' for this reason. In the patient described above, the insulin concentration was low. The extent of the metabolic disturbance is usually less severe in NIDDM than in IDDM, and ketoacidosis (see below) is not usually a feature of NIDDM. The presence of ketones on the breath would therefore also support a diagnosis of IDDM.

IDDM affects both sexes equally, but there is a slightly earlier peak in age of onset in girls than boys. It is more prevalent in Caucasians than non-Caucasians, and more prevalent in people living in the Northern hemisphere than the Southern hemisphere. There is a higher incidence of first diagnoses in winter than summer. The frequency of the disease has been increasing during the last 60 years. This is probably in part due to dietary factors and increased obesity. Only approximately 15% of diabetic patients suffer from IDDM (<0.3 % of the population). The majority of diabetics suffer from NIDDM, although other rare forms of diabetes exist.

There is evidence for a genetic predisposition, particularly to IDDM. In identical twins, there is a 30–50% concordance for IDDM. The HLA genes on chromosome 6 are associated with the condition, and a number of rare predisposing genetic mutations have recently been identified. However, other factors are important (see below).

IDDM is an immune-mediated disease. Circulating antibodies to cytoplasmic proteins of the β-cell are present in most patients, although these particular antibodies may be a secondary phenomenon as they disappear early in the disease. Evidence for a more direct involvement of antigens that react with intracellular enzyme proteins, such as glutamic acid decarboxylase and tyrosine phosphatase is emerging. There is also strong evidence for defects in cell-mediated immunity in IDDM. Studies in first-degree relatives of children with IDDM, who have a higher than normal risk of developing the disease, have demonstrated islet antibodies in the circulation in the first few years of life, i.e. years before diagnosis, and this could also prove to be a useful tool in predicting the disease.

The aetiology of IDDM is largely unknown, although in some cases it may be due to a viral infection. Viruses that have been implicated are Coxsackie B virus, mumps and rubella. Evidence has also been reported, which implicates environmental toxins. (It has been known for many years that alloxan and strepto-zotocin can cause β-cell necrosis and diabetes in rodents.) One candidate is nitrosamines, found in some smoked foods, which have been shown to be toxic to pancreatic β-cells in animals. Bovine serum albumin present in cow's milk has also been implicated; antibodies to this protein are more common in the blood of diabetic than non-diabetic patients, and they cross-react with a peptide known as p69, which is often present on the surface of β-cells during infectious episodes.

Apart from the symptoms mentioned in the patient above (listlessness, weight loss, polyuria, polydipsia, Kussmaul breathing), vomiting and abdominal discomfort, mental confusion and coma, and tachycardia and hypertension can also be present. Secondary complications in IDDM are neuropathy (sensory and motor), retinopathy, nephropathy, and cardiovascular defects such as ischaemic heart disease, cerebrovascular disease, peripheral vascular disease and renal failure.

The absorptive state

In the absorptive state, the nutrients entering the blood from the gastrointestinal tract are hexose sugars and amino acids. The liver is the first port of call for these absorbed nutrients. It takes up a large fraction of the nutrients, thereby altering the composition of the blood before it circulates to the rest of the body. The nutrients remaining in the blood are taken up by adipose tissue, muscle and other tissues. Lipids are absorbed from the small intestines into the lymph as components of chylomicrons (ch. 8). They enter the venous blood at the thoracic duct, and are then metabolized and stored in adipose tissue.

Fate of absorbed carbohydrate

Absorbed carbohydrate consists of glucose, galactose and fructose. However, the liver converts fructose and galactose to glucose and then releases glucose into the blood. It is expedient therefore, to consider absorbed carbohydrate as glucose. Figure 9.1 illustrates the various fates of glucose during the absorptive state.

A large fraction of the absorbed glucose enters the various cells of the body, where it is used for the production of energy. During the absorptive state, glucose is the main fuel for most tissues of the body, which utilize it by glycolysis, the citric acid cycle and other pathways. The rest of the absorbed glucose is used to provide stores of energy for later use during the post-absorptive (fasting) state (see below). The tissues that store most of the body's energy are liver, adipose tissue and muscle. Glucose is taken up by all of these tissues in the absorptive state.

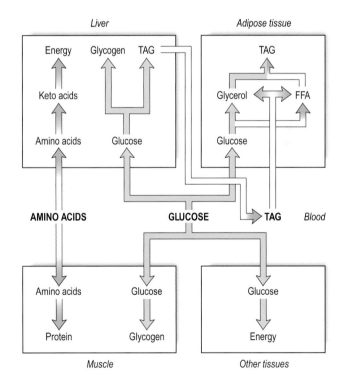

Fig. 9.1 Energy metabolism in the absorptive state. TAG, triacylglycerol; FFA, free fatty acids.

Some of the glucose taken up by the liver is converted to glycogen that is then stored in the liver, and some is converted to triacylglycerol. The glucose provides both the glycerol and the fatty acid moieties of triacylglycerol. Some of the triacylglycerol synthesized in the liver is stored there, but most is released into the blood as a component of very low density lipoproteins. Very little glucose and fat is utilized for energy in the liver itself. (The liver's main source of energy in the absorptive state is amino acids, see below.)

Another fraction of the blood glucose enters skeletal muscle where it is converted to glycogen for storage in the muscle. A further fraction enters adipose tissue, where it is converted to fatty acids and α-glycerol-phosphate, which are used in the synthesis of triacylglycerol. The α-glycerol-phosphate pathway for triacylglycerol synthesis is outlined in Chapter 8.

In summary, during the absorptive phase, glucose is used for energy production by most tissues of the body, and the excess is stored in muscle and liver as glycogen, and in adipose tissue as fat. These relationships are outlined in Figure 9.1.

Various inherited disorders of carbohydrate metabolism have been characterized, where either glycogen storage is excessive, or abnormal glycogen is produced (see Box 9.1). These conditions are due to defects in enzymes involved in glycogen metabolism.

Fate of blood triacylglycerol

Absorbed triacylglycerol is carried in the lymph as droplets partially coated with protein, known as chylomicrons (see Ch. 8). The triacylglycerol synthesized from glucose in the liver is released to circulate in the blood, but as components of very low density lipoproteins. The blood enters the adipose tissue where the lipids present in both very low density lipoproteins and chylomicrons, are hydrolysed to fatty acids and glycerol by a lipoprotein lipase present in the endothelial surfaces of the capillaries. Most of the fatty acids produced are taken up into the adipose cells (adipocytes) by passive diffusion, although a small fraction circulates to other tissues. The glycerol produced is either taken up by the adipose tissue cells or transported to other tissues. In adipocytes, the fatty acids and glycerol are reconstituted to triacylglycerol via the α-glycerol phosphate pathway (see Ch. 8), and stored in the cells. Thus, during the absorptive state, triacylglycerol in adipose tissue arises from three sources; absorbed glucose, very low density lipoproteins released from the liver, and dietary triacylglycerol present in chylomicrons. These relationships are summarized in Figure 9.1.

Adipose tissue is abundant in the body, and widely distributed in subcutaneous, perirenal, mesenteric and other regions. An adipocyte contains a small amount of cytoplasm, which surrounds a large lipid droplet. There is very little water present in adipose cells. Lipid has a very low density. It provides a very efficient storage form of energy; 1 g of triacylglycerol contains more than twice as many calories as 1 g of glycogen or protein. Moreover, a 70 kg man has approximately 15 kg triacylglycerol that provides 135 000 kcal of energy, but only approximately 0.2 kg of glycogen, providing only 800 kcal of energy.

Box 9.1 Glycogen storage disorders

Most glycogen storage diseases are autosomal recessive disorders. They are caused by enzyme defects that lead either to accumulation of glycogen, or to an abnormality in the structure of glycogen. Glycogen is synthesized in liver or muscle. Some defects are restricted to liver and some to muscle.

Defects in liver enzymes

- *Phosphorylase or phosphorylase kinase* (see fig. 9.9). A defect in either of these enzymes leads to hepatomegaly and hypoglycaemia; the prognosis is good
- *Phosphorylase 6 kinase*. The defect leads to hepatomegaly, hypoglycaemia and fatiguability
- *Debranching enzyme*. The defect leads to an abnormal structure of liver and muscle glycogen. The clinical features are similar to those for glucose-6-phosphatase deficiency (see below)
- *Branching enzyme*. A defect in this enzyme results in abnormal structure in liver glycogen. The clinical features are hepatomegaly and cirrhosis, and death in the first 5 years of life
- *Glucose 6-phosphatase* (Von Gierke's disease, see fig. 9.8). In this disease, the defect leads to hepatomegaly (enlarged liver), ketototic hypoglycaemia, stunted growth, obesity and hypotonia. Liver, intestine and kidney are affected. There is a high mortality rate.

Defects in muscle enzymes

- *Phosphorylase* (McArdle's disease). The symptoms are muscle cramps and myoglobinuria after exercise. The life-span is normal
- *Phosphofructokinase* (see fig. 9.8). The clinical features are similar to those seen in phosphorylase deficiency (see above)
- *Lysosomal acid α-glucosidase*. A defect in this enzyme leads to cardiomyopathy and heart failure, and death in infancy. Liver, muscle and heart tissues are affected.

Fate of absorbed amino acids

In the absorptive state, a fraction of the absorbed amino acids is taken up by the liver (Fig. 9.1) and converted to ketoacids that are oxidized via the citric acid cycle and other pathways. Ketoacids are the liver's main source of energy in the absorptive state. Excess ketoacids can be converted to triacylglycerol in the liver. The conversion of amino acids to ketoacids involves deamination, with the formation of ammonia that is converted to urea in the liver. The urea is released from the liver into the blood, and subsequently secreted by the kidneys.

Amino acids that are not taken up by the liver enter other tissues, such as muscle, where they are utilized for protein synthesis. Muscle is quantitatively the most important tissue in this respect. Protein is not a particularly labile source of energy, but it is broken down and used for energy during prolonged fasting.

Insulin

Insulin has a central role in the control of metabolism. If it is injected, the absorptive state is duplicated, and if its plasma concentration is very low, as in untreated IDDM, the pattern of metabolism that predominates is an exaggerated version of that seen in the post-absorptive state. Insulin is a polypeptide (MW 6000), consisting of two peptide chains that are connected together by two disulphide bridges (Fig. 9.2). The prohormone precursor of insulin is a single peptide chain (MW 9000) known as proinsulin, which is converted to insulin by proteolytic cleavage. This results in the removal of a peptide, known as C peptide. In the prohormone, C-peptide connects the two peptide chains of insulin (Fig. 9.2). Both insulin and the C peptide are stored in granules in the β-cells of the pancreas. C peptide is secreted with insulin in a ratio of 1:1, but C peptide, unlike insulin that is removed from the blood by the liver, is excreted in the urine. Its concentration in the urine can be used to assess an individual's ability to secrete insulin. It has no established biological function.

The release of insulin into the blood is stimulated by eating and inhibited by fasting, and insulin is largely responsible for promoting the pattern of metabolism seen in the absorptive state. High levels of glucose and amino acids in the blood (as when a meal is being processed) are the primary stimuli for insulin secretion. The hormone acts on most tissues of the body, but muscle, adipose tissue and liver are quantitatively the most important. However, some tissues, such as brain and erythrocytes, which are obligatory utilizers of glucose for fuel, are not sensitive to insulin.

Control of insulin secretion

Insulin is a protein hormone secreted by the islets of Langerhans in the pancreas. It is released by exocytosis in response to raised intracellular Ca^{2+} concentrations. The second messengers involved include cAMP, but intracellular inositol trisphosphate, and diacylglycerol, which activates protein kinase C, are also increased. The release of insulin from the pancreas is controlled to a large extent by the concentration of glucose and amino acids in the blood perfusing the pancreas. Other factors, such as hormones and neurotransmitters, potentiate or inhibit the effects of the blood nutrients on insulin secretion.

Control by glucose

The secretion of insulin in response to an increase in blood glucose is under feedback control (Fig. 9.3). After a meal the blood glucose increases as it is absorbed from the gastrointestinal tract. This results in stimulation of insulin secretion from the β-cells of the islets of Langerhans. These cells respond to both the actual glucose concentration, and the rate of change of glucose concentration in the blood. The effect is due to the

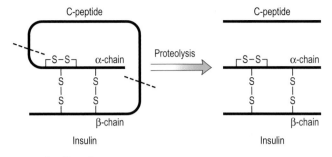

Insulin prohormone

Fig. 9.2 Proteolytic processing of the insulin prohormone to insulin and C-peptide.

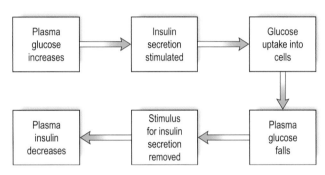

Fig. 9.3 Feedback control of insulin release.

uptake and intracellular metabolism of glucose in the β-cells. Glucose is transported into these cells via the GLUT2 transporter. The enzyme glucokinase which catalyses glucose 6 phosphate formation from glucose, the rate-limiting step in glycolysis (see Fig. 9.8), is a key mediator in the β-cells. However 3-carbon compounds such as glyceraldehyde, which are intermediates formed downstream from glucose-6-phosphate in the glycolytic pathway, are potent stimulators of insulin release. The secretory mechanism depends on the generation of ATP via glucose metabolism. ATP closes an ATP-sensitive K^+ channel, and this results in depolarization of the cell, causing a voltage-dependent Ca^{2+} influx. Elevated intracellular Ca^{2+} then causes insulin exocytosis.

Insulin lowers blood glucose by promoting its uptake into cells (see below). Thus as the concentration of insulin in the blood rises, the concentration of glucose falls and the stimulus for insulin secretion is removed. As a consequence, the concentration of insulin falls. The feedback control of insulin secretion by plasma glucose is summarized in Figure 9.3.

The concentration of plasma insulin normally parallels the rise and fall in the levels of plasma glucose. This is illustrated in Figure 9.4A that shows the results of a glucose drink in a fasting individual. Concentrations of glucose above 5 mmol/L are effective in increasing insulin release. The response to an oral glucose load (glucose tolerance test) is used to diagnose diabetic states, where the fasting glucose concentration is not sufficiently raised

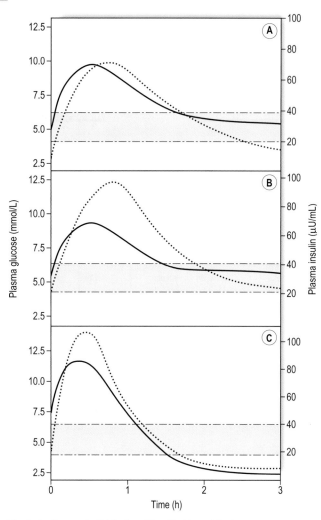

Fig. 9.4 Glucose (solid line) and insulin (dotted line) responses to a carbohydrate meal in (A) a normal individual, (B) an obese individual and (C) an individual with reactive hypoglycaemia. The shaded areas show the normal range for fasting plasma glucose concentration.

to give a clear diagnosis on its own (Case 9.1: 3). In obese individuals there is a slower uptake of glucose into cells after a meal, and an exaggerated insulin response to the increase in plasma glucose (Fig. 9.4B). The plasma insulin concentration rises to a higher level than in people of normal weight.

The glucose tolerance test may also be used to diagnose hypoglycaemic states. After a high carbohydrate meal, the concentration of plasma glucose may rise rapidly. This causes a rapid secretion of insulin from the β-cells, with an earlier and higher peak than after a more balanced meal. This results in a rapid fall in plasma glucose to levels that may be lower than normal (hypoglycaemia). This effect is exaggerated in some individuals, whose β-cells produce an excessive insulin response to the rise in plasma glucose. They are said to have 'reactive hypoglycaemia' (Fig. 9.4C). Various symptoms result from hypoglycaemia, including tremor, hunger, weakness, uncoordinated movements, blurred vision and impaired

Insulin-dependent diabetes mellitus: 3

Diagnosis and treatment

Tests that may be performed to assess the diabetic status of an individual include plasma and urine glucose, plasma insulin, and plasma and urine ketone bodies. Glucose and ketone bodies in blood and urine can be measured by automated colorimetric procedures and insulin by radio-immunoassay. In untreated IDDM blood and urine glucose concentrations are high and plasma insulin concentration is very low, or undetectable. In severe cases, plasma and urine ketone concentrations are high.

Glucose tolerance test in IDDM and NIDDM

The diabetic status of an individual can be assessed by an oral glucose tolerance test, although this is rarely necessary in IDDM because of the presence of a markedly raised blood glucose concentration and glucosuria. For the glucose tolerance test the patient fasts overnight and then drinks a solution containing 75 g of glucose in 250–300 mL of water. A 'fasting' sample of blood is obtained immediately prior to the glucose load and then further blood samples are obtained at 30-min intervals thereafter, for 3 h. Figure 9.5 shows the results of such a test in a normal individual, a patient with IDDM, and a patient with NIDDM. In a normal individual the fasting plasma glucose concentration is usually within the range 3.5–7.0 mmol/L. After an oral glucose load it increases to reach a peak between 30 and 60 min and returns to normal by 2 h. In both of the diabetic patients, the fasting concentration of glucose was abnormally high, but it was highest in the patient with IDDM. After the glucose load, the

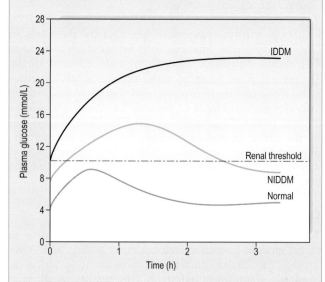

Fig. 9.5 Glucose tolerance curves in a normal subject, a subject with IDDM, and a subject with NIDDM. The renal threshold for glucose reabsorption in the kidney tubules and glucose excretion in the urine is indicated.

**Insulin-dependent diabetes
mellitus: 3 (continued)**

plasma glucose concentration increased to a very high level in both patients but it was highest in the patient with IDDM, and remained higher for longer than in the patient with NIDDM.

Treatment of IDDM

IDDM is treated by subcutaneous injections of insulin. If inadequate insulin is administered, the patient may become comatose as a result of ketoacidosis, electrolyte imbalance and dehydration (see Case 9.1: 5). However, an overdose of insulin can also lead to coma due to hypoglycaemia. Therefore the amount of insulin administered must be carefully adjusted to bring the blood glucose concentration back to normal. Figure 9.4C shows the changes in plasma glucose following an oral glucose load in a person with reactive hypoglycaemia, a condition in which there is hypersecretion of insulin. The response resembles that seen in an individual who has been injected with too much insulin.

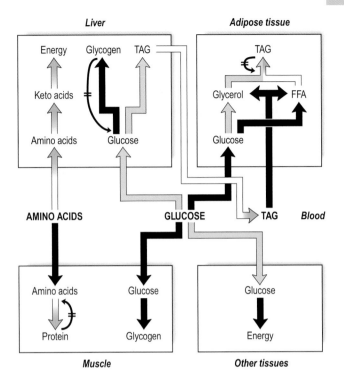

Fig. 9.6 Control of energy metabolism by insulin in the absorptive state. The bold arrows indicate the pathways and uptake mechanisms stimulated by insulin, and the arrows crossed out indicate the pathways inhibited by insulin. TAG, triacylglycerol; FFA, free fatty acids.

mental ability. Such people need to control their blood glucose levels by limiting their intake of carbohydrates, and eating small meals at frequent intervals. Patients who have undergone gastrectomy can have similar symptoms due to rapid entry of food into the small intestine. (This situation is discussed in Ch. 3.)

Control by amino acids

Insulin secretion is also controlled by the levels of amino acids in the blood. Thus, after a high protein meal, which results in a high level of amino acids, insulin secretion is increased. The most potent amino acids in this respect are arginine, leucine and alanine. The mechanism whereby these amino acids exert this effect first involves their transport into the β-cells. The anionic amino acids depolarize the membrane and open voltage-gated Ca^{2+} channels. The resulting Ca^{2+} influx then stimulates insulin secretion.

Control by other hormones

Glucagon stimulates insulin release and somatostatin inhibits it. Glucagon is produced by the α-cells and somatostatin by the D cells in the pancreas (see Ch. 5). The actions of these hormones on insulin release from the pancreatic β-cells may be local paracrine effects, or they may act locally via the blood in the islet capillaries.

Oral administration of glucose causes a greater increase in blood insulin levels than the same glucose load injected into the blood. The mere presence of food in the gastrointestinal tract elicits an increase in insulin secretion (known as the 'incretin effect'). This indicates that insulin secretion is controlled by factors originating in the gastrointestinal tract (the enteroinsular axis). The duodenal hormones

cholecystokinin (CCK), gastric inhibitory peptide (GIP), and glucagon-like peptide 1 (GLP-1) may be responsible. These hormones are all secreted when a meal is being processed in the gastrointestinal tract (see Chs 4 and 5).

Control by nerves

The islets of Langerhans are innervated by both parasympathetic and sympathetic nerves. Stimulation of the vagus (parasympathetic) nerve fibres that innervate the β-cells potentiates insulin release via acetylcholine acting on muscarinic receptors. It is phospholipase C-mediated and involves Ca^{2+} uptake into the β-cells. Stimulation of the sympathetic nerves inhibits insulin release via noradrenaline acting on $α_2$-adrenergic receptors on the islet β-cells.

Actions of insulin in the absorptive state

The actions of insulin during the absorptive state are indicated in Figure 9.6. It acts on membrane receptors in many cells to promote the uptake of glucose, amino acids, K^+, Mg^{2+} and PO_4^{3-}. In addition it stimulates or inhibits rate-limiting steps in many pathways involved in energy metabolism. It directly stimulates the entry of glucose into muscle and adipose tissue, but not liver. This is a primary action of insulin. However, an increase in intracellular glucose speeds up the reactions in which it is utilized, via the mass action effect due to the increased supply of the reactant. These are secondary effects of insulin. Thus glucose oxidation, and lipid and glycogen synthesis are all stimulated in insulin-sensitive tissues when blood insulin concentration increases because more glucose enters the cells.

In addition to the secondary effects of insulin on metabolism, it also exerts primary effects on metabolism by directly stimulating rate-limiting reactions in a variety of pathways. It stimulates key reactions involved in the utilization of glucose for energy production via the citric acid cycle, and in its utilization for the synthesis of glycogen and triacylglycerol. At the same time it inhibits glycogenolysis, gluconeogenesis and lipolysis.

Insulin also directly stimulates the uptake of amino acids into muscle and other tissues. This results in increased synthesis of protein by a mass action effect. In addition it directly inhibits the breakdown of protein.

The overall effect of insulin in the absorptive state is to provide glucose for utilization as energy, to promote the storage of excess carbohydrate and fat in forms (which can be used later to provide calories in the post-absorptive state and to increase protein synthesis (Fig. 9.6).

The insulin receptor

Insulin binds to a receptor in the cell membrane of insulin-responsive tissues. The receptor is a transmembrane glycoprotein with both extracellular and cytoplasmic faces. Figure 9.7 shows the effects of activation of the receptor by insulin. It is a tetramer composed of two α- and two β-subunits. The α-subunit is situated on the extracellular face of the membrane. Insulin binds to a site on the α-subunit. The β-subunit spans the membrane, but most of it comprises a tail on the intracellular face. Each α-subunit is bound to a β-subunit by a disulphide bridge, and the two αβ-dimers are joined extracellularly through the α-subunit by another disulphide bridge. The receptor is a tyrosine kinase enzyme. When it is not bound to insulin, it is enzymatically inactive, but when it combines with insulin, a conformational change occurs, which results in the exposure of three intracellular phosphorylation sites on the β-subunit tail. These sites can be autophosphorylated, using ATP as the substrate, and this results in activation of the enzyme. The phosphorylated receptor kinase can then activate tyrosine residues on various intracellular proteins, known as insulin receptor substrate (IRS) proteins. When these proteins become phosphorylated they in turn phosphorylate a number of intracellular kinases and phosphatases. These activated enzymes then stimulate glucose and amino acid uptake, and a number of rate-limiting reactions in various metabolic pathways. These actions determine the net direction of those pathways. However, activation of the receptor also suppresses the levels of intracellular cAMP, which results in suppression of various catabolic processes as well as gluconeogenesis (see below). The nature of all the post-receptor events stimulated by insulin has not been fully elucidated. After activation of the receptor, it is endocytosed, and either degraded, or recycled.

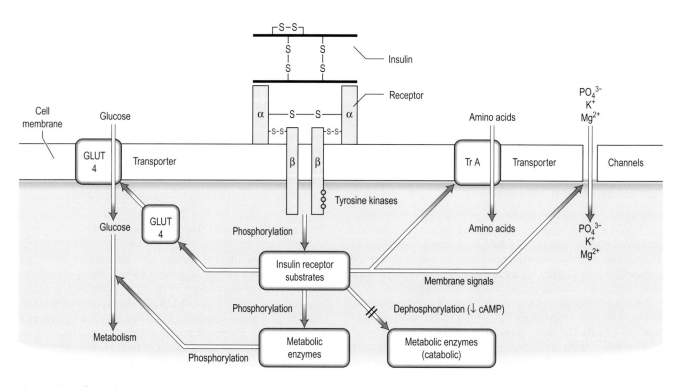

Fig. 9.7 The effects of activation of its receptor by insulin. GLUT4, hormone-sensitive GLUT4 glucose transporter; Tr A, amino acid transporter A.

Glucose entry into cells

Basal glucose uptake in muscle and adipose tissue is via the GLUT1 transporter. However, facilitated glucose transport involves GLUT4, which is an insulin-sensitive transporter. This transporter is bound to endosomes in the cytosol, and it cycles between the cytosol and the cell membrane (Fig. 9.7). When insulin concentration in the blood is low, most of the transporters reside in the cytosol, bound to the endosomes. Activation by insulin of its receptor stimulates the translocation of the transport-ers from the cytosol into the membrane. This event may involve the formation of phosphatidylinositol phosphates produced by the action of phosphatidylinositol-3-kinase, one of the enzymes that are activated by the receptor tyrosine kinase. In addition insulin increases the synthesis of the GLUT4 transporter, and possibly also its activity. At low insulin concentrations, glucose transport is the rate-limiting step in the utilization of glucose. After a meal, when high concentrations of insulin are present, glu-cose transport into cells can be stimulated up to 20-fold. Reactions in the intracellular metabolic pathways then become rate-limiting for the utilization of glucose.

Glycolysis

Insulin increases the utilization of glucose via glycolysis by increasing the synthesis of a number of the enzymes involved (Fig. 9.8). It increases the synthesis of liver glu-cokinase, phosphofructokinase and pyruvate kinase, enzymes which catalyse key steps in the pathway. In addi-tion it inhibits the synthesis of glucose-6-phosphatase and fructose-1,6-bisphosphatase which catalyse reactions which oppose the utilization of glucose via glycolysis.

Glycogen synthesis

An increase in glucose in cells stimulates glycogen syn-thesis by a mass action effect, but insulin also stimulates glycogen synthesis directly, by stimulating the activity of glycogen synthase, the rate-determining enzyme of the pathway. In addition, insulin promotes the synthesis of glucokinase in liver (but not muscle), which catalyses the formation of glucose-6, phosphate (see above). These actions enable more glucose to enter the glycogenic path-way in liver. In addition insulin inhibits hepatic glu-cose-6-phosphatase thereby inhibiting the release of free glucose into the blood.

Triacylglycerol synthesis

Figure 9.6 indicates the effect of insulin on the synthesis of triacylglycerol from glucose in adipose tissue. It stimu-lates fatty acid synthesis from glucose by activating sev-eral of the enzymes involved in the pathway, including pyruvate dehydrogenase which catalyses the conversion of pyruvate to acetyl CoA in the mitochondrion. Acetyl CoA is then directed to fatty acid synthesis, because insulin activates acetyl CoA carboxylase that diverts the acetyl CoA to the synthesis of fatty acid in the cytosol.

Inhibition of glycogenolysis, lipolysis and gluconeogenesis

Insulin suppresses the mobilization of body energy stores. It inhibits glycogen and triacylglycerol breakdown and gluconeogenesis by decreasing the level of intracellular cAMP. cAMP is a second messenger which activates an intracellular cascade, which leads to phosphorylation of enzymes involved in key steps in the catabolic pathways. Figures 9.9 and 9.10 outline the intracellular cascades involved in glycogenolysis and lipolysis. cAMP phos-phorylates a protein kinase which then phosphorylates critical enzymes involved in these pathways. Thus, lower-ing the levels of cAMP by insulin, causes a reduction in the

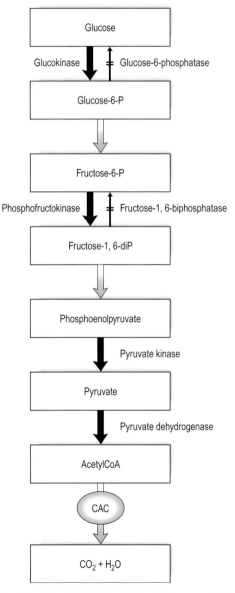

Fig. 9.8 Control of glycolysis by insulin. The bold arrows indicate the enzymes whose synthesis is stimulated by insulin, and the crossed arrows indicate those whose synthesis is inhibited by insulin.

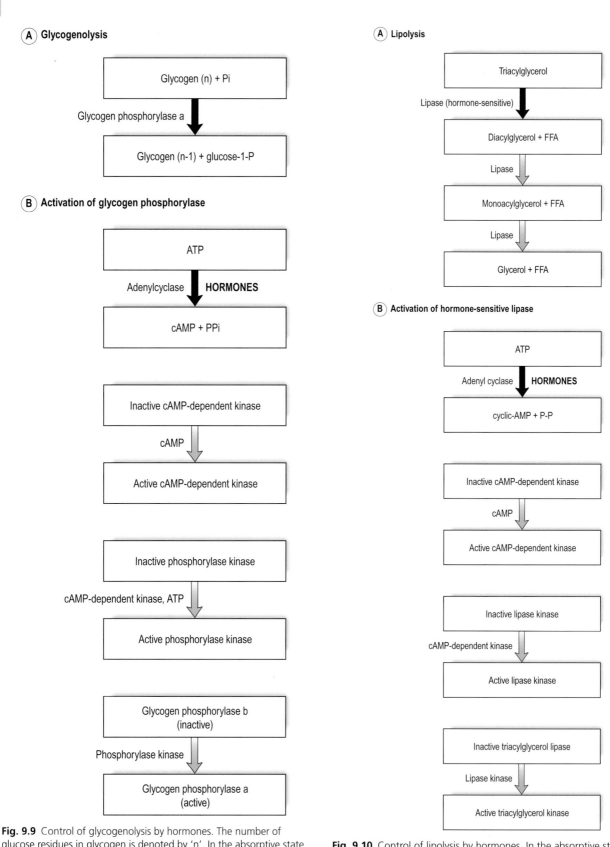

Fig. 9.9 Control of glycogenolysis by hormones. The number of glucose residues in glycogen is denoted by 'n'. In the absorptive state the formation of cAMP (bold arrows) is inhibited by insulin. In the post-absorptive state it is stimulated by adrenaline, glucagon, growth hormone, and cortisol.

Fig. 9.10 Control of lipolysis by hormones. In the absorptive state the formation of cAMP (bold arrows) is inhibited by insulin. In the post-absorptive state it is stimulated by adrenaline, glucagon, growth hormone, and cortisol.

activity of the protein kinase, and this leads to decreased activity of these key enzymes and suppression of the metabolic pathway. Insulin decreases cAMP via activation of a membrane-associated phosphodiesterase that hydrolyses it to 5′AMP.

Amino acid transport and protein synthesis

Insulin facilitates the uptake of amino acids into cells via the amino acid transporter A, a sodium-dependent carrier that transports neutral amino acids and imino acids. Insulin controls the synthesis of mRNA for many specific proteins, increasing some and suppressing others. It stimulates the synthesis of mRNA for certain enzymes involved in glycolysis and represses the synthesis of mRNA for others that are involved in gluconeogenesis. It also stimulates DNA synthesis, cell division and cell differentiation. The mechanisms involved in these actions of insulin are not fully understood.

Insulin sensitivity

The magnitude of the effects produced by insulin depends not only on its concentration in the plasma, but also on the sensitivity of the tissues to it. The responsiveness of tissues to insulin varies even in normal individuals. Thus, for example, habitual exercise increases tissue sensitivity to insulin. It is pertinent to note here, however, that glucose is taken up into muscle during acute exercise by an insulin-independent mechanism, which has not yet been elucidated, although it may partly depend on the increase in plasma β-endorphin that occurs during exercise as this peptide stimulates glucose uptake in muscle.

Insulin sensitivity is decreased in obese individuals, leading to abnormally slow uptake of glucose into tissues after a meal (Fig. 9.4B). Relatively high amounts of insulin are secreted in response to the resulting elevated plasma glucose. The elevated insulin tends to maintain the fasting concentration of plasma glucose within the normal range. The mechanisms underlying changes in insulin sensitivity in obesity are not clear.

Post-absorptive state

Some tissues, such as brain and erythrocytes, can only survive if glucose is delivered to them for fuel. They cannot initially utilize other nutrients to any significant extent. Lack of glucose causes brain damage, coma and death within minutes. During the post-absorptive state when glucose is not being absorbed from the gastrointestinal tract, the plasma levels of glucose are maintained within a physiological range. This is brought about in two ways. First, glucose is generated by glycogen breakdown, glycogenolysis and gluconeogenesis. Second, many tissues can utilize substrates other than glucose, such as fatty acids, for energy provision. This spares the available glucose for the tissues that are obligatory utilizers of it. However, in starvation, when the blood glucose falls slowly, the nervous system is able to adapt after a few days to use ketones as a source of energy (see Case 9.2: 1 and 2). In IDDM where insulin is deficient (see Case 9.1: 4) and in NIDDM where the tissues are insensitive to insulin (see Box 9.2), the metabolic state resembles the post-absorptive state.

Glucose-supplying reactions

The reactions that supply glucose to the blood during the post-absorptive state are outlined in Figure 9.12. During the post-absorptive state, glycogen stored in the liver is broken down to glucose, which is liberated into the blood. Muscle glycogen is also broken down in the absorptive state, but muscle lacks glucose-6-phosphatase (the enzyme which converts glucose 6 phosphate to free glucose), and so in muscle glucose-6-phosphate is broken down to lactate and pyruvate, which are released into the blood. These metabolites are taken up by the liver and then converted to glucose (via gluconeogenesis, see below), which is liberated into the blood. The stores of glycogen in liver and muscle can amount to 600–800 g in the post-absorptive state. This source of glucose is sufficient to meet the energy needs of the body for approximately only 4 h.

In any prolonged period of fasting, the stored glycogen is used up and gluconeogenesis becomes the more important process for generating glucose and maintaining the plasma glucose concentration. Lactate provides one substrate for gluconeogenesis, but in prolonged fasting, amino acids derived from protein in muscle, and taken up by the

---

Case 9.2 Starvation: 1

A round-the-world yachtsman was blown off course and his boat sank. He managed to get into the yacht's dinghy and to retrieve a large container of drinking water from the boat. After 7 weeks without food, he was rescued by a passing liner. His water supply had lasted out, but he was weak and emaciated.

Consideration of this case history provokes the following questions:

- Which metabolic processes would have been occurring to enable this man to maintain his plasma glucose levels? Would his plasma insulin levels be normal?
- Would the man's acid–base status be disturbed? Would he be excreting glucose and ketone bodies in his urine? Is it likely that acetone would be detectable on his breath?
- Would the man's plasma glucagon levels to be high or low?
- What treatment would be recommended for the starving yachtsman? Would it be advisable for him to drink a concentrated solution of glucose?

Metabolism in starvation

Plasma glucose

It is important that the yachtsman's plasma glucose concentration does not fall too far because the nervous system is an obligatory utilizer of glucose during the initial phase of fasting. Later, it can adapt to utilize keto acids.

The metabolic processes that would have been occurring to enable this man to maintain his plasma glucose concentration are:

- Glycogenolysis in liver
- Glycogenolysis in muscle, which would provide glucose indirectly via lactate production
- Gluconeogenesis in liver, which would provide glucose from amino acids lactate and glycerol.

The rescued man's plasma insulin concentration would be at the basal level, as it is largely controlled by plasma glucose concentration, which would have been maintained within physiological limits.

Energy provision

The man's energy provision for tissues that are not obligatory users of glucose would be mostly from stores of body fat. Fatty acids derived from triacylglycerol in adipose tissue would provide a large part of the energy requirements of most other tissues. Ketone bodies derived from fatty acids, would be utilized for energy in liver. He would be unlikely to be excreting glucose and ketone bodies in his urine, but acetone could probably be detected on his breath.

The man's plasma glucagon concentration would be high initially, as low glucose stimulates glucagon secretion from the pancreatic α-cells. However, after a few days of fasting it returns to normal. Thus in this man, the levels of glucagon would not be elevated.

Acid–base status

The starving man would probably have a metabolic acidosis due to the production of ketone bodies and fatty acids, but respiratory and renal compensation would be occurring.

Treatment

It would not be advisable for this man to drink a concentrated solution of glucose because it would pass too quickly into the small intestine and cause osmotic diarrhoea, and he could become dehydrated. The rapid absorption of glucose could cause him to suffer from a rebound hypoglycaemia, and possibly fainting. However, isotonic or hypotonic solutions would help. He should probably drink isotonic fluid containing some glucose for a while.

Metabolic state

In untreated IDDM, when insulin concentrations are very low, plasma glucose concentration is high because the uptake of glucose into muscle, adipose tissue and other tissues is impaired, and the utilization of glucose for energy provision and glycogen and fat synthesis, is reduced. Insulin also inhibits glycogenolysis and lipolysis, so these catabolic processes occur at an increased rate in its absence. Increased glycogenolysis in liver results in glucose release into the blood. Increased glycogenolysis in muscles results in lactate release, which is used by the liver for glucose production by gluconeogenesis. Increased lipolysis results in fatty acids and glycerol being released into the blood. The glycerol is taken up and used to produce glucose via gluconeogenesis. Thus these processes all result in further increases in blood glucose, and exacerbate the hyperglycaemia.

Fatty acids formed in the adipose tissue are released into the blood and taken up by various tissues and oxidized to acetyl CoA. In IDDM, if the levels of fatty acids are excessive, acetyl CoA production in the liver exceeds the capacity of the citric acid cycle to oxidize it and the excess is converted to ketone bodies (Fig. 9.11). These are released into the blood, resulting in high concentrations of plasma ketone bodies and ketosis. Metabolic acidosis results from the high concentrations of (acidic) ketone bodies and fatty acids in the blood plasma (see Case 9.1: 5).

Amino acid uptake into tissues is also reduced in IDDM, due to very low insulin levels, and protein breakdown is increased. This results in an excessive conversion of amino acids to glucose via gluconeogenesis in the liver. Thus, the overall effect of these metabolic disturbances is elevated levels of glucose, ketone bodies and fatty acids in the plasma.

Comparison with post-absorptive state

The pattern of metabolism in untreated IDDM is an exaggeration of that seen in the post-absorptive state. Insulin levels are low, glucose and amino acid uptake into tissues is reduced,

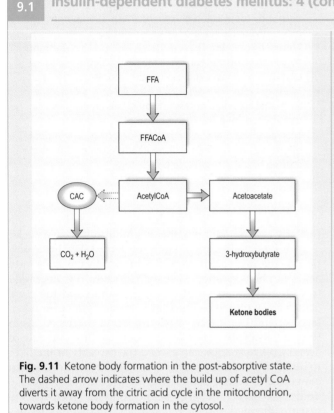

Fig. 9.11 Ketone body formation in the post-absorptive state. The dashed arrow indicates where the build up of acetyl CoA diverts it away from the citric acid cycle in the mitochondrion, towards ketone body formation in the cytosol.

and glycogenolysis, lipolysis, gluconeogenesis and protein breakdown increase. These events result in increases in plasma glucose, plasma fatty acids and ketone bodies. Furthermore, in diabetes mellitus, in spite of the presence of hyperglycaemia, there are increases in many of the hormones associated with the post-absorptive state, including plasma catecholamines, glucagon, cortisol and ACTH, and sometimes growth hormone. Increases in secretion of these hormones accompany various types of stress, and they are probably partly due to activation of the sympathetic nervous system. Thus, for example, stimulation of the preganglionic sympathetic nerves to the adrenal medulla causes the release of adrenaline into the blood, and stimulation of the sympathetic nerves to the α-cells of the pancreas causes release of glucagon. However, in IDDM, the predominating mechanism causing the release of these hormones (which are normally suppressed by hyperglycaemia) is largely unknown.

In non-diabetic subjects, in the post-absorptive state, the plasma glucose and ketone bodies do not normally exceed the threshold for reabsorption in the kidney, so metabolites do not appear in the urine.

Box 9.2 Non-insulin-dependent diabetes mellitus

In the UK, non-insulin-dependent diabetes mellitus (NIDDM) is known to affect approximately 2% of the population, and surveys of adults show that in at least another 2% the condition is present, but undiagnosed. It affects more men than women (ratio 3:2), and is much more prevalent in ethnic minority groups, especially those originating from the Indian subcontinent (typically 7%). Obesity and lack of physical exercise are predisposing factors for NIDDM. Thus the incidence of NIDDM is increasing in the Western world, as more people are becoming obese and more are following sedentary lifestyles. In both NIDDM and IDDM there is a predisposition to vascular disease and hypertension, high cholesterol, high very low density lipoproteins (VLDL), neuropathy, retinopathy and nephropathy. It may be pertinent that some of these problems, for example hypertension, are associated with obesity even in non-diabetic individuals. (The differential diagnosis of NIDDM is discussed in Case 9.1: 3.)

Defects

In NIDDM, insulin secretion is eventually impaired, although the plasma concentration may be initially normal or even increased in response to the hyperglycaemia. As the disease progresses, the β-cells become less responsive to increases in plasma glucose, and the β-cell mass may eventually be diminished by up to 40% (whereas in IDDM these cells are completely destroyed).

A further serious defect in NIDDM is that tissues such as liver, muscle and adipose develop insulin resistance. The resistance involves not only glucose uptake into muscle and adipose tissue, but also the metabolic actions of insulin, such as its effects to stimulate glycogen synthesis in muscle and liver and to inhibit lipolysis in adipose tissue. In consequence, circulating glucose and plasma free fatty acids are increased. In most cases, insulin binds normally to its receptor but insulin signalling in the cell is attenuated. The mechanism is unknown. In a few cases of NIDDM there is a structural abnormality of the receptor or a known intracellular protein. The metabolic defects are similar to those seen in IDDM (see Case 9.1: 4) but they are usually less severe. Thus, ketosis is not usually present.

Treatment

NIDDM can often be controlled if the patient follows a healthy, calorie-restricted diet and a more active lifestyle. These measures increase tissue sensitivity to insulin. If they are insufficient, oral drugs are used. These include:

- *Sulphonylureas.* These drugs stimulate insulin secretion by binding to a component of the ATP-sensitive K^+ channel in the β-cell membrane, and directly closing it. They are therefore only effective in patients with

Box 9.2 Non-insulin-dependent diabetes mellitus (continued)

a functioning β-cell mass. A potentially serious side-effect is hypoglycaemia because the action of many sulphonylureas can persist for over 24h. They may also promote weight gain. Tolbutamide is a relatively short-acting sulphonylurea

- *Meglitinides*. These drugs also stimulate insulin secretion by closing the ATP-sensitive K^+ channel in the β-cells. They are short-acting, and promote insulin secretion in response to meals
- *Biguanides*. Metformin is a useful biguanide drug that increases insulin sensitivity, and reduces hepatic glucose

output by suppressing gluconeogenesis. It does not induce hypoglycaemia or cause weight gain
- *Thiazolidinediones*. These drugs promote insulin resistance by an unknown mechanism. They reduce hepatic glucose output and enhance glucose uptake into tissues
- *Intestinal enzyme inhibitors*. Inhibitors of α-glucosidase, such as acarbose, suppress carbohydrate absorption, thereby reducing the rise in blood glucose that accompanies meal consumption. Side-effects are osmotic diarrhoea and flatulence due to undigested carbohydrate passing into the colon (see Ch. 7).

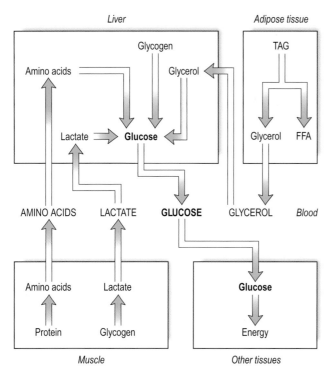

Fig. 9.12 Glucose-supplying reactions in the post-absorptive state. TAG, triacylglycerol; FFA, free fatty acids.

liver, are quantitatively the most important substrate for the generation of glucose via gluconeogenesis. Glycerol derived from triacylglycerol in adipose tissue, and taken up by the liver is also converted to glucose via gluconeogenesis.

Glucose-sparing reactions

Most of the energy requirement of the body during the post-absorptive state is derived via glucose-sparing reactions that utilize the energy stored as triacylglycerol during the absorptive state. Fat is broken down in adipose tissue to glycerol and free fatty acids, which are released into the blood. The glycerol is used for gluconeogenesis in liver (see above), but the fatty acids are taken up by

many other tissues and oxidized to CO_2 and water via the fatty acid oxidation pathway and the citric acid cycle.

In the post-absorptive state the liver takes up a portion of the fatty acids from the blood. In the liver fatty acids can be converted to acetyl CoA which is degraded to CO_2 and water by fatty acid oxidation and the citric acid cycle, with the production of energy. However when large quantities of fatty acids are being produced, as in the post-absorptive state (or diabetes mellitus) the rate of acetyl CoA formation can exceed the capacity of the liver to utilize it via the citric acid cycle. The acetyl CoA is then converted to ketone bodies (Fig. 9.13). Some of the ketone bodies are used for energy purposes in the liver, and the rest are liberated into the blood, taken up by other tissues and utilized via the citric acid cycle (after conversion to acetyl CoA). The ketone bodies are acetone, acetoacetate and β-hydroxybutyrate. The production of acetone during the fasting state accounts for the distinctive breath odour of fasting people and patients with IDDM (see Case 9.1: 5). Thus, the liver uses ketone bodies for energy production and ceases to use amino acids during the post-absorptive state, thereby sparing them for gluconeogenesis. Thus ketone body production is also a means of supplying extrahepatic tissues with fuel during fasting. Some ketone bodies are weak acids, i.e. acetoacetic acid and β-hydroxybutyric acid, and in pathological conditions such as diabetes mellitus, where there is excessive fat utilization, excessive ketone body production can result in severe acidosis (see Case 9.1: 5).

Thus in the post-absorptive state, fatty acids and ketone bodies are provided to tissues which can utilize them for energy during fasting, sparing the glucose for tissues such as the nervous system, which is dependent on it. The energy provided during the post-absorptive state by glycogenolysis and gluconeogenesis provides about 800 kcal/day, which is the equivalent of approximately 180 g glucose/day. However, the average adult needs between 2000 and 3000 kcal/day. Thus, most energy is provided by substrates other than glucose (i.e. largely free fatty acids and ketone bodies). Most adults have enough energy stored in triacylglycerol in adipose tissue to supply sufficient fuel to enable them to survive without food for several weeks.

Diabetic ketosis and fluid and electrolyte disturbances

Diabetic ketoacidosis is the first presentation of IDDM in 20–30% of patients. In these individuals, insulin levels are usually below the levels of detection. Mortality from ketoacidosis is 2–5% in developed countries. Ketoacidosis can be precipitated in patients with IDDM by a number of factors, including infections, neglect of insulin medication, and myocardial infarction, but in many cases the precipitating factor is unknown.

Lipolysis increases in untreated IDDM. This is due to the absence of insulin, and the presence of elevated plasma glucagon, catecholamines, cortisol and growth hormone (see Case 9.1: 4). Increased lipolysis leads to increased production of ketone bodies (hyperketonaemia). The consequent high plasma concentrations of the keto acids, β-hydroxybutyrate and acetoacetate, cause metabolic acidosis. The increase in plasma H^+ ions results in stimulation of the rate of breathing which partially readjusts the blood pH (see the companion volume *The Respiratory System*). The kidneys are also involved in compensatory adjustments for acidosis by excreting H^+ ions (see the companion volume *The Renal System*). In untreated clinical ketoacidosis, these compensatory mechanisms are not sufficient to maintain the pH within the normal physiological range (i.e., 7.25–7.45).

In ketoacidosis, ketones as well as glucose are lost in the urine as the threshold for reabsorption in the kidney proximal tubules is exceeded. The presence of these solutes in the urine causes an osmotic diuresis (polyuria). The increased flow of urine causes dehydration and thirst (polydipsia), which are exacerbated by increased water loss via the lungs (as a consequence of hyperventilation). Although vasopressin (ADH), the hormone which stimulates water reabsorption, is released from the posterior pituitary in response to the increased osmolarity of the blood and the reduced blood volume, the osmotic diuretic effect prevails.

Furthermore, the increased level of glucose and ketone bodies in the plasma causes water to pass out of the cells of the body, down the osmotic gradient, into the plasma. This helps to maintain the plasma volume. However, as the polyuria causes the plasma volume to become more severely decreased, renal perfusion declines. This results in further elevation of plasma glucose.

In ketoacidosis the plasma Na^+ concentration is usually normal or low. This is partly because of the osmotic effect of plasma glucose drawing water out of the cells, but also because the hormone aldosterone is released from the adrenal cortex into the blood, in response to the reduced extracellular fluid volume. This hormone decreases Na^+ excretion by increasing its reabsorption in the kidney tubules, and opposes the effect of decreased insulin and elevated glucagon.

Total body K^+ also falls in diabetic ketoacidosis. Insulin normally increases K^+ uptake into cells (see above), and when the plasma concentration of insulin is low, the plasma concentration of K^+ increases. A net loss of K^+ from cells of the body occurs in ketoacidosis as intracellular K^+ is exchanged for H^+ from the blood, and K^+ is consequently lost in the urine. Treatment of ketoacidosis involves administration of insulin, fluid and electrolytes.

The causes of some of the symptoms in individuals with ketoacidosis are not entirely clear. The weight loss is partly due to loss of fluid in the urine, and partly to loss of muscle and adipose tissue mass, as a consequence of increased proteolysis and lipolysis, respectively. The mental confusion and coma are partly attributable to the acidosis and dehydration, but other factors such as cerebral hypoxia, are probably also involved. The cause of the abdominal discomfort and vomiting is unclear.

Control of the post-absorptive state

The onset of the pattern of metabolism in the post-absorptive state is due to both the decline in insulin concentration in the plasma and the increase in the concentrations of a number of other hormones. These hormones include adrenaline, glucagon, cortisol, growth hormone, TSH and ACTH. They are all released either directly or indirectly, in response to low blood glucose.

When the blood glucose concentration falls, the main stimulus for insulin release is removed and the insulin concentration falls. Thus, the major stimulus for glucose uptake into tissues and for synthesis of energy stores is abolished. The inhibitory effect of insulin on glycogenolysis and lipolysis is also abolished. Thus, the pattern of metabolism occurring in the absorptive state is effectively suppressed. The pattern of metabolism in untreated IDDM resembles the post-absorptive state (see Case 9.1: 4).

The overall effect of the hormones that control metabolism in the post-absorptive state is to increase plasma levels of glucose, by inhibiting glucose uptake in tissues, and by stimulating glycogenolysis and gluconeogenesis. They also stimulate processes that lead to the provision of alternative energy substrates. Thus, they promote both glucose-supplying reactions and glucose-sparing reactions. These effects are summarized in Figures 9.14 and 9.15. Thus, the effects of this group of hormones oppose the actions of insulin and facilitate the post-absorptive state. The plasma concentrations of many of these hormones are also increased in IDDM (see Case 9.1: 4).

Release of hormones in the post-absorptive state

Adrenaline is released from the adrenal medulla by activity in the preganglionic sympathetic nerves that innervate it. Sympathetic nerves are stimulated by low blood

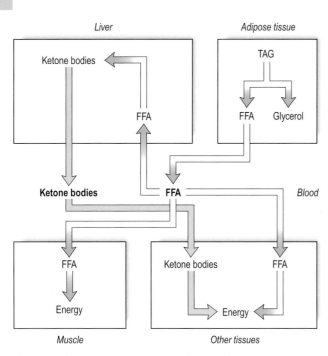

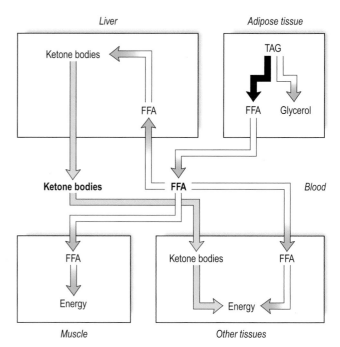

Fig. 9.13 Glucose-sparing reactions in the post-absorptive state. TAG, triacylglycerol; FFA, free fatty acids

Fig. 9.15 Effect of hormones on glucose-sparing reactions in the post-absorptive state. The bold arrow indicates the stimulation of lipolysis by adrenaline, glucagon and growth hormone in the post-absorptive state. The effect of cortisol on lipolysis is permissive.

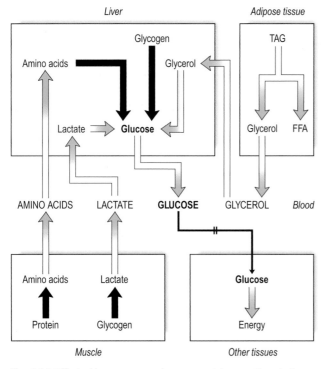

Fig. 9.14 Effect of hormones on glucose-supplying reactions in the post-absorptive state. The bold arrows indicate the pathways that are stimulated, and the crossed arrow indicates inhibition of glucose uptake by cortisol and growth hormone. In liver, glycogenolysis is stimulated by adrenaline and glucagon and gluconeogenesis from amino acids is stimulated by glucagon and cortisol. In muscle glycogenolysis is stimulated by adrenaline.

glucose. For this reason, low blood glucose precipitates the symptoms associated with activation of the sympathetic nervous system, such as an increase in anxiety levels and palpitations. Many individuals experience these symptoms in the late afternoon when the blood sugar concentration tends to be low.

Glucagon is produced by the α-cells of the islets of Langerhans. Its release is regulated by the concentration of plasma glucose. Low plasma glucose stimulates glucagon release and high blood glucose inhibits it. Thus, blood glucagon concentrations are high during the post-absorptive period. The release of growth hormone from the pituitary is also stimulated by low blood glucose. This is possibly due to activation of glucoreceptors in the hypothalamus, which results in the release of growth hormone releasing factor (GHRF) that, in turn, acts on the pituitary to stimulate the release of growth hormone. An increase in plasma glucose inhibits growth hormone release. Other pituitary hormones are also secreted in response to low blood glucose via an effect on the hypothalamus to cause secretion of releasing factors which act on the pituitary cells to stimulate the secretion of the hormones. Thus, low blood glucose causes the release of corticotrophin releasing factor (CRF) from the hypothalamus. This in turn stimulates the release of ACTH from the pituitary. Thus ACTH is increased in the blood during the post-absorptive state. ACTH in turn causes the release of hormones such as cortisol from the adrenal cortex. Table 9.1 lists some of the hormones that are released in the post-absorptive state, in response to low blood glucose.

Table 9.1 Hormones secreted in the post-absorptive state

Hormone	Origin
Glucagon	α-cells of the pancreas
Adrenaline	Adrenal medulla
Cortisol	Adrenal cortex
Growth hormone	Anterior pituitary
Adrenocorticotropin (ACTH)	Anterior pituitary
Thyroid stimulating hormone (TSH)	Anterior pituitary

The hormones listed are collectively responsible for the pattern of energy metabolism that pertains in the post-absorptive state. They are all secreted either directly, or indirectly, in response to low blood glucose.

Table 9.2 Control of the post-absorptive state

Effect	Adrenaline	Glucagon	Growth hormone	Cortisol
Plasma glucose	↑	↑	↑	↑
Glucose uptake			↓	↓
Glyco-genolysis	↑	↑		
Gluco-neogenesis		↑		↑
Plasma FFA (Lipolysis)	↑	↑	↑	↑

Effects of some of the hormones, released in the post-absorptive state on aspects of energy metabolism, which result in either increases in blood glucose, or the provision of energy substrates (FFA, free fatty acids) that spare glucose for the tissues dependent on it for their energy requirements.

Actions of hormones in the post-absorptive state

Effects on glucose-supplying reactions

The effects of hormones on glucose-supplying metabolic pathways in the post-absorptive state are shown in Figure 9.14. Growth hormone and cortisol inhibit the uptake of glucose by reducing the number of GLUT4 transporters in the cell membrane. For this reason, patients with growth hormone producing tumours can develop diabetes. Moreover, in diabetic animals, removal of the pituitary, which secretes growth hormone, reduces the severity of diabetes.

Adrenaline and glucagon stimulate glycogen breakdown to glucose in liver, with the liberation of glucose into the blood. In addition, adrenaline, but not glucagon, stimulates glycogen breakdown to lactate and pyruvate, in muscle. These products are released into the blood, taken up by the liver, and converted to glucose via gluconeogenesis, and the glucose is then released into the blood. The action of these hormones on glycogen breakdown is via stimulation of the rate-limiting step that is catalysed by phosphorylase. This increases the concentration of cAMP that activates a kinase, which in turn activates phosphorylase kinase, leading to activation of phosphorylase itself (Fig. 9.9). In addition, cortisol also stimulates glucose-6-phosphatase resulting in increased release of glucose into the blood. Furthermore, glucagon and cortisol stimulate gluconeogenesis from amino acids in liver. Cortisol also stimulates the breakdown of protein to amino acids in liver.

Effects on glucose-sparing reactions

Figure 9.15 shows the effects of hormones on glucose-sparing metabolic pathways in the post-absorptive state. Adrenaline, glucagon and growth hormone stimulate lipolysis in adipose tissue, thereby increasing the free fatty acid concentration in the plasma. Cortisol has a permissive effect on lipolysis, i.e. it has no effect by itself but it potentiates the effects of adrenaline, glucagon and growth hormone. The sympathetic nerves to adipose tissue are also stimulated by low blood glucose. These nerves release mainly noradrenaline that, like adrenaline, increases lipolysis in adipose tissue. The effects of adrenaline and noradrenaline are exerted on the rate-limiting step in the lipolysis pathway, i.e. the hydrolysis of triacylglycerol to diacylglycerol and free fatty acid, which is catalysed by the 'hormone-sensitive' lipase. The effect of these hormones involves an increase in the intracellular concentration of cAMP that triggers an intracellular cascade of reactions (Fig. 9.15) similar to that seen for the activation of phosphorylase (see above). The subsequent hydrolysis of diacylglycerol to monoacylglycerol and free fatty acid, and of monoacylglycerol to glycerol and free fatty acid, by other lipases, is extremely rapid. Table 9.2 summarizes the effects of hormones to control glucose-supplying and glucose-sparing reactions in the post-absorptive state.

THE COLON

10

Chapter objectives

After studying this chapter you should be able to:

1. Understand the functioning of the large intestine.

2. Understand the consequences of disease of the large intestine.

Introduction

The colon is the last 150cm or so of the gastrointestinal tract. It is a tube of approximately 6cm in diameter that extends from the ileum to the anus. Its main function is to store faecal material, and regulate its release into the external environment. It also absorbs water and electrolytes from the chyme, with the result that the faecal material becomes more solid as it passes through the colon. In addition it produces a thick mucinous secretion, which lubricates the passage of the faecal material through it. It also provides an environment for bacteria, some of which synthesize an important part of the vitamin requirement of the body.

Disease of the colon can result in diarrhoea, or constipation, or both. In this chapter, Hirschsprung's disease will be used to illustrate the importance of the motor function of the colon. It is a condition in which there is an absence of intramural ganglion cells from the wall of the colon, usually in a distal region (Case 10.1: 1).

Anatomy

The arrangement of the large intestine and its associated structures is shown in Figure 10.1. It can be divided into various regions: the caecum, the ascending colon, the transverse colon, the descending colon, the sigmoid colon and the rectum. The rectum is the portion beyond the sigmoid colon. The lumen of the colon becomes narrower towards the rectum. The lumen of the rectum, which is wider, provides a reservoir for faecal material, prior to defecation.

The caecum forms a blind-ended pouch below the junctions of the small intestine and the large intestine. The appendix is a small finger-like projection from the end of the caecum. It has no known function in the human. It has a thick wall, and a very narrow lumen that often collects debris.

In the large intestine, the outer longitudinal smooth muscle layer is arranged in three prominent bands, known as taeniae coli. These bands are shorter than the other coats of the colon. There is also a segmental thickening of the circular smooth muscle. Together these features impart a sacculated appearance to the organ. It has no villi (only projections). Its coat is therefore smoother than that of the small intestine, and the consequence of this is that the surface area of the colon is only one-thirtieth that of the small intestine.

The anal canal is the terminal portion of the rectum. It begins at a region where the rectum suddenly becomes narrower. The surface of the upper portion of the anal canal exhibits a number of vertical folds, known as anal (or rectal) columns (Fig. 10.2). These folds are relatively more pronounced in children than in adults. The depressions between the anal columns are known as anal sinuses. The sinuses end abruptly at the lower ends of the columns (the dentate line) where there are small crescent-shaped folds of mucosa oriented around the

Case 10.1 Hirschsprung's disease: 1

A newborn infant was observed to have a distended abdomen. He had passed very little meconium in the 2 days since he had been born. The doctor examined the infant's rectum by inserting a finger. The examination revealed that the rectum was empty. However, when the doctor withdrew her finger, there was a gush of meconium, and decompression of the abdomen. The obstruction reoccurred within a day or so. By this time, the child had started to vomit excessively. The symptoms were relieved by an enema. A biopsy of the rectum was performed and Hirschsprung's disease was diagnosed. An abdominal operation was arranged. The surgeon removed the distal large bowel and sutured the remaining colon to the lower rectum. The child made a good recovery, and his symptoms disappeared.

After examining the details of this case, the following questions arise:

- Why was the infant's abdomen distended, and why had he passed no meconium since he was born?
- What is the defect in this condition, and what causes it? What did the biopsy reveal?
- Why was it necessary to resect a segment of the infant's intestine?
- How does this abnormality affect motility in the colon?
- How does the abnormality affect defecation?

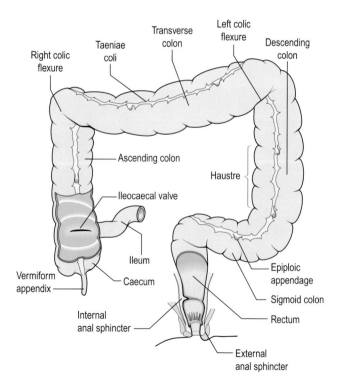

Fig. 10.1 Anatomical features of the large intestine.

wall. These folds are termed anal valves. The anal canal is surrounded by sphincter muscle that controls the release of faecal material. The internal sphincter is a thickening of the circular layer of the muscularis externa. The external sphincter, which consists of several parts, is composed of striated muscle. The arrangement of the sphincters is shown in Figure 10.2.

Innervation

The ascending colon and most of the transverse colon are innervated by the parasympathetic vagus nerve. Beyond that the pelvic nerves innervate the colon. These are the sacral outflow of the parasympathetic nervous system. Figure 10.3 illustrates the extrinsic innervation of the large intestine. The cholinergic parasympathetic nerves synapse with neurones in the intramural plexi. They also synapse directly on the smooth muscle of the colon and the internal anal sphincter. Excitatory cholinergic neurones are also present in the ganglia of the submucosal and myenteric intramural plexi. In Hirschsprung's disease intramural ganglion cells are absent from the myenteric and submucosal plexi (Case 10.1: 2).

The colon is also innervated by adrenergic sympathetic nerves from the lower thoracic and upper lumbar segments of the spinal cord. These nerves synapse with inhibitory nerves in the intramural plexi. They also synapse directly with the smooth muscle of the colon and internal anal sphincter. The external anal sphincter is innervated by somatic motor fibres in the pudendal nerves. It is controlled both reflexly and voluntarily.

Contraction of the levator ani, an external skeletal muscle, constricts the lower end of the rectum. Contraction of another external skeletal muscle, the puborectal muscle that is attached to the external side of the wall of the anal canal, pulls the upper canal forward. This produces a sharp angle between the rectum and the anal canal, and prevents faeces from entering the anal canal, until defecation is initiated. The levator ani and the puborectal muscles are innervated by somatic motor fibres in the pudendal nerve.

Terminals of afferent sensory nerve fibres are present in the mucosa, submucosa and muscle layers of the colon. The colon is fairly insensitive to painful stimuli but it is very sensitive to changes in pressure. Stretching of the colon as a consequence of overdistension results in abdominal pain, but removal of lesions, such as polyps, from the lining of the colon can be achieved painlessly without anaesthetic. There is a profusion of sensory nerve fibres in the wall of the anal canal. Some of these are sensitive to touch, some to cold, some to pressure, and some to friction.

Histology

As in other regions of the gastrointestinal tract, the wall of the large intestine is composed of four layers: the mucosa, the muscularis externa, the submucosa and the serosa (Fig. 10.5A).

The mucosa contains numerous straight tubular glands that extend through the full thickness of the mucosa (Fig. 10.5B). The surface epithelium of the mucosa and glands consists of simple columnar epithelial cells. The predominant cell type is the columnar absorptive cell. This cell has a thin striated border on its apical surface. In many respects, it resembles the enterocytes of the small intestine. Its main function is to absorb ions and water. However, some nutrients are also absorbed, especially in

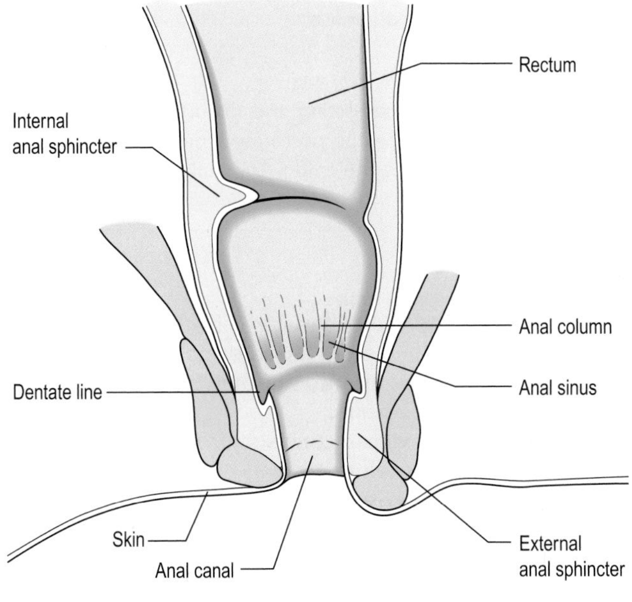

Fig. 10.2 Structure of the anal canal.

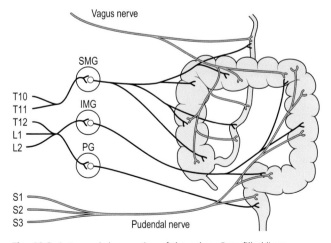

Fig. 10.3 Autonomic innervation of the colon. Grey-filled lines indicate parasympathetic nerves, and solid black lines indicate sympathetic nerves. T10, T11, T12, thoracic segments; L1, L2, lumbar segments; S1, S2, S3, sacral segments, of the spinal cord. SMG, superior mesenteric ganglion; IMG, inferior mesenteric ganglion; PG, pelvic ganglion.

Defect, diagnosis and treatment

Defect

Hirschsprung's disease, also known as congenital megacolon (enlarged abdomen), is a familial disease that affects one in 5000 live births. It is more common in males. There is an association with Down's syndrome. The genetic mechanism is not fully understood, but it involves multiple chromosomal deletions. A similar condition (acquired megacolon) can arise later in life, from a variety of causes (Fig. 10.4).

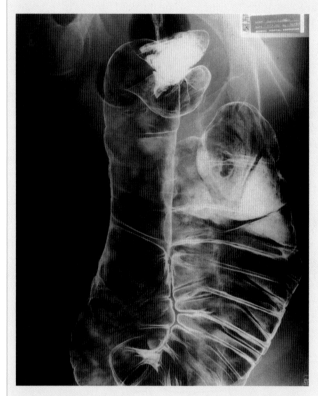

Fig. 10.4 An abdominal X-ray showing a grossly dilated colon filled with gas (megacolon). The mucosa has been coated with barium.

In Hirschsprung's disease, intramural ganglion cells are absent from the myenteric and submucosal plexi, usually in a segment of the distal colon. This is due to a defect in embryonic development, involving the arrest of the caudal migration from the neural crest, of the cells that are destined to become ganglion cells of the intramural plexi. Examination of biopsy specimens reveals an absence of ganglion cells from the affected segment. Excitatory and inhibitory neurones are missing. The segment involved is of variable length, in a region extending from the anal canal proximally up the colon. The lumen becomes narrowed in the aganglionic segment, due to tonic contraction of the smooth muscle. The passage of faecal material is obstructed at this narrowed segment and it accumulates in the region proximal to the aganglionic segment. Usually the normal reflex relaxation of the internal anal sphincter in response to distension of the rectum cannot be elicited in this condition. Because the aganglionic segment creates an obstruction to faecal flow, the proximal large bowel becomes chronically distended, giving rise to the name 'megacolon'.

Diagnosis

The normal reflex relaxation of the internal anal sphincter in response to distension of the rectum usually cannot be elicited in this condition.

A well-known finding in Hirschsprung's disease is an elevated level of acetylcholinesterase in the narrowed segment. This is indicative of an abnormality of the cholinergic innervation. Diagnosis of Hirschsprung's disease is by barium enema and biopsy showing an absence of ganglion cells. In cases where the diagnosis is unclear, a histological frozen section of the region can be stained for the enzyme to see if the levels are elevated, to aid the diagnosis.

Treatment

Surgery is effective in correcting the disturbance of motility. Various procedures can be performed, depending on the extent of involvement of the colon. They all involve removal of the aganglionic segment.

the proximal colon. There are also goblet cells. These are more numerous in the colon than in the small intestine. They produce mucus, which lubricates the intestine and coats the faecal material, which becomes increasingly more solid as it passes through the colon. This enables it to move along easily. There are also undifferentiated cells, and sparsely distributed APUD cells of various types that secrete hormones into the blood (see Ch. 1). The lamina propria, muscularis mucosa of the colon, and submucosa are similar in the small and large intestines. Nodules of lymphatic tissue are present in the mucosa, and these

usually extend into the submucosa. In the region of the junction between the rectum and the anal canal, the muscularis mucosa breaks up into bundles, and further down the anal canal it disappears.

The muscularis externa consists of circular and longitudinal layers of smooth muscle, as elsewhere in the gastrointestinal tract. However, in the large intestine (except for the rectum) the outer longitudinal layer appears to be incomplete. It is arranged in three bands, known as taeniae coli. However, between these bands there is actually a very thin sheet of longitudinal muscle. In the rectum,

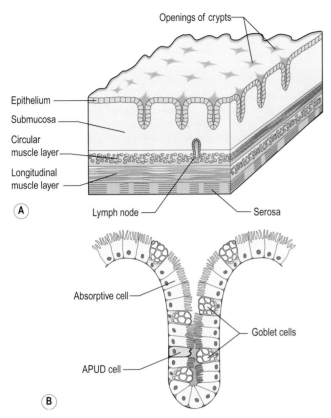

Fig. 10.5 Structure of the wall of the colon. (A) Layers present. (B) Cell types in the epithelium.

Labels: Openings of crypts, Epithelium, Submucosa, Circular muscle layer, Longitudinal muscle layer, Lymph node, Serosa, Absorptive cell, Goblet cells, APUD cell

the outer longitudinal muscle is a uniformly thick layer (as in the small intestine) and this presumably aids defecation. The inner layer of the muscularis externa consists of circular rings of smooth muscle, which allow effective peristalsis as is the case in the small intestine.

The submucosa is similar to that present elsewhere in the gastrointestinal tract. The outer layer is a typical serosa, except where it is in direct contact with other structures (as on much of its posterior surface), when its outer layer is an adventitia.

Ulcerative colitis is a fairly common disease of the large intestine which usually starts in the rectum, and may extend proximally. It is an inflammatory condition where the mucosa becomes ulcerated (Case 10.2: 1 and 2).

Appendix

The appendix is a narrow, tube-like structure. Its wall resembles that of the colon, except that it has a complete layer of outer longitudinal muscle, and numerous lymph nodules, in the mucosa and submucosa, which disrupt the muscularis mucosa, giving it the appearance of isolated lengths of smooth muscle. The appendix is the commonest source of intra-abdominal sepsis (appendicitis). This condition can be life-threatening if the appendix ruptures, thereby allowing the sepsis to spread within the peritoneal cavity (peritonitis). This occurs when the appendix

becomes obstructed. An abscess forms within it, resulting in a secondary inflammatory process within the wall. This inflammation can result in thrombosis of the blood vessels (appendicular artery and vein) supplying it. The loss of blood supply leads to gangrene and perforation of the appendix. It is the absence of any secondary blood supply to the appendix (that could prevent gangrene) that makes appendicitis such a dangerous condition.

Anal canal

In the submucosa of the anal columns are the terminal ramifications of the superior rectal artery and veins. The numerous veins in this region are longitudinal, and thin-walled. They can become dilated and convoluted, to produce a condition known as haemorrhoids or piles.

Case 10.2 Ulcerative colitis: 1

A 22-year-old woman, who had, for the past 2 years, been experiencing intermittent attacks of diarrhoea and rectal bleeding, visited her general practitioner. She said each attack lasted for several weeks, but there was complete remission of the symptoms between attacks. During the attacks she experienced lower abdominal cramps and sometimes felt feverish. The general practitioner thought the symptoms could be explained by the presence of a number of different conditions, including infection, irritable bowel syndrome and ulcerative colitis, and she decided to send the patient to see a specialist. The patient was referred to an outpatient clinic, and subjected to sigmoidoscopy (direct visual examination of the rectum and distal sigmoid colon) and a radiographic examination of her abdomen. The provisional diagnosis of ulcerative colitis was made on the basis of the finding of inflamed and bleeding mucosa. A rectal biopsy specimen was taken during the procedure, and sent to the pathology laboratory to confirm the diagnosis. A blood sample was taken for determination of plasma electrolytes, blood haemoglobin and plasma albumen. The patient was prescribed aminosalicylate and corticosteroids, and these drugs ameliorated the symptoms of the disease within a week or so.

After studying this case history, we should consider the following questions:

- What would the sigmoidoscopy and radiography probably have shown?
- Why were the patient's plasma electrolytes determined?
- Why was the patient's haemoglobin determined?
- Why was the patient's plasma albumen concentration determined?
- What could be the cause of the diarrhoea, and frequent bowel movements?
- What is the rationale for treating this patient with corticosteroids?

THE COLON

THE DIGESTIVE SYSTEM   175

Defect, diagnosis and treatment

Defect

Ulcerative colitis is a fairly common condition in which the mucosa of the colon is ulcerated and diffusely inflamed (Fig. 10.6). It is the most common cause of bloody diarrhoea in the Western world. It affects both men and women and is most common in people aged 20–40 years. In many ways, the condition resembles Crohn's disease, although the latter more commonly affects the small intestine, while in ulcerative colitis, the distal colon and rectum are always affected.

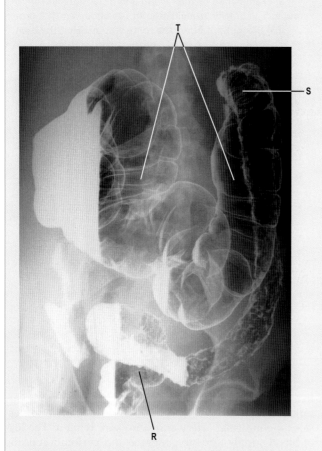

Fig. 10.6 Ulcerative colitis. An X-ray of the large bowel in which the mucosa has been coated with barium (a double contrast barium enema). The normal mucosal folds are seen in the transverse colon (T). The ulcerated mucosa extends from the splenic flexure (S), to the rectum (R).

Histological findings show that the inflammation is restricted to the mucosa and (to a lesser extent) the submucosa. Near the tips of the crypts are accumulations of polymorphonuclear cells (crypt abscesses). The epithelial cells in the crypts show evidence of degeneration (mucosal atrophy). Ulceration of the mucosa may also be evident. The aetiology of this disease is unknown, although it has been variously ascribed to infection, and to an abnormality of the immune system.

The damaged mucosa cannot absorb water and ions adequately, and this results in diarrhoea. Frequent bowel movements can result from large volumes of diarrhoea, but may also be due to colonic or rectal irritability in this condition.

Diagnosis

The patient's abdomen may be distended, but the anus is usually normal. At sigmoidoscopy, the mucosa of the colon would probably be seen to have a smooth, glistening pink surface. Radiography would show dilation of the colon, and may reveal an irregular mucosa, indicative of mucosal atrophy. It may also show foreshortening of the colon and loss of haustration. A barium enema may reveal fine ulceration.

The patient's plasma electrolytes were determined because loss of Na^+ and K^+ from the colon could lead to dehydration (reduced ECF), hyponatraemia and hypokalaemia. Loss of HCO_3^- could lead to metabolic acidosis. Her haemoglobin was determined because mucosal ulceration results in chronic loss of blood from the colon which can lead to iron-deficiency anaemia. Her plasma albumen concentration was determined because chronic protein losses from the colon can occur in this condition.

Treatment

This patient was treated with oral aminosalicylate. This is broken down to 5-aminosalicylate by bacteria in the colon. Its mode of action is presumed to be anti-inflammatory and it is usually effective in inducing remission. Corticosteroids (usually rectal prednisolone) also have a powerful anti-inflammatory action and are used in all types of inflammatory disease. They reduce the redness and swelling and also the degree of dilatation of blood vessels, thereby reducing fluid exudation. Their predominant effect is to reduce the inflammatory response to mucosal ulceration.

In severe cases, surgery is required to prevent perforation and secondary peritonitis. This usually involves an ileostomy, and removal of the colon and the rectum. Surgery for ulcerative colitis is curative because, unlike in Crohn's disease, the disease is limited to the large bowel.

The mucosa of the upper part of the anal canal is similar to that of the large intestine, with straight, tubular glands. Numerous goblet cells are found throughout the epithelium. In the region of the anal sinuses, are anal glands. Most of these extend into the submucosa, but some extend into the muscularis externa. They are branched, straight, tubular glands containing mucous cells. The duct of each gland consists of stratified columnar epithelium. It opens into the anal crypt, which is a small depression in the mucosa. If a duct becomes occluded, the glands can become infected, creating perianal abscesses. The epithelium of the lower portion of the anal canal is stratified squamous epithelium. In the intermediate zone between the simple columnar epithelium of the upper canal, and the stratified squamous epithelium of the lower region, there is a variable amount of stratified columnar epithelium. The stratified squamous epithelium of the lower area is continuous with that of the skin. In the skin of the circumanal region are large apocrine glands known as circumanal glands.

The key function of the anal canal is that performed by the sphincter, which comprises an internal (smooth muscle) ring and an outer (striated muscle) ring. This sphincter, which is under both autonomic and somatic nerve control, enables defecation to occur (see below).

Functions

Secretion

The large intestine secretes a thick mucinous secretion, with a high content of K^+ and HCO_3^- ions. The electrical potential across the mucosa, set-up by the entry of Na^+ into the cell (see below) is partly responsible for driving the transport of K^+ ions into the lumen, through the tight junctions. Other, as yet unclear, mechanisms may also be involved in the secretion of K^+ ions in the colon. HCO_3^- ions are secreted in exchange for Cl^- ions (Fig. 10.7).

Secretion of the colon is stimulated by distension, and by mechanical irritation of the walls. Secretomotor neurones from the submucosal and myenteric nerve plexi stimulate secretion, probably via the release of acetylcholine and vasoactive intestinal peptide (VIP). Stimulation of the parasympathetic pelvic nerves also elicits secretion. This is directly via synapses on the epithelial cells, and indirectly via synapses with neurones in the intramural plexi. Stimulation of the sympathetic nerves suppresses secretion in the colon via adrenaline and somatostatin release. For this reason, somatostatin analogues can be administered to treat secretory diarrhoea (see Ch. 7).

Absorption and digestion

Ions and water

The absorption of ions and water occurs mainly in the proximal region of the colon. The net absorption of

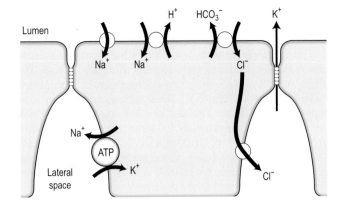

Fig. 10.7 Absorption and secretion of ions in the epithelial cell of the colon.

Na^+ and Cl^- occurs by mechanisms similar to those in the ileum. However, in the colon the transport of Na^+ across the luminal membrane occurs via an electrogenic Na^+ channel. This produces an electrical potential of about 30 mV (lumen negative) across the mucosa.

The electrical potential caused by Na^+ absorption, promotes the secretion of K^+ into the lumen (see above), but K^+ is also absorbed in the distal colon, where the transport is via exchange with H^+ ions. The latter is an active process, involving an anionic exchange mechanism similar to that for H^+/K^+ exchange in the stomach.

The absorption of water and ions is under both neural control via the enteric nerve plexi, and hormonal control. Aldosterone increases net water absorption in the colon by stimulating the synthesis of the electrogenic Na^+ channel in the luminal membrane of the epithelial cell, and increasing the number of Na^+,K^+-ATPase molecules in the basolateral membrane. Glucocorticoids also stimulate the transport of Na^+ ions by increasing the number of ATPase pumps (hence the fluid retention seen in patients taking prednisolone and other steroid medication), and angiotensin stimulates the absorption of water and Na^+ in the colon. Vasopressin (antidiuretic hormone, ADH) decreases water absorption.

In ulcerative colitis, the damaged mucosa cannot absorb ions and water adequately and this results in diarrhoea (Case 10.2: 2).

Products of bacterial action

The human body is composed of approximately 10^{14} cells, but only 10% of these are human cells. The rest are microbial cells that colonize the body surfaces and the gastrointestinal tract. The gastric acid of the stomach destroys most microflora, and the stomach and small intestines are only sparsely colonized by them. Most of the flora that colonize the gastrointestinal tract, reside in the large intestine. A large number of bacteria are lost in the faeces, and human faeces contain approximately 10^{11} bacteria/g. More than 99% of the bacteria in faeces are rod-shaped, non-sporing, anaerobes. Apart from anaerobic bacteria, lactobacilli and coliforms also colonize the large intestine. The colonic microflora population is so complex, that most of the bacteria are yet to be typed.

The bacteria in the large intestine synthesize certain vitamins that are required by the body. These are vitamins of the B complex, including thiamin, riboflavin, vitamin B_{12} and vitamin K. The synthesis of vitamin K is especially important because the average diet does not contain enough for normal blood clotting. In fact animals bred in germ-free conditions develop clotting defects. The vitamins are probably absorbed by passive diffusion in the large intestine. Vitamin K is fat-soluble, and therefore may be absorbed fairly readily. A small proportion of the synthesized vitamins may be refluxed into the small intestine, and absorbed in that region.

Intestinal bacteria also have digestive actions. Thus they convert primary bile acids to secondary bile acids, and deconjugate conjugated bile acids. The lipid solubility of these substances is greater than that of the primary bile acids, and a proportion of them are absorbed passively in the colon. Colonic bacteria also convert bilirubins to urobilinogens. The reactions involved are described in Chapter 6.

Absorption of drugs

Some drugs can be administered via the rectum. Thus anti-inflammatory drugs can be used in this way to treat the rectal mucosa in ulcerative colitis. However, this route can also be used for drugs that produce systemic effects. It is used following abdominal surgery, in patients suffering from vomiting, or who require analgesia. In such patients absorption from the small intestine can be unreliable.

Motility

The motor function of the large intestine serves both to mix the contents of the lumen, and to propel them towards the anus. The chyme entering the large intestine is semi-liquid, but water is absorbed from it, and the residual matter gradually becomes solid, as it passes along the colon. A major function of the distal large bowel (particularly the rectum) is to store faecal material. The passage of the luminal contents through the stomach and small intestine usually takes less than 12h, but the residue from a meal can remain in the large intestine for over a week. However, normally 80% has been extruded by the end of the 4th day. The expulsion of material from the colon is highly variable, being under both autonomic and somatic control.

Mixing

Mixing or kneading of the contents of the large intestine is due to contractions of the circular muscle. These contractions result in the formation and reformation of sacs, known as haustrae, and this type of segmental motility is known as haustration. The rectum is more active in segmental contractions than the colon.

Propulsion

Propulsion of material in the large intestine is affected by segmental propulsion, peristalsis and peristaltic mass movements.

Segmental propulsion involves sequential haustration. Several segments may contract simultaneously, propelling the contents along. Although this can result in the material being propelled in both directions, it is usually pushed in the caudad direction. Material is displaced through several haustrae, approximately every 30min.

Peristalsis involves waves of contraction which travel towards the anus, pushing the contents slowly along. At rest, these waves travel at approximately 5cm/h, but the speed increases to approximately 10cm/h after a meal. Peristaltic mass movements involve the simultaneous contraction of large segments of the ascending and transverse colon, which can propel the contents one-third to three-quarters of the length of the colon in a few seconds. There are also additional peristaltic movements in the descending colon that deliver the faecal material into the rectum.

Effect of food

Ingested material can affect motility in the large intestine in two ways. First, food that contains large amounts of indigestible material causes stimulation of mechanoreceptors in the walls of the colon, resulting in its rapid transit through the large intestine. This is how 'fibre' in the diet prevents constipation. Second, some substances (e.g. laxatives) stimulate chemoreceptors in the walls of the colon to stimulate motility.

Distension

The volume of faeces entering the colon can be increased if fibre is ingested. Fibre consists of polymeric substances such as cellulose, hemicelluloses, pectins, gums, mucilages, and lignins. Most of these are polysaccharides, although lignin is a phenyl propane polymer. These substances are found in bran, fruit and vegetables. Western diets are low in fibre compared with diets in many other parts of the world such as rural Africa, and the relative lack of fibre in the diet may account for the higher prevalence of many diseases of the large intestine in Western populations than in other populations.

These diseases include:

- Constipation
- Diverticular disease
- Haemorrhoids
- Polyps (adenomatous)
- Cancer of the colon
- Irritable colon.

Adding fibre to the diet prevents or remedies constipation, eases haemorrhoids, and relieves the symptoms of diverticular disease. It is interesting in this respect, that Seventh Day Adventists, living in the USA, who are predominantly vegetarian, have a very low incidence of cancer of the colon.

Adding fibre to the diet prevents constipation partly because it increases the bulk of the material entering the colon. This increases the stimulation of the smooth muscle, and decreases the transit time for the passage of material through the colon. Moreover, polysaccharides, such as cellulose, take up water and swell to form gels. This makes the faeces softer, and more easily moved through the colon and anus. Haemorrhoids are caused in constipated individuals who strain to defecate. Thus, dietary fibre relieves this condition, by reducing the need for straining during defecation. The reasons for the other beneficial effects of fibre are not clear. However, it is possible that constipation leads to the accumulation of carcinogens and other toxins that may cause cancer and inflammatory disease respectively. Thus adding fibre to the diet could (in theory) help to prevent these conditions developing, by preventing constipation, and diluting any toxins. Intestinal gas can also stimulate motility in the colon, mainly via causing distension. The gases that can be present include carbon dioxide, hydrogen, oxygen, methane and nitrogen. These gases do not smell. The odour associated with expelled gas is due to traces of other substances, such as ammonia, hydrogen sulphide, indole, skatole, short chain fatty acids and volatile amines. A normal individual releases approximately 500 mL of gas per day. The gases are partly swallowed air, but they can also be derived from substances in the food, or be produced in the lumen by neutralisation of gastric acid, or by bacterial fermentation processes. They can also arise via diffusion from the blood.

Laxatives

Some ingested substances stimulate motility in the colon via activation of chemoreceptors. An example of such a compound is senna bisacodyl. The increase in motility is mediated via the myenteric plexus. This plexus can be damaged by prolonged high doses of laxatives. Thus long-term use of these agents will reduce their efficacy.

Emotions

The effect of emotions on colonic motility has been studied in patients who have been provided with a colostomy. It has been shown that anger and resentment increase motility, whilst depression decreases it. The mechanisms involved are not clear, but they presumably involve autonomic nerves.

Control of motility in the colon

The smooth muscle cells of both the longitudinal layer and the circular layer exhibit spontaneously oscillating

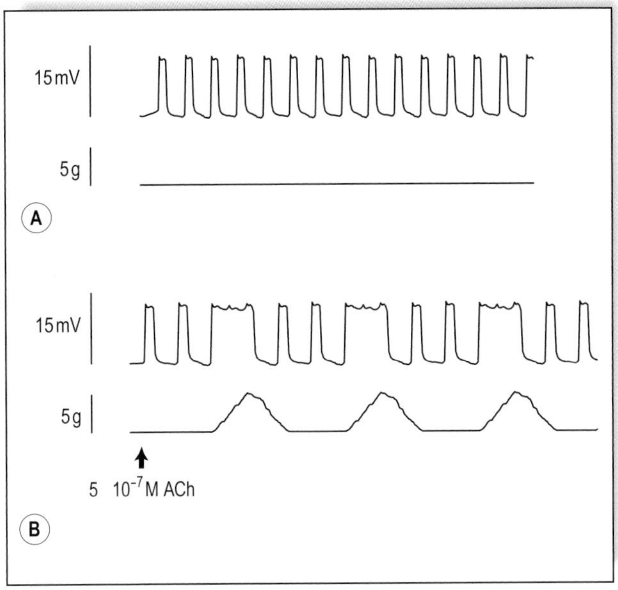

Fig. 10.8 Oscillating membrane potential (upper traces) and contractile activity (lower traces) in the circular smooth muscle of the colon. (A) Unstimulated muscle. (B) The effect of acetylcholine (ACh) (added at the arrow).

membrane potentials. In the longitudinal layer the amplitude of the oscillations sometimes reaches the threshold level for action potential generation, resulting in spontaneous contractions of the muscle. In the circular layer, however, contractions do not usually occur unless the muscle is stimulated by nerves, which release transmitters such as acetylcholine, in the vicinity of the pacemaker cells. Acetylcholine increases the time course of the slow wave oscillations, and these longer waves elicit contractions (Fig. 10.8).

Haustration and segmentation are occurring most of the time, although they are not perceived. However the frequency of these movements diminishes during sleep. They are spontaneous contractions that are modified by various factors, such as stretch that increases the strength of the contractions (see Ch. 1). Other factors that control colonic motility include extrinsic autonomic nerves, intrinsic nerves in the intramural nerve plexi and hormones.

Nervous control

Motility in the colon is controlled by intrinsic nerves of the intramural plexi and by extrinsic autonomic nerves. Figure 10.9 illustrates these pathways. Intrinsic nerves that release acetylcholine or substance P stimulate motility, and intrinsic nerves that release purines, VIP and nitric oxide (NO) inhibit it. The importance of the intrinsic nerve plexi to the normal functioning of the colon is illustrated by the problems that occur in Hirschsprung's disease (Case 10.1: 3) and Chagas disease (trypanosomiasis). Both conditions are characterized by an absence of intramural ganglion cells in a narrowed region of the colon.

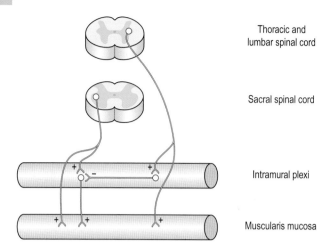

Thoracic and
lumbar spinal cord

Sacral spinal cord

Intramural plexi

Muscularis mucosa

Fig. 10.9 A simplified scheme for the control of motility in the colon.

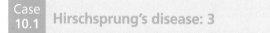

Case 10.1 Hirschsprung's disease: 3

Motility

The importance of the intramural nerves in the control of motility in the colon becomes clear from the symptoms of Hirschsprung's disease. Loss of the ganglionic cells from a segment of the large bowel disrupts the coordinated propulsive activity of the organ, leading to severe constipation. Both excitatory and inhibitory neurones are affected.

An absence of excitatory cholinergic ganglion cells prevents segmental contractions and coordinated propulsion from taking place. However, the parasympathetic cholinergic fibres from the sacral spinal cord innervate the muscle directly and their activity results in sustained contraction, because modification of the contractile activity by inhibitory interneurones in the plexi can no longer take place. (Furthermore, the adrenergic sympathetic nerve fibres can no longer act via inhibitory interneurones to augment the inhibition of the cholinergic nerves in the plexi.) Thus, effective relaxation of the circular muscle is lost. Moreover extrinsic sympathetic nerves also synapse directly on smooth muscle, and activation of the α-receptors on the smooth muscle cells by these nerves produces excitation and increased muscle tone. Thus both parasympathetic and sympathetic extrinsic influences lead to sustained tonic contraction of the smooth muscle in the aganglionic segment. The presence of the contracted segment results in blockage of the colon.

Hirschsprung's disease is a congenital abnormality, while the defect in Chagas disease is due to trypanosome parasites (*Trypanosoma cruzi*) which infest the wall of the intestines. The parasites produce a toxin that destroys the intramural ganglion cells, leading to symptoms similar to those seen in Hirschsprung's disease.

Extrinsic autonomic nerves are also involved in the control of the colon. They synapse with neurones in the plexi to modulate the effects of the intrinsic innervation, and they innervate the smooth muscle directly. Stimulation of the parasympathetic nerves increases motility, both via the interneurones and via their direct action on the muscle. Stimulation of the sympathetic nerves inhibits motility via the interneurones in the plexi, but their direct action on the muscle causes increased contraction (Fig. 10.9). α-Adrenergic receptors are present at the synapses of sympathetic nerves, both in the plexi and on the muscle. The inhibitory interneurones in the plexi, which the sympathetic nerves synapse, are not adrenergic (see above).

Reflex control

Distension of some regions of the colon causes relaxation in other parts. This is the colono-colic reflex. In addition other regions of the gastrointestinal tract can reflexly influence colonic motility. Thus a marked increase in motility in the large intestine occurs three to four times a day due to the gastro-colic reflex. This reflex is a response to food in the stomach, and it usually coincides with the ileo-gastric reflex (see Ch. 7). The gastro-colic reflex depends on the parasympathetic innervation of the colon, but the hormones gastrin and cholecystokinin (CCK) may also be involved.

Defecation

Defecation (see fig. 10.10) is a reflex response to the sudden distension of the walls of the rectum resulting from mass movements in the colon moving the faecal material into it. The reflex response has four components:

- Increased activity in the sigmoid colon
- Distension of the rectum
- Reflex contraction of the rectum
- Relaxation of the internal and external anal sphincters (which are normally closed).

Figure 10.10 illustrates the process of defecation.

Control of defecation

The caudal extremity is under nervous control. Defecation is basically an intrinsic reflex mediated by impulses in the internal nerve plexi, which is reinforced by an autonomic reflex that is transmitted in the spinal cord. The reflex is integrated via the defecation centre in the sacral spinal cord. However, defecation is also influenced by signals from higher centres. Figure 10.11 illustrates the pathways involved in the neural control of defecation. When faeces enter the rectum, distension of the wall activates pressure receptors. These send afferent signals that spread through the myenteric plexus to initiate peristaltic waves in the descending and sigmoid regions of the colon, and the rectum. These waves of contraction force the faeces towards the anus. As the wave

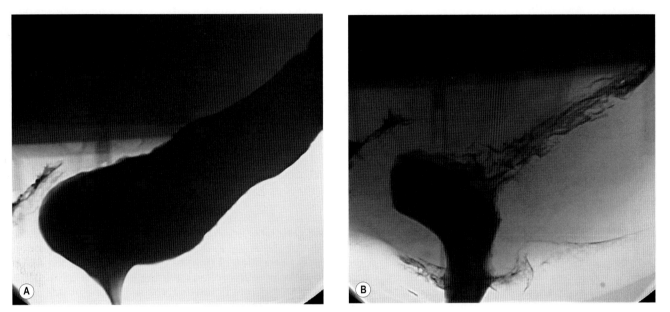

Fig. 10.10 An X-ray showing a rectum filled with contrast (barium) (A) before and (B) during contraction/defecation.

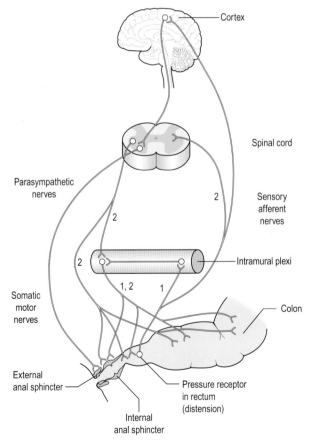

Fig. 10.11 A simplified scheme illustrating the neural control of defecation. The basic reflex operates via the intramural plexi, and the spinal parasympathetic reflex reinforces the basic reflex. Control is also exerted by the conscious brain. 1, components of the basic reflex; 2, components of the spinal sympathetic reflex.

Cortex

Spinal cord

Parasympathetic
nerves

2

Sensory
afferent
nerves

2

2

Intramural plexi

1, 2   1

Somatic
motor
nerves

Colon

External
anal sphincter

Pressure receptor
in rectum
(distension)

Internal
anal sphincter

Case
10.1

Hirschsprung's disease: 4

The defecation reflex

The loss of reflex inhibition of the internal anal sphincter in Hirschsprung's disease illustrates the importance of the intramural nerves in the reflex control of defecation. The innervation of the internal sphincter is defective in this condition and there is a fluctuating but continuous contraction of the sphincter (this process is sometimes referred to as 'sampling'). The normal relaxation response of the sphincter muscle to distension of the rectum does not occur. This is because its relaxation normally depends on the presence of inhibitory fibres in the intramural plexi. Hence secondary relaxation of the external sphincter does not occur and defecation does not occur.

The basic defecation reflex in response to distension of the rectum depends on the transmission of afferent impulses to the intramural nerve plexi, and efferent impulses from these plexi to the muscle of the rectum and internal anal sphincter, to cause reflex contraction of the rectum and relaxation of the internal anal sphincter. This basic reflex cannot be operational if the ganglion cells are absent. Moreover the anal sphincter is innervated directly by parasympathetic cholinergic and sympathetic α-adrenergic nerve fibres. The activity in the extrinsic nerves normally reinforces the basic reflex via synapses with neurones in the plexi. However in Hirschsprung's disease these influences cannot occur, and both the direct parasympathetic and the direct sympathetic innervation of the sphincter muscle cause contraction of the sphincter. In Hirschsprung's disease the sphincter remains contracted.

The response of the external anal sphincter is normal in Hirschsprung's disease as the somatic motor innervation is not affected.

approaches the anus, the sphincters are inhibited, and they relax. The external sphincter that is innervated by somatic motor nerves is under voluntary control. If the external sphincter is relaxed voluntarily when the faeces are pushed towards it, defecation will occur.

This intrinsic reflex is augmented by an autonomic reflex. This involves parasympathetic nerve fibres in the pelvic nerves arising from the sacral spinal cord, which innervate the terminal colon. Thus activation of pressure receptors by distension of the rectum sends afferent impulses to the spinal cord (as well as to nerves in the intramural plexi). This results in impulses being transmitted in the parasympathetic nerve fibres to the descending colon, the sigmoid colon and the rectum. The parasympathetic signals intensify the peristaltic waves, and augment the effect of the intrinsic neurones to cause increased motility, contraction of the rectum, and relaxation of the internal and external anal sphincters. Thus the parasympathetic reflex converts the weak intrinsic reflex to a powerful reflex. In Hirschsprung's disease the innervation of the internal anal sphincter is defective, resulting in loss of reflex inhibition of the sphincter (Case 10.1: 4).

The sacral control centre also coordinates the other effects which accompany defecation, including a deep inspiration, closure of the glottis, and contraction of the abdominal muscles, which forces the faeces downwards and extends the pelvic floor, so that it pulls outward on the anus to expel the faeces. The reflex normally initiates contraction of the external anal sphincter, which temporarily prevents defecation. The conscious mind then takes over, and either it inhibits the external sphincter to cause relaxation and allow defecation to occur, or it keeps it contracted it so that defecation is resisted. Pain inhibits relaxation, and this results in straining. If this becomes chronic it leads to dilation of the haemorrhoidal veins ('piles'), and may even prolapse the rectum through the anal canal. Interestingly rectal prolapse is also seen in weightlifters, in whom the process of repeated lifting requires straining against a contracted external sphincter.

The sensation of fullness of the rectum and the desire to defecate often follows the ingestion of a meal. If the urge to defecate is resisted, the sensation subsides, and the sphincters regain their normal tone. Therefore the reflex reactions to distension of the colon are transient.

The frequency of defecation, and the time of day when it is performed is a matter of habit. In two-thirds of healthy individuals it is between five and seven times a week.

In the human adult, approximately 150 g of material are eliminated per day. Of this 150 g, two-thirds are water and one-third is solids. The solids are normally mostly undigested cellulose, bacteria, cell debris, bile pigments and some salts. There is a high content of K^+ ions in the faeces, relative to the concentration in the fluid entering the colon, because K^+ is secreted by the walls of the colon. The brown colour of faeces is due to the presence of stercobilin and urobilin (see Ch. 6). The odour is caused mainly by traces of other substances, including products of bacterial fermentation (see above).

GASTROINTESTINAL PATHOLOGY

11

Chapter objectives

After studying this chapter you should be able to:

1. Provide an overview of gastrointestinal disease.

2. Give an insight into the relative clinical importance, in terms of incidence and clinical import, of the different disorders.

3. Explain the features of the more common disorders in terms of disruption of the normal function.

Introduction

Understanding normal body function is the foundation of clinical practice. In this book the normal anatomy, physiology and histopathology of the gastrointestinal tract has been applied to explain why different clinical conditions manifest their specific signs and symptoms. In the first 10 chapters, clinical examples of diseases have been selected to highlight specific aspects of physiological gastrointestinal function. The final chapter provides an overview of gastrointestinal pathology and its manifestations.

The diseases described in this chapter are addressed anatomically under the headings: the oral cavity, the oesophagus, the stomach, the duodenum, the pancreas, the liver and biliary tract, the small bowel and the large bowel. In addition to these sections, three other clinical areas are addressed separately. These are:

1. Cancer of the gastrointestinal tract, which is the commonest cause of death from digestive tract disorders.

2. Abdominal pain, which is one of the most frequent causes of acute presentation to the health service.

3. Gastrointestinal surgery, which provides further insight into the functional importance of the components of the digestive tract.

Gastrointestinal malignancy

In the Western world, malignancy of the gastrointestinal tract accounts for approximately 10% of all deaths and 40% of deaths from cancer. Effective and even curative treatment is available for these tumours if they are diagnosed at an early stage. For these reasons, malignancies of the gastrointestinal tract must be considered at an early stage in the diagnostic process for any patient presenting with gastrointestinal symptoms (Table 11.1).

A number of general factors will influence the clinician as to the likelihood of any symptom being due to an underlying malignancy:

- The age of the patient
- The duration of symptoms
- The progression of symptoms
- Identifiable aetiological factors
- A family history of malignancy.

Solid tumours, including gastrointestinal cancers, occur in patients with increasing frequency with advancing years. They are rarely diagnosed in patients under the age of 50 years, but thereafter rapidly increase in frequency into the seventh decade of life. Symptoms may start in an insidious fashion, but often progress over a period of weeks or months. This is in contrast to acute infection, which often has a sudden onset of symptoms, or chronic inflammatory conditions, which commonly display periods of exacerbation and remission.

Table 11.1 Common gastrointestinal cancers

Site	Cases per annum (England and Wales)	Presenting symptoms
Large bowel	35 000	Alteration in bowel action
Stomach	10 000	Indigestion, epigastric pain
Pancreas	10 000	Jaundice, back pain, steatorrhoea
Oesophagus	8000	Regurgitation, difficulty in swallowing (dysphagia)
Liver (hepatoma)	500	Features of chronic liver disease. A history of alcohol abuse or hepatitis

Some 40% of all deaths from cancer in the Western world are attributable to gastrointestinal malignancy. Most early symptoms are due to the abnormal function of the organ.

Environmental factors may also alert the clinician to the underlying diagnosis. Thus, a history of prolonged alcohol intake and chronic liver disease can alert the clinician to the possibility of a primary liver tumour (hepatoma).

The importance of dietary intake in causing gastrointestinal malignancies has long been recognized. In the Indian subcontinent chewing beetle nut is known to predispose to oral cancer, ingestion of pickles and salted fish in Japan is associated with an increased incidence of gastric cancer, and the high animal fat, low roughage diet of the Western world predisposes to colorectal cancer. More recently it has been recognized that many gastrointestinal malignancies develop because of an underlying inherited genetic predisposition.

Genetic predisposition may influence up to one-third of all colorectal cancer. In patients who are already predisposed to an inherited colorectal tumour, the tumours will tend to occur at an earlier age than in the general population. In addition, the tumours may be multiple because the predisposition affects all the cells in the large bowel mucosa. A clinical history from the patient may reveal first-degree relatives affected by the same tumour, because they are usually inherited in an autosomal dominant fashion. The genetic defects that have led to the predisposition pertain to fundamental cellular functions. It is usual for these patients to be at risk of developing more then one type of tumour, and so a history of several different tumours in the same patient would also lead to the suspicion of an underlying inherited predisposition.

The most common tumours of the gastrointestinal tract affect its mucosal lining. These cells are presumed to be most at risk because of their high rate of proliferation. Moreover, these cells are constantly subjected to injury by ingested carcinogens. By comparison, tumours of the muscle wall, connective tissue, lymphatics or serosal surface of the bowel (peritoneum) are rare. The vast majority of gastrointestinal tumours are tumours of the glandular structures (adenocarcinomas), that develop from the glandular cells of the mucosal lining of the gastrointestinal tract. In the clinical setting, if a metastatic tumour deposit is identified, histological features of an adenocarcinoma would alert the clinician to look for a primary tumour in the digestive tract.

Symptoms of gastrointestinal malignancy

It is helpful to categorize symptoms of malignant disease into three groups:

- Symptoms due to primary disease
- Symptoms due to secondary disease
- Symptoms due to non-metastatic manifestations of malignancy.

Primary disease

The symptoms of malignant disease of the gastrointestinal tract will depend upon the site and function of the part of the gastrointestinal tract that is affected. Carcinoma of the oesophagus will usually present with difficulty in swallowing (dysphagia), whereas adenocarcinoma of the colon will usually manifest with symptoms of a change of bowel habit. In addition to symptoms of disordered function, the site of the pain may also help to localize the tumour. Pancreatic adenocarcinoma often presents with back pain because of the retroperineal position of the pancreas, where a tumour of the liver may be associated with pain in the right side of the upper abdomen because of a localized inflammatory response in the overlying peritoneum (Fig. 11.1).

Secondary disease

One of the features of malignancy is the ability of the tumour to spread from the site of primary disease. This spread may occur via the lymphatics, the bloodstream or through the peritoneal cavity (transcoelomic spread). The lymphatic drainage follows its arterial blood supply. Consequently, tumours of the stomach, small bowel or large bowel can spread via the lymphatics to the root of the coeliac artery, superior mesenteric artery, and inferior mesenteric artery respectively. As these lymph nodes are deep inside the abdominal cavity such spread is often initially undetected. The tumour may spread further up the thoracic chain and manifest as a swelling in the supraclavicular lymph nodes in the neck. Because the thoracic duct drains into the veins on the left side of the neck, an enlarged lymph node in the left supraclavicular region is always suspicious of lymphatic spread from an underlying gastrointestinal malignancy.

The venous drainage from the gastrointestinal tract is via the portal vein to the liver. For this reason gastrointestinal malignancies commonly develop blood-borne metastases

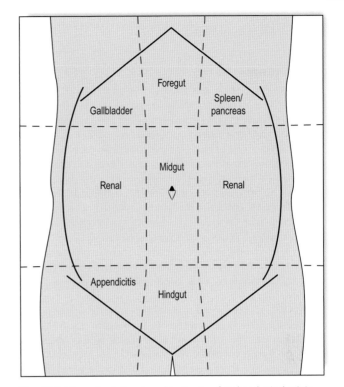

Fig. 11.1 Visceral pain is referred to its site of embryological origin. Parietal pain is more localized and is derived from inflammation of the overlying parietal peritoneum. The pointing pain in the right iliac fossa in appendicitis is typical of parietal pain.

in the liver. Abdominal examination may reveal enlargement of the liver in the right sub-costal region and affected individuals may occasionally present with symptoms of pain or jaundice.

Non-metastatic manifestations of malignancy

Malignancy, particularly in its advanced stages, is associated with an increased metabolic rate. This is due in part to the rapid cell division and tumour growth, and also due to secreted proteins released from the tumour. This catabolic state results in loss of body weight and, in its advanced stages, visible loss of muscle mass. This can occur in the presence of a normal dietary intake, and is one of the most common non-metastatic manifestations of malignancy. A further common finding is anaemia, due to bone marrow suppression. Because gastrointestinal malignancies usually disrupt the epithelial lining, which protects the gastrointestinal tract from injury, blood loss from the gastrointestinal tract is also common. The blood loss may be chronic and is often not clinically apparent. As the iron stores are depleted, red blood corpuscle maturation becomes impaired. An iron-deficient anaemia develops, in which the red blood cells are smaller (microcytic) and contain a reduced haem component (hypochromic).

Colorectal cancer: 1

Colon cancer

A 60-year-old woman presented to her general practitioner (GP) because of gastrointestinal symptoms. On direct questioning she said that the frequency of her bowel action had increased over the preceding weeks. In addition she had noticed some traces of blood in her stool on two occasions. She also complained that the consistency of her stool had changed and that she had not passed a formed stool in the preceding 6 weeks. No other person in the family had suffered any recent gastrointestinal upset and she had not suffered similar symptoms in the past. On specific questioning, she informed her GP that her father had died from colorectal cancer.

On examination, the GP found the patient to be anaemic, and her clothes were loose, indicating she had recently lost weight. Examination of her abdomen revealed an enlarged liver.

The GP was concerned that she may have an underlying colonic cancer and referred her to the hospital for further investigation. The consultant arranged a barium enema and a CT (computerized tomography) scan of her liver. The barium enema revealed a narrowing in the colon consistent with a carcinoma. The CT scan of the liver revealed a single metastasis in the right lobe. The diagnosis was explained to the patient and arrangements were made for surgery. At operation a left hemicolectomy was performed. This involved removal of the sigmoid and descending colon with its blood supply, and subsequent anastomosis of the splenic flexure to the recto-sigmoid junction. In addition, the right lobe of the liver, containing the metastasis, was removed.

Following operation, the patient made a slow but steady recovery. She returned to a normal diet on the 6th postoperative day. She did not become jaundiced following her operation.

Common gastrointestinal malignancies

In the Western world over half of deaths are accounted for by diseases of the cardiovascular system. The next most frequent cause of death is that of malignancy, which accounts for approximately 40% of all deaths. Gastrointestinal malignancies account for over 30% of all deaths from cancer, some 60 000 deaths per annum in England and Wales alone. Unfortunately, although early tumours can often be cured by surgery, most patients present after the disease has spread and as a consequence, treatment is less likely to be curable. The reserves of function in the gastrointestinal tract are such that radical resection of large sections is still compatible with a full and active life.

Table 11.2 Oesophageal cancer

Symptom	Mechanism
Difficulty in swallowing (dysphagia)	The tumour may encase the oesophagus leading to narrowing or infiltration of the mucosal coat resulting in impaired motility
A history for many years of painful swallowing	It can develop following longstanding oesophagitis in the lower oesophagus
Weight loss	This may be due to alteration in diet secondary to difficulty in swallowing
Respiratory symptoms	Problems with swallowing will usually predate the development of metastatic disease. The patient may have symptoms from local infiltration of the organ such as the bronchi or trachea

Carcinoma of the oesophagus

Carcinoma of the oesophagus affects approximately 5/100 000 of the population per annum. Two-thirds of the tumours are squamous carcinomas and the rest are adenocarcinomas. This reflects the epithelial lining of the oesophagus, which is of squamous type. Adenocarcinomas are usually localized to the distal third of the oesophagus and probably develop from ectopic gastric mucosa.

The classical symptom is of difficulty in swallowing (dysphagia). The symptoms are slowly progressive, with patients describing difficulty in swallowing solids and often having altered their diet to compensate. Oesophageal tumours may enlarge into the lumen, but more often, will infiltrate diffusely along and around the oesophageal wall (Table 11.2). The tendency for these tumours to grow along the wall of the oesophagus makes complete surgical resection difficult. Furthermore, the lack of a serosal covering to the oesophagus enables direct extension of the tumour into the mediastinum. Involvement of the adjacent trachea and bronchi will result in respiratory problems. The oesophagus and rectum are the only two parts of the gastrointestinal tract that are not covered by a peritoneal coat, and tumours in these two locations commonly invade surrounding local structures. Spread into the lymphatic system may manifest with a palpable supraclavicular lymph node, and spread into the portal venous system results in the development of liver metastases. Because tumours of the oesophagus do not usually invade the lumen of the oesophagus, dysphagia is a late feature and as a consequence the tumour is rarely curable. Only 6% of patients survive for 5 years.

A number of aetiological factors are known to be associated with this tumour. The most frequent of these are heavy alcohol intake and smoking. These factors probably account for much of the variation in instance seen across

Colorectal cancer: 2

Treatment

Alteration in bowel habit is a common symptom of colonic cancer. It can be due to partial obstruction of the lumen of the large bowel or be the result of ulceration of the mucosal surface. Ulceration can also give rise to the symptoms of intermittent bleeding.

Colorectal cancer clusters in families in up to 20% of cases and so a family history of this disease is not uncommon in affected individuals. This is believed to be genetically determined, although the molecular basis in most families is not understood. Non-metastatic manifestations of gastrointestinal malignancies are more common in advanced disease and include weight loss and anaemia. The patient may have also been anaemic because of chronic gastrointestinal bleeding.

The GP was suspicious that the enlarged liver was due to metastatic disease, and in the light of the patient's large bowel symptoms the GP felt that a colorectal cancer was the most likely diagnosis. A double-contrast barium enema outlines the lining of the bowel, and infiltration by neoplasm creates a rigid narrowing that is easily visualized (Fig. 11.2). Computerized tomography is a useful way of defining abnormal areas of tissue in solid organs like the liver. The increased vascularity of metastatic tumours makes these easy to visualize on a CT scan (Fig. 11.3).

Surgical treatment required removal of the primary tumour, the draining lymph nodes, and the single metastasis in the liver. Because blood-borne metastases from colonic cancer preferentially spread to the liver, resection of these advanced tumours can still be curative for selected cases. It is important to exclude other sites of metastatic disease before undertaking such a procedure. The second most common site of spread from colonic tumours is the lung, which is why the chest X-ray was reviewed prior to surgery.

Normal bowel function following segmental resection of the colon would be expected. No impairment of liver function would be anticipated following a limited resection so jaundice or fat malabsorption would not be anticipated.

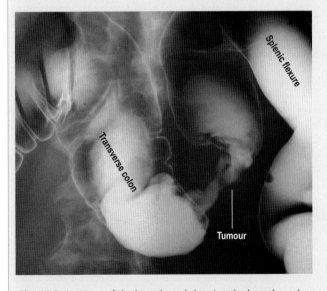

Fig. 11.2 An X-ray of the large bowel showing the large bowel lined with a coating of barium. A large tumour is visible at the splenic flexure. This encircles and narrows the lumen, creating the typical 'apple core' appearance.

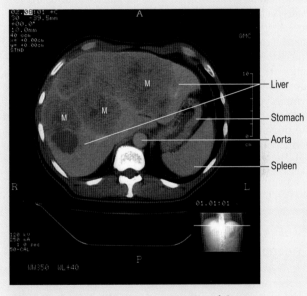

Fig. 11.3 A CT scan showing a cross-section of the upper abdomen. Multiple opacities are seen in the liver due to blood-borne metastases (M) from a primary colonic cancer.

different populations. A further interesting aetiological factor is that of acid reflux. Chronic oesophagitis associated with an incompetent gastro-oesophageal sphincter causes damage to the mucosa in the lower third of the oesophagus. This chronic injury appears to predispose to the development of adenocarcinoma in the lower third of the oesophagus. These different aetiological factors all result in a chronic injury to the oesophageal mucosa which over a period of time can lead to neoplastic change.

Gastric carcinoma

Gastric carcinoma (Table 11.3) is exceptional, in that its incidence has been in steady decline for the last 30 years, while other gastrointestinal tumours have increased in frequency with increased longevity. Despite this, it remains the third most common cause of death from gastrointestinal tumours in Western countries, and is a major health issue in Japan and Chile. Variation in populations

Table 11.3 Gastric cancer

Aetiology	The storage function of the stomach makes it particularly susceptible to ingested toxins and dietary factors that can contribute to malignant change
Symptoms	
Bleeding	Ulceration of the tumour results in exposure of the submucosal vessels
Abdominal distension	Gastric tumours often spread from the serosal surface of the stomach creating peritoneal metastases. Leakage of extracellular fluid occurs in association with these lesions and gives rise to ascites
Weight loss	This is more a feature of advanced disease in gastric cancer because the tumours do not usually prevent the passage of ingested food (unlike oesophageal cancer)

is believed to be due to local environmental, mainly dietary, factors. Recognized dietary factors include spiced foods, dietary nitrates, as well as smoking and alcohol. *Helicobacter pylori* infection, which is known to predispose to peptic ulcer disease, has also been implicated in gastric carcinomas. Conditions injurious to the gastric mucosa, such as pernicious anaemia and atrophic gastritis, are also associated with an increased incidence of subsequent neoplastic change. Symptoms due to the primary gastric tumour either arise as a consequence of ulceration of the mucosa, or from diffuse infiltration of the muscular wall. The ulcerating lesion has been classified as 'intestinal', whereas widespread infiltration of the muscle is classified as 'diffuse' type. Ulcerating tumours may present with pain from the injury to the mucosa, bleeding from erosion into underlying blood vessels, or peritonitis from perforation of the ulcer allowing gastric contents to leak into the peritoneal cavity. In contrast, diffuse gastric cancer often presents with a more insidious onset. The infiltrating nature of this tumour leads to a constricted stomach with a grossly thickened wall (lienitis plastica). The nature of diffuse-type cancer mitigates against successful surgical resection. Unfortunately many gastric cancers present at an advanced stage. Patients may have an enlarged liver and associated jaundice due to blood-borne metastases. The disease may spread through the stomach wall onto the peritoneum causing ascites. In these situations the tumour is incurable.

Tumours of the pancreas

In common with other gastrointestinal tumours, the majority of tumours of the pancreas are adenocarcinomas developing from the exocrine component of the organ. Because of the high concentration of endocrine cells in the pancreas, they are also the commonest site for endocrine tumours and account for 15% of pancreatic neoplasms. The site of the tumour in the pancreas and the nature of the cell type involved in the tumour will determine its presenting symptoms.

Adenocarcinomas often present with insidious symptoms of unexplained back pain and weight loss. Weight loss is particularly marked in pancreatic cancer, perhaps because of malabsorption compounding the catabolic effects of the tumour. The non-specific nature of these symptoms can delay diagnosis and as a consequence, these tumours are often unresectable. Tumours that involve the head of the pancreas may present earlier

---

Case 11.2 Adenocarcinoma of the pancreas: 1

Adenocarcinoma of the pancreas

A 70-year-old man presented to his GP with symptoms of vague upper abdominal pain, which he had noticed over the preceding weeks. From the clinical history, the doctor noted that the patient was a smoker. He suspected the symptoms may be due to peptic ulcer disease and prescribed a course of H$_2$ antagonists. The patient returned after 2 weeks without resolution of his symptoms. On this occasion, the patient declared that the pain had spread to his back. The doctor considered the symptoms may be due to gallstones and arranged an ultrasound scan of the gall bladder. The ultrasound scan confirmed stones in the gall bladder, but also suggested that there was a degree of dilatation of the common bile duct. The serum bilirubin level was checked and was found to be elevated. These findings suggested that there was an obstruction at the lower end of the common bile duct and the GP referred the patient to a gastroenterologist.

At the hospital, the patient underwent further investigations including blood glucose, CT scan of the upper abdomen including the pancreas, and endoscopic retrograde pancreatography (ERCP). His serum glucose was found to be mildly elevated, and the CT scan demonstrated a lesion in the head of the pancreas which was compressing the common bile duct. At ERCP, cytology brushings were taken from the pancreatic duct, which subsequently supported the diagnosis of adenocarcinoma at the head of the pancreas. During the same procedure, a short plastic tube (stent) was placed into the common bile duct to allow free drainage of bile from the liver.

Unfortunately, the tumour was found to be encasing the superior mesenteric artery and curative resection was not possible, as it would require division of the blood supply to the small bowel. Nonetheless, the patient's symptoms from obstructive jaundice were relieved with the stent and pain control was achieved by injection of the nerves in the coeliac plexus.

because of obstruction to the common bile duct. The commonest symptoms are progressive jaundice due to obstruction of the bile duct, and steatorrhoea due to obstruction of the pancreatic duct and malabsorption of fat. Some early tumours of the head of the pancreas may be curable with radical surgery. The rarer endocrine tumours of the pancreas will often present with symptoms due to hypersecretion of hormones. An insuloma or glucagonoma may present with hypoglycaemia or diabetes, respectively, whereas a gastrinoma will present with intractable peptic ulceration and diarrhoea (Zollinger–Ellison syndrome).

It has long been recognized that pancreatic cancer is associated with maturity-onset diabetes. It was believed that the injurious process that caused diabetes resulted in subsequent tumour development. However, more recent studies have shown that pancreatic adenocarcinomas may secrete an anti-insulin factor that can cause diabetes, and removal of the tumour can be associated with restoration of normal glucose control. This could provide a future mechanism for earlier diagnosis of this increasingly common condition.

Acute abdominal pain

Diagnosis of the cause of acute abdominal pain is one of the more challenging aspects of clinical medicine. Because of the lack of a somatic sensory nerve supply, identifying the diseased organ and the nature of the pathology requires a clear understanding of the anatomy, innervation and physiological function of the different gastrointestinal structures. There are two sources of intra-abdominal pain. Pain may arise from stimulation of the autonomic afferent nerves innervating the abdominal organs. This results in poorly localized abdominal discomfort that manifests

---

Case 11.2 Adenocarcinoma of the pancreas: 2

Treatment

Abdominal pain that is localized to the upper abdomen can be caused by any structure derived from the foregut. This would include conditions affecting the stomach, gall bladder, or pancreas. Pancreatic diseases may involve the coeliac plexus which lies in close proximity and results in pain that also radiates through to the back.

Investigation of the upper abdomen frequently identifies gallstones, but these are often asymptomatic and may not be the cause of the pain. The bile duct passes through the head of the pancreas before entering the duodenum, and as a consequence tumours in this area can compress the duct and obstruct the flow of bile from the liver. This results in (obstructive) jaundice. The bile duct and pancreatic duct can be visualized by endoscopy. The tissue of the pancreas is best demonstrated by a CT scan of the upper abdomen (see Fig. 4.6). At ERCP, cells that have been shed into the ducts can be sampled for microscopic evidence of neoplastic change (cytology). Because tumour tissue is generally friable this provides a useful method of diagnosis in less accessible tumours. A rigid plastic tube can be placed into the bile duct at endoscopy to relieve the obstruction (Fig. 11.4).

The superior mesenteric artery passes just posterior to the neck of the pancreas. This vessel supplies the whole of the midgut. It has to be preserved or the small bowel will be devascularized. If a tumour is involving this artery, surgical excision is impossible. Pain from advanced disease of the pancreas is often due to involvement of the nearby coeliac plexus of autonomic nerves. Injection of this region can safely obliterate the nerves and so help to reduce the pain.

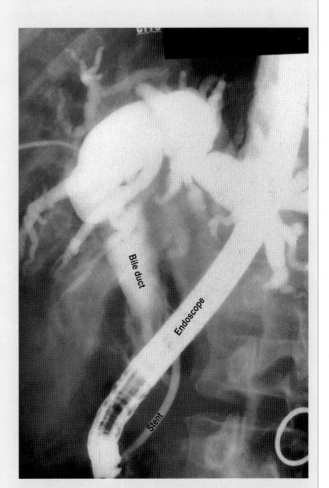

Fig. 11.4 A radio-opaque stent has been placed in the common bile duct using an endoscope, which has been passed via the stomach into the duodenum. The grossly dilated bile ducts have been made visible by the injection of contrast via the stent.

in the region of the corresponding somatic afferent nerve root. This is known as referred pain. Because the gastrointestinal tract is derived embryologically from a mid-line structure, pain is referred to the mid-line, usually anteriorly. This is typified by inflammation of the appendix, which derives its autonomic nerve supply from the level of T10 (along with the rest of the midgut). Pain is therefore referred to the peri-umbilical region, which is innervated by somatic sensory nerves that enter the spinal cord at the same level (T10). Pain from the large bowel also refers to the mid-line, but to the infra-umbilical region. Pain from foregut structures (stomach and duodenum) is referred to the central upper abdominal region (epigastrium, see Fig. 11.1).

The second type of abdominal pain is due to inflammation of the overlying parietal peritoneum. This has its own somatic innervation and, therefore, results in well-localized pain over the area of inflammation. This is referred to as peritonism. In the case of appendicitis, pain moves from the peri-umbilical region to the right lower abdomen region (right iliac fossa) once the inflammatory process in the appendix penetrates through the serosal surface resulting in secondary inflammation of the overlying parietal peritoneum (Fig. 11.1).

The speed of onset of the pain can also help determine the nature of the organ involved. Very muscular structures with a narrow lumen will quickly cause severe pain if they become acutely distended (such as the ureter). Thin-walled distensible structures will, however, give rise to a pain of more insidious onset (gall bladder). Pain due to distension is initially due to stimulation of stretch receptors. As a consequence, the pain is often cyclical in nature (colic). This contrasts with pain from inflammation of tissue, which gives rise to a persistent pain (such as pancreatitis).

Surgical resections

Most major surgical resections performed on the gastrointestinal tract are for the treatment of cancer. The fact that, following most procedures, patients are able to continue a normal and active life without nutritional support demonstrates the considerable amount of redundancy in the digestive system, and also its ability to adapt even after radical resections.

Major surgical resection of the oesophagus is undertaken for oesophageal carcinoma, when the disease is localized. Although this operation is rarely curative it provides remarkably good symptomatic relief from pain and obstruction, allowing the patient to return to a largely normal

---

Case 11.3 Acute appendicitis: 1

Case history

A 20-year-old man called out his GP complaining of severe lower abdominal pain. On enquiry, the patient described a pain that had started insidiously and was initially centred around his umbilicus. He had first noticed it when he got out of bed, but had thought nothing of it. When he arrived at work, the pain started to become more severe. He could not get comfortable and was unable to eat lunch. The pain shifted to the right lower abdomen and started to prevent him from walking. He returned home early and despite going to bed the pain persisted.

On examination, the GP found the patient to have pyrexia and a tachycardia. Palpation of his abdomen revealed tenderness localized to the right lower quadrant. The pain was made worse on releasing pressure (rebound tenderness). The GP also tested the patient's urine but found no evidence of protein or blood. He contacted the local hospital which admitted the patient and as his symptoms and signs had not improved, proceeded to arrange for him to undergo an appendectomy. At operation the small bowel and omentum were adherent to an inflamed, swollen, necrotic appendix. Postoperatively, the patient made a rapid recovery and was able to return home on the third postoperative day.

Case 11.3 Acute appendicitis: 2

Pathophysiology

The pain from the appendicitis often starts in the peri-umbilical region. As a midgut structure it derives an autonomic nerve supply from the level of T10, which is referred to the umbilicus. Once the inflammatory process in the wall of the appendix reaches the serosal surface, it causes secondary inflammation of the overlying peritoneum. This results in somatic pain, which becomes localized to the right iliac fossa. Any stretching of the peritoneum, which may be caused by movement or by palpation, will result in pain localizing to the right lower quadrant. This inflammatory process also produces reactive changes in the overlying structures such as the small bowel and omentum, which become adherent. The inflammatory exudate, which is seen at operation as a purulent fluid in the peritoneal cavity, contains large numbers of white blood cells. Patients commonly describe a loss of appetite. This is believed to be due to the triggering of the ileo-gastric reflex, which impairs gastric emptying. In addition there is a protective 'ileus', which reduces the peristaltic activity of the small bowel.

The appendix has an end artery supply, and inflammation through the wall of the appendix can easily result in thrombosis of the blood supply. This can cause gangrene in the wall and result in perforation of the appendix. Delaying the diagnosis and treatment of appendicitis is a common cause of peritonitis, because of perforation of the appendix wall. The doctor checked the patient's urine for evidence of a urinary tract infection which may have mimicked the symptoms of appendicitis. As there were no red blood cells or protein in the urine, a urinary tract infection was regarded as unlikely.

diet. Most tumours of the oesophagus involve the lower two-thirds. Removal of this portion of the oesophagus is possible. Restoration of continuity can be achieved by mobilization of the stomach, which is brought into the chest and connected to the remaining oesophagus in the upper thorax. This is possible because the blood supply of the stomach is so plentiful that the right gastric vessels can be divided and the blood supply sustained on the left gastric artery. If a more radical resection of the oesophagus is required then a length of small bowel can be placed in the chest to be joined from the throat to the stomach. This requires re-anastomosis of the arterial supply and venous drainage as the superior mesenteric vessels (supplying the small bowel) are insufficiently long to reach into the upper thorax.

Replacement of the oesophagus will result in loss of normal peristalsis and so the patient will need to sit upright when eating. In addition there will be impairment of the motility and storage capacity of the stomach because of division of the vagal nerves. This requires the patients to eat smaller and more frequent meals to sustain their nutrition. This minor lifestyle adaptation is usually all that is required.

Removal of the antrum and pylorus of the stomach can be undertaken for the complications of peptic ulcer disease and occasionally for carcinoma of the stomach. This portion of the stomach mucosa contains the majority of the gastrin-secreting G cells, and as a result, resection dramatically reduces acid secretion in the stomach. In addition, there is loss of the pyloric control of gastric emptying and reduced storage capacity. The stomach remnant can be reconnected to the proximal duodenum or the upper jejunum. This results in premature release of chyme from the stomach, in advance of the release of digestive juices from the gall bladder and pancreatic duct. The main consequence of this is impaired fat absorption and sometimes osmotic diarrhoea from incomplete digestion. Patients can usually control these symptoms by simple modification of their diet. The functional consequences of the loss of gastrin are not usually clinically apparent. An interesting, but relatively rare, complication of this operation is paradoxical hypoglycaemia following meals. The patient complains of symptoms of sweating and feeling faint soon after meals. This is due to inappropriate release of insulin from the pancreas in response to ingestion of food, but in advance of sufficient absorption of glucose from the gastrointestinal tract to counterbalance the insulin release.

Gastric carcinoma may require total gastrectomy in an attempt to cure the disease. In this case, the jejunum is brought up to connect with the oesophagus, and the distal (the fourth part of) duodenum is re-joined to the jejunum more distally (Fig. 11.5). This anatomical rearrangement is necessary because the alkaline secretions from the gall bladder and pancreas would cause severe ulceration of the unprotected oesophageal mucosa if allowed to come into direct contact with it. Loss of the whole stomach does significantly impair the storage capacity of the digestive tract. As a consequence, the patients must eat more frequent and smaller meals to maintain nutrition. Loss of acid secretion, pepsinogen and gastrin, all have surprisingly little effect

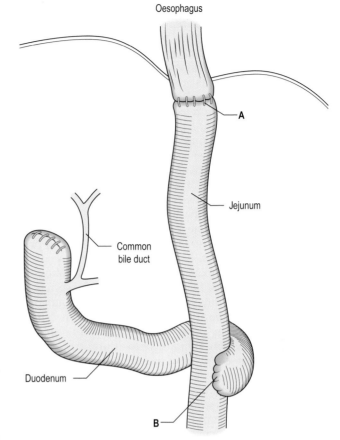

Fig. 11.5 The anatomical arrangement following a total gastrectomy usually performed for a carcinoma of the stomach. The proximal jejunum (A) is joined to the oesophagus. The bile and pancreatic juice is directed away from the oesophagus by rejoining the fourth part of the duodenum to the mid-jejunum (B).

on gastrointestinal function. However, loss of intrinsic factor does require replacement therapy by subcutaneous injection of vitamin B_{12}.

Removal of the gall bladder (cholecystectomy) is one of the most common abdominal procedures performed in the Western world. The gall bladder is removed by division of the cystic artery and cystic duct, but the common bile duct is left intact to enable free drainage of bile from the liver into the duodenum. Loss of the storage reservoir for bile salts results in adaptation of bile salt present in the liver. Following surgery, the bile is present in higher volumes from the liver and is released continuously into the duodenum at a slow rate. On ingestion of a fatty meal, liver bile release increases rapidly which compensates for the lack of a gall bladder, and patients are able to tolerate meals with even a high fat content. There is an interesting secondary effect from this operation and that is the increased rate of bile uptake from the ileum into the enterohepatic circulation. This results in a higher proportion of secondary bile acids because of the increased circulation of the bile. There is some evidence to suggest that this may have a potentially carcinogenic effect on the large bowel and there is an association with an increased incidence of colorectal cancer.

Resection of the pancreas is a technically challenging procedure carried out both for inflammatory diseases of the pancreas (pancreatitis) and also for pancreatic cancer. Most pancreatic tumours arise in the head of the pancreas. When they are diagnosed at an early stage they can be treated successfully by removal of the head and neck of the pancreas. Because the pancreas receives a joint blood supply with the duodenum, it is safer to remove the duodenum together with the head of the organ. This requires the common bile duct, tail of the pancreas, and stomach, to be re-joined with a loop of jejunum (Fig. 11.6). Safely joining the bowel to the pancreas is a hazardous procedure. This is partly because the tissue of the pancreas is soft and friable but also because activated digestive enzymes released from the pancreas interfere with the healing process at the anastomosis. Following this major procedure, patients will have impaired fat and protein metabolism. This is not usually due to insufficient pancreatic secretion, but rather to premature stomach emptying without coordinated secretion from the pancreas and liver. It can be partially overcome by preservation of the pyloric sphincter (pylorus-preserving Whipple's procedure).

Total pancreatectomy is in one respect a safer operation, because anastomosis to the remaining pancreas is not required. It does, however, involve loss of all endocrine and exocrine secretions from the pancreas. For satisfactory digestion of food, it is necessary to add pancreatic enzyme supplements to the diet. In addition, these patients are diabetic, and because there is loss of both insulin and glucagon, control of their diabetes is especially difficult, sometimes referred to as brittle diabetes.

Liver resection is being undertaken with increasing frequency, particularly for the treatment of metastases from colorectal cancer. Gastrointestinal tumours most commonly metastasize via the portal venous system to the liver, making this a common site for metastatic disease. The ability of the liver to cope with even major resections is remarkable. It is perfectly feasible to remove 75% of the liver and still retain normal function of the organ. This is in part due to its regenerative properties. These were recognized even by the Ancient Greeks. The God Prometheus was punished by Zeus, who ordered him to be tied to a rock and have an eagle eat his liver. Prometheus was said to have survived this repeated insult because of the regenerative capacity of the liver.

The redundant capacity of the small bowel and its ability to adapt, even after major resection, is similarly noteworthy. As a consequence, satisfactory digestive and absorptive capacity is present, even if 60% of the ileum and jejunum are removed. Nutritional support via intravenous feeding (parenteral nutrition) may be required if more then 75% of the ileum and jejunum are removed. This is an unusual situation and is usually only required after a vascular catastrophe when the blood supply from the superior mesenteric artery is lost, and the embryological midgut cannot survive on the collateral circulation from the coeliac and inferior mesenteric arteries. Following such a resection,

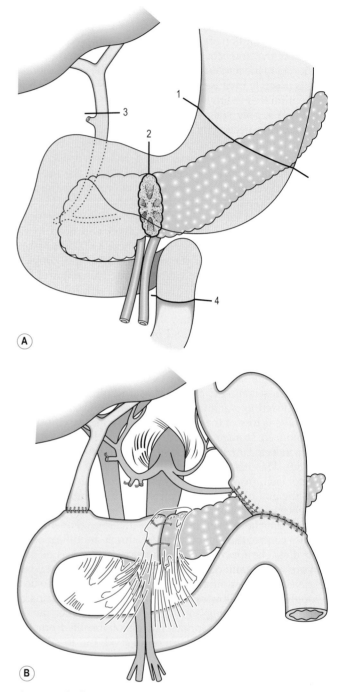

Fig. 11.6 The foregut anatomy (A) before and (B) after a partial pancreaticoduodenectomy (Whipple's resection). The stomach antrum is divided (1) along with the head of the pancreas (2) common bile duct (3) and the fourth part of the duodenum (4). The specimen is removed and the proximal jejunum joined to the stomach, bile duct and body of pancreas as shown. The operation is usually done for a carcinoma of the head of the pancreas.

there is insufficient residual digestive and absorptive function to sustain life. In addition, the patient will lose considerable quantities of fluid (up to 7 L/day), which also need to be replaced. It is possible to markedly reduce the secretion by the use of omeprazole (a proton pump inhibitor), which reduces gastric juice secretion, and as a consequence of the higher pH of the chyme, also reduces secretions in the duodenum. Long-acting somatostatin analogues, such as octreotide, inhibit pancreatic secretion and can also help to control the fluid and salt loss. Despite these measures intravenous fluid and nutritional support are required. Segmental resections of the small bowel are frequently and safely performed for conditions such as Crohn's disease. These segmental resections rarely result in any significant loss of physiological function.

The large bowel is a common area of surgical pathology in the gastrointestinal tract. The most common conditions are inflammatory disorders, such as ulcerative colitis and neoplasia, both of which involve the lining of the large bowel. Colorectal carcinoma is usually treated by surgery. This is both to prevent the life-threatening complications of obstruction and perforation and to attempt to cure the disease. Treatment involves a segmental resection of the large bowel along with its arterial blood supply. The arterial blood supply is taken in order to remove the draining lymph nodes into which tumours commonly spread. As long as the anal canal is left intact it is possible to reconnect the two bowel segments, reconstituting intestinal continuity. This results in little change in gastrointestinal function unless the rectum is removed, in which case there is loss of the storage capacity, and a more frequent bowel action. The major function of the large bowel is water absorption and any remaining colon quickly adapts to overcome the loss of function of the resected segment.

Ulcerative colitis, when it requires surgical intervention, usually affects the lining of the whole of the large bowel. As a consequence, surgical treatment involves removal of the colon and rectum from the caecum to the anal canal. Despite the radical nature of this resection, it is still possible to restore continuity by joining the terminal ileum to the anus. The terminal ileum is reconstructed to form a new reservoir to replace the rectum. Most patients can maintain continence following this procedure. There is considerable adaptation of the small bowel, which reduces its secretions and increases the fluid absorption. As a consequence, although patients will not pass formed stools, they will usually only open their bowels three to four times a day. Remarkably, the adaptation of the small bowel is such that even in this extreme situation salt and water loss is controlled and dietary supplements are rarely required. There may be an increased loss of bile acids because of loss of absorption in the terminal ileum and large bowel. This can lead to persistent diarrhoea, but is controllable by oral chelating agents which bind the bile salts and so reduce their osmotic potential.

Mouth and oropharynx

The primary function of the mouth and oropharynx is to initiate the digestive process by chewing and producing salivary secretions, to convey food from the mouth into the oesophagus, and simultaneously to prevent aspiration

Table 11.4 Parotid disease

Presentation	Cause	Mechanism
Parotid swelling		
Painful	Infection	Ascending bacterial infection from the mouth, via the parotid duct
	Calculus	Parotid duct obstruction results in secondary inflammation in the obstructed gland. The pain is exacerbated by eating which stimulates secretion from the gland
Painless	Tumour	Usually involves the superficial portion of the gland, but malignant tumours can invade the facial nerve which passes through the gland. This will result in weakness of the facial muscles on that side

of oral contents into the respiratory tract. The digestive function of this part of the gastrointestinal tract is not essential and its impairment has few nutritional consequences. Functional impairment in safely transporting food into the oesophagus can, however, have serious consequences in terms of both nutrition and acute respiratory complications.

A wide range of benign and malignant conditions can affect the mouth and oropharynx. Any painful condition can inhibit the patient from eating, including problems with dentition or other infections of the oral mucosa. Painless causes include weakness of the facial muscles, impairing chewing and swallowing. The commonest cause of this is a vascular injury to the contralateral cerebral hemisphere.

An acute cerebral vascular injury commonly damages the motor area, resulting in contralateral facial weakness, impaired mastication, and dribbling. Injury to the cranial nerves, particularly the glossopharyngeal nerve, will impair swallowing and can result in aspiration of food into the trachea, because of loss in sensation to the posterior third of the tongue and oropharynx. Damage to the hypoglossal nerve will impair tongue movement but actually has little effect on the ability to swallow. A viral infection of the facial nerve can cause ipsilateral paralysis of the facial muscles (Ramsay Hunt syndrome), as can idiopathic paralysis (Bell's palsy). The process of mastication is not impaired as these muscles are innervated by the mandibular nerve.

The salivary glands are another common site of disease. Examples of parotid disease are shown in Table 11.4. A painful swelling of the cheek may be due to an acute bacterial infection of the parotid gland. These infections usually ascend from the mouth via the parotid duct. Drainage from the duct may be impaired by the formation of stones (calculi). Obstruction of the parotid

Table 11.5 Oesophageal disease

Condition	Clinical features	Mechanism
Varices	Massive gastrointestinal haemorrhage, and haematemesis	Portal hypertension results in dilation and engorgement of the veins communicating between the portal and systemic circulation. Spontaneous haemorrhage occurs because of the raised venous pressure
	Features of cirrhosis	Chronic liver disease is associated with morphological changes in the hepatic architecture. This occludes venous drainage into the inferior vena cava and results in portal hypertension
Infection	Associated with impaired immunity	The squamous epithelium of the oesophagus provides effective protection against infection. This can be impaired by immunosuppression
	Infection is often by organisms that are not normally pathogenic	Impaired immunity results in overgrowth of organisms that are commonly present in the oropharynx such as *Candida* (a yeast) or herpes simplex viruses
Oesophageal pouch (diverticulum)	The patient is usually elderly and complains of regurgitation of 'old' food	Weakness in the wall of the upper oesophagus allows the mucosa to bulge through the muscle coat. Because this sac is not enclosed by muscle it cannot contract, so food can collect in it

duct can result in secondary inflammation and swelling of the gland. The symptoms are exacerbated by eating, because this stimulates the secretion of the obstructed gland. A painless swelling of the cheek may be due to an underlying parotid tumour. Because the facial nerve passes through the parotid gland, malignant tumours often involve the branches of the facial nerve, and this is a further cause of unilateral facial weakness.

Oesophagus

Disorders of the oesophagus can be divided into motor disorders and mucosal disease (Table 11.5), though the two can co-exist. In the majority of cases motor disorders are incompletely understood. Failure to relax the lower end of the oesophagus and the lower oesophageal sphincter (LOS) results in a functional obstruction. This is known as achalasia. This unusual condition usually manifests in adult life. Oral contrast can be swallowed and X-ray imaging will demonstrate a grossly dilated proximal oesophagus. A second disorder of peristalsis is known as diffuse oesophageal spasm. In this condition, peristalsis is dysfunctional throughout the length of the oesophagus. Failure of peristalsis in both of these conditions results in regurgitation of food. Most conditions can be helped by smooth muscle relaxants. An oesophageal pouch is also thought to be a motor disorder of the oesophagus. The diverticulum occurs between the cricopharyngeus muscle and the pharyngeal constrictor muscles. A congenital weakness in the wall of the oesophagus allows the mucosa to bulge through the muscle coat creating a sac in which food can collect. The condition is thought to develop because of failure of the cricopharyngeus muscle to relax on swallowing. Food that collects in the pouch can regurgitate into the mouth and pass into the airway (aspiration). A large pouch may be visible in the neck, and itself can impair swallowing because of pressure on the oesophagus.

Table 11.6 Oesophagitis

Aetiology	Reflux of gastric content into lower oesophagus
	Failure to clear luminal contents into the stomach
Symptoms	*Mechanism*
Pain	Inflammatory changes in the lower oesophageal mucosa
Dysphagia	Secondary fibrosis and narrowing of the lower oesophagus
	Impaired motility due to damage to underlying smooth muscle
Regurgitation	Blockage of the lumen. This may result from secondary neoplastic change
Weight loss	More common in the presence of neoplastic change
Investigation	
Endoscopy	Allows direct visualization of the mucosa and biopsy for histological assessment
Barium swallow	Allows visualization of the level of an obstruction, and also shows function of peristalsis

Mucosal disorders of the oesophagus are widespread in the population; the most common of these is reflux oesophagitis (Table 11.6). Reflux of gastric contents and failure to promptly clear the lumen results in chronic irritation to the lower oesophageal mucosa. The squamous epithelium is not designed to be an effective barrier to extreme shifts in the pH. Reflux oesophagitis is a chronic inflammatory process mediated by acid and pepsin from the stomach as well as bile from the duodenum, and can result in ulceration of the mucosa and secondary fibrosis in the muscle wall. The latter leads to narrowing of the lower oesophagus. It is believed that secondary changes in the mucosa may occur, with metaplasia of the squamous epithelium into columnar epithelium (Barrett's oesophagus). This is considered a premalignant condition and regular endoscopic surveillance is undertaken in these patients. Ulceration of the lower oesophagus associated with oesophagitis may also lead to haemorrhage. This is unusual and major haemorrhage is more commonly associated with peptic ulcer disease or varices of the lower oesophagus.

Oesophageal varices are due to portal hypertension. This is a common complication of cirrhosis of the liver which causes obstruction to the portal blood flow. The porto-systemic anastomoses at the lower end of the oesophagus become massively dilated in response to the raised venous pressure. These veins are thin-walled and bleed easily. Bleeding can be massive and life-threatening. The associated liver disease can complicate the situation because of impairment of coagulation. Optimal management requires occlusion of the veins by endoscopic ligation or sclerotherapy.

Infections of the oesophagus are surprisingly rare; the squamous epithelium is a highly effective barrier. Nonetheless, in the presence of impaired immunity, or obstruction and secondary stasis, infection can occur. Candidal fungal infection, seen as white plaques in the oesophagus, is a common infecting organism, particularly if patients have been on long-term antibiotics. Viral infections are also seen in the immunocompromised patient, notably herpes simplex and cytomegalovirus.

Stomach and duodenum

The most common clinical conditions in the stomach and duodenum involve the mucosa. The common benign conditions include acute and chronic gastritis, and peptic ulcer disease. Malignant disease in the stomach is an important site for gastrointestinal malignancy, but interestingly is relatively rare in the duodenum, as is the case for the rest of the small bowel. This observation indicates that the common aetiological factors involved in the development of peptic ulcers may differ from those that predispose to gastric cancer.

Acute gastritis is an inflammatory injury to the mucosa of the stomach, which is usually due to the ingestion of toxic substances such as drugs or bacteria in food. It is probably most commonly seen following alcohol ingestion. The condition is self-limiting and does not usually progress to chronic ulceration. Chronic gastritis, like other conditions that result in longstanding injury to the bowel mucosa, predisposes to malignant change. The aetiology of chronic gastritis is multifactorial but is best documented in pernicious anaemia. This is a familial disorder with a history of an affected relative in 30% of patients. Serum antibodies against gastric parietal cells and intrinsic factor are commonly found. Intrinsic factor antibody causes B_{12} deficiency. The condition is increasingly common in older patients who may present with (megaloblastic) anaemia or even neurological disorders

Table 11.7 Peptic ulcer disease

Aetiology	*Helicobacter* infection of the mucosa impairs the protective mechanisms and allows secondary damage from the acid environment
Symptoms	*Mechanism*
Epigastric pain	Inflammatory reaction to chemical injury to the mucosa, notably hydrochloric acid and pepsin
Bleeding	Erosion of the submucosa exposes the underlying blood vessels which are then vulnerable to damage and secondary haemorrhage
Sudden severe epigastric pain	Further damage to the deeper muscle layers of the wall leads to fibrosis and ischaemia. If this is allowed to progress the ulcer can erode through the serosal surface leading to life-threatening peritonitis
Profuse vomiting	This is occasionally seen in chronic ulcers in the pyloric region and the duodenum because of the narrow lumen. Large ulcers in this region can cause obstruction to the outlet of the stomach

caused by a lack of vitamin B_{12}. Approximately 1 in 12 affected patients will develop a carcinoma of the stomach, and for this reason, regular surveillance endoscopy of the stomach is performed.

The reason some patients with acute mucosal ulceration may progress to chronic peptic ulcer disease has been a field of extensive investigation because of the high prevalence of this condition (Table 11.7). Environmental and genetic factors have been implicated. It has been shown that patients with duodenal ulcers tend to have a high basal level of acid secretion in the stomach. However, the overlap between the normal range and that seen in patients with peptic ulcer disease is considerable. A major development in understanding this condition followed the discovery of *H. pylori*. This organism is resistant to acid secretion and so can proliferate in the mucosa of the stomach and the duodenum. A strong association between this infection and chronic ulceration has now been established. Historically, the treatment of peptic ulcer disease has centred on reducing acid secretion either by surgical or medical means in order to minimize the mucosal damage. Modern therapy, however, focuses on clearing *Helicobacter* infection by the use of antibiotics. This treatment has been shown to result in a high percentage of ulcer healing and, importantly, a low incidence of recurrence of the disease. Historically, peptic ulcer disease was one of the most common reasons for intestinal surgery. The advent of medical therapy has revolutionized the management of this condition and surgery is now largely restricted to the treatment of complications from peptic ulcer disease. Because of the erosive nature of these ulcers, they can result in catastrophic gastrointestinal haemorrhage, or perforation of the ulcer into the peritoneal cavity. These complications still require surgical intervention.

Hepatobiliary disease

Disorders of the hepatobiliary system include both diseases of the biliary tree and diseases affecting hepatocytes (Table 11.8). Diseases that primarily involve the hepatocytes impair liver function. This causes reduced production of serum proteins including albumin, and as a consequence leakage of fluid into the extracellular space by osmosis (oedema). The patient also develops an impaired immune status, resulting in a susceptibility to a range of infections. Derangement of the hepatocyte organization can obstruct the drainage of the portal vein into the inferior vena cava and so produce a rise in pressure in the portal venous system. The combination of reduced protein production and raised portal pressure causes fluid to collect inside the abdominal cavity (ascites).

Disorders of the biliary tree can result in blockage of drainage of the bile into the duodenum. This manifests as jaundice. Chronic obstruction of bile flow can also produce (secondary) damage to the hepatocytes because of back pressure in the biliary system. It will primarily cause obstructive jaundice, which manifests with skin pigmentation, pale stools (due to the lack of bilirubin), and dark urine (due to the excretion of excess bilirubin by the kidneys).

Disorders of the biliary tree

The commonest disorder to affect the biliary tree is gallstone disease. This affects over 5% of the adult population in Britain. While these stones remain in the gall bladder, they can be asymptomatic. Obstruction of flow of bile from the gall bladder into the common bile duct will, however, result in biliary colic when the gall bladder attempts to contract, and secondary infection in the gall bladder due to stasis (cholecystitis). If the stones pass into the common bile duct they often lodge at the narrowing created by the ampulla of Vater, where the duct enters the duodenum. In this position they also obstruct the flow of bile from the liver and result in obstructive jaundice. This results in dark-coloured urine because of reflux of conjugated bile into the systemic circulation, and pale stools because of the absence of bile pigment in the faeces, as well as the classic yellow pigmentation of the skin, most easily seen in the sclera of the eyes. Common bile duct stones may, in addition, interfere with the flow of secretions from the pancreas, and cause acute pancreatitis. An interesting aspect of pain from the gall bladder is discomfort in the right shoulder. This is because it is partly derived embryologically from the diaphragm and shares its autonomic innervation via the phrenic nerve. These nerves enter the spine at the level of C4, along with sensory fibres from the shoulder tip.

The management of complications from gallstone disease is largely surgical. It involves the removal of any stones from the biliary tree in addition to removal of the gall bladder. In the Western world, the vast majority of gallstones form primarily in the gall bladder. In the Far East, where infections of the biliary tract are more common, the formation of stones primarily in the hepatic duct around the porta hepatis creates considerable management problems because of their inaccessible position.

Obstruction to the flow of bile may result from fibrosis in the wall of the biliary tree. This is a rare disorder known

Table 11.8 Hepatobiliary disease

Condition	Features	Mechanism
Gallstones	Right-sided abdominal pain and shoulder tip pain	Gallstones may obstruct the flow of bile from the gall bladder. Pain is referred to the shoulder tip because of the level of autonomic innervation (C4). Abdominal tenderness is due to inflammation of the overlying parietal peritoneum
	Fever	The stagnant bile becomes infected (cholecystitis)
	Jaundice	Gallstones may pass from the gall bladder and lodge at the ampulla of Vater. This will obstruct the flow of bile from the liver
Acute hepatitis	Right upper quadrant pain	Swelling of the liver stimulates nerves in the liver capsule and overlying peritoneum
	Bleeding and bruising	Impaired coagulation results from failure to manufacture proteins required for the clotting cascade
	Reduced level of consciousness	Toxins build up in the systemic circulation because of failure of detoxification and excretion in the liver
Chronic hepatitis	History of previous liver damage	Most patients have suffered a clinical attack of acute hepatitis. Occasionally this is subclinical and passes unnoticed. This has been seen in hepatitis C infection from infected blood transfusions
Chronic liver disease (cirrhosis)	Jaundice	Failure to excrete bilirubin
	Oedema (fluid collecting in the extracellular space), swollen ankles, ascites	Failure of protein production reduces intravascular osmotic pressure and allows fluid to leak into the extracellular space

as primary sclerosing cholangitis. It is occasionally seen in association with inflammatory bowel disease, especially ulcerative colitis, and for this reason is believed to be of immunological aetiology. The chronic and progressive obstruction of the flow of bile results in secondary damage to the hepatocytes. There are currently no effective treatments for this chronic inflammatory disorder and, if progressive, liver transplantation can be required.

Hepatocellular disease

Conditions that result in primary damage to hepatocytes result in acute hepatitis. This can be due to infections, usually viral (hepatitis A and B for example), or damage by drugs such as paracetamol, or by toxins such as alcohol. This can result in a range of presentations from mild sub-clinical liver injury to massive liver necrosis and hepatic failure. Any acute hepatitis can result in long-standing liver cell damage (chronic hepatitis). Progressive chronic liver cell injury results in disordered liver architecture associated with fibrosis and regenerative nodules. This is known as cirrhosis. This is an irreversible state resulting in impaired hepatic function encompassing bilirubin excretion, protein manufacture including immune function, and detoxification of drugs. This gives rise to the classic stigmata of chronic liver disease. Two important sequelae of cirrhosis are portal hypertension and liver cell tumours (hepatoma). The only therapeutic option for advanced cirrhosis is liver transplantation.

Nutrients from the gastrointestinal tract are transported via the venous system into the portal vein, which drains directly into the liver. Derangement in the liver architecture, commonly caused by cirrhosis, results in obstruction to the blood flow and a rise in portal venous pressure. This results in opening up of the collateral venous pathways and enlargement of the spleen (splenomegaly). The enlarged spleen traps circulating platelets leading to thrombocytopenia (low blood platelet levels). Collateral veins open up around the falciform ligament, leading to the appearance of dilated veins around the umbilicus (caput medusae). The clinically important collateral pathway is the communication between the left gastric vein and azygous vein in the lower oesophagus. These dilated veins in the lower oesophagus (varices) are fragile and can burst spontaneously, leading to life-threatening haemorrhage. As the bleeding is often accompanied by thrombocytopenia and deranged clotting (because of the underlying cirrhosis), this can exacerbate the bleeding problem. Treatment requires ligation or sclerosis of the dilated veins, which can often be achieved endoscopically via the oesophagus. In the acute setting, direct balloon compression of the veins may be required. This is done using a specially designed tube (Minnesota tube), which can be passed from the mouth into the stomach.

The commonest malignant tumours of the liver in the West are metastatic cancer, often from primary cancers elsewhere in the gastrointestinal tract. Primary malignant tumours of the liver (hepatoma) are usually seen on a background of cirrhosis. These patients have a particularly poor prognosis as the reserves of liver function are often not sufficient to allow safe resection of the primary tumour. Transplantation of the liver, in the presence of a hepatoma and cirrhosis, is hazardous. This is because immunosuppression, required to prevent rejection of the transplant, will result in rapid tumour progression, if there is any residual disease.

Pancreas

Disorders of exocrine function of the pancreas are an important cause of malabsorption because of the central role of this organ in the digestion of fat and protein. Inappropriate activation of digestive enzymes in the pancreas can result in destruction of the organ with potentially catastrophic consequences. This secondary destructive process results in severe unrelenting epigastric pain, which usually radiates through to the back. The most important endocrine functions of the pancreas are the production of insulin and glucagon. Destruction of these islet cells results in diabetes. The pancreas has considerable reserves of function and destruction of over 70% of the organ is required before clinical manifestation of diabetes or malabsorption becomes apparent.

Acute pancreatitis is a medical emergency, resulting in autodestruction of the organ (Table 11.9). This process can be precipitated by bile duct stones, which disrupt free drainage of the pancreatic duct, or by acute alcohol ingestion, which is toxic to the organ.

The clinical presentation is often seen in middle-aged women (due to gallstone disease) and young men (following excessive alcohol ingestion). The destructive process results in severe upper abdominal pain, and is commonly associated with vomiting as a consequence of irritation of the overlying stomach. The autolysis causes a massive fluid and protein shift into the extracellular space, depleting the intravascular volume. This can lead to poor perfusion of the kidneys (renal failure), leakage of fluid into the lungs (pulmonary oedema), and generalized hypotensive shock. The key to treatment is prompt and rapid intravenous fluid replacement.

Chronic pancreatitis is a related disorder, usually caused by excessive longstanding alcohol ingestion. In this disease, the destruction of the pancreas is a slow and progressive disorder. Patients gradually develop steatorrhoea because of fat malabsorption, and diabetes because of injury to the islet cells. The destruction of the pancreatic tissue results in secondary calcification in the organ and cystic changes that are presumed to be due to obstruction of drainage of the small ductules in the gland. Successful management is largely reliant upon the patient ceasing to take alcohol.

Cystic fibrosis is a condition that is inherited in an autosomal recessive fashion, where both parents are carrying one defective gene. It is due to failure of the chloride pump at the duct cell surface. Before the genetics of the disease were fully understood, the diagnosis relied upon excessive sodium and chloride being found in the

Table 11.9 Acute pancreatitis

Aetiology	Autodigestion of the pancreas by secreted enzymes. Caused by toxic damage (e.g. alcohol) or by obstruction of secretions (e.g. gallstones)
Symptoms	
Epigastric pain	Local inflammation process damages autonomic nerves from the coeliac plexus
Vomiting	Local irritation of the stomach, which overlies the pancreas
Systemic damage	
Shortness of breath	There are massive fluid shifts into the extracellular space due to inflammatory injury and local release of digestive enzymes. Fluid leaks into the lung extracellular space and into alveoli (pulmonary oedema)
Hypotension	Loss of fluid from the vascular space. This results in underperfusion of many organs including the kidneys
Investigations	
Serum amylase	Inappropriately released into the system from the damaged pancreatic cells
CT scan	This will demonstrate swelling and destruction of the pancreatic gland and surrounding tissue
ERCP	This enables the pancreatic and bile ducts to be visualized and can demonstrate gallstones stuck at the ampulla of Vater (see Fig. 11.4). Stones can also be removed at this procedure

patients' sweat. Because this is such an important cellular mechanism, the consequences are widespread (Table 11.10). Newborn babies may be born with acute constipation due to meconium obstruction in the large bowel; this is known as meconium ileus. They may also have a failure in lung expansion because of difficulty in clearing secretions. This problem continues throughout life. Secretory problems in the pancreas result in obstruction of the duct and late pancreatic failure as well as the development of adult onset cirrhosis of the liver. The management of this condition has progressed rapidly over the last decade. Identification of the cystic fibrosis gene enables detection of carriers of the affected gene. Life expectancy has been prolonged by aggressive chest physiotherapy to help with secretory problems in the lungs, and respiratory failure can now be treated by lung transplantation. Gene therapy trials are now underway for this condition.

Small bowel conditions

The primary function of the small intestine is to absorb fluid and nutrients that are ingested. Tumours of the small intestine are surprisingly rare given the size of the organ, and as a consequence, the most common conditions affecting the small bowel are concerned with alterations of function. The key functional unit in the small bowel is the mucosa, and malabsorption is invariably due to conditions that are injurious to the mucosal lining. These can be broadly divided into infective and non-infective causes (Table 11.11).

Improvements in living standards and hygiene in the Western world have reduced the frequency and clinical importance of gastrointestinal infections. An acute history of nausea, vomiting and diarrhoea of sudden onset, often affecting a number of family members, implicates an infective cause. A range of viruses, bacteria, protozoa or toxins can be implicated. Diagnosis can often be made by culture of the liquid diarrhoea. Key to the successful management of acute infections is the replacement of salts and fluid by the oral route, or, if necessary, the intravenous route. Blood-stained diarrhoea is most likely to be due to a bacterial organism, such as *Salmonella*, and will benefit from appropriate antibiotic therapy. Most infections in Britain today are due to viruses or toxins, and are self-limiting. Cholera remains a major killer worldwide, although improvements in water supply and sewerage have helped to control this infection. *Salmonella* remains an important bacterial infection even in the West, and in the 1990s, reports of infection by poultry products received considerable media attention. Chronic subclinical infections can occur, usually in the biliary tree. As a consequence, members of the public who handle food and food products continue to be a source of outbreaks of this infection.

Crohn's disease

The cause of chronic symptoms of diarrhoea can be more difficult to ascertain. Crohn's disease provides a good example of chronic small bowel disease (Table 11.12). Although it is relatively rare, with an incidence in the UK of approximately 1 in 10 000, Crohn's disease is a chronic condition with periods of remission and exacerbation, and patients are frequent presenters to the health services. They develop classical symptoms of diarrhoea and abdominal pain, associated with weight loss. It can be genetically determined, and mutations in the CARD15 gene (encoding for the NOD2 receptor) have been shown to cause the disease in some families. This protein is involved in the inflammatory response and is believed to alter the response to some infective/inflammatory stimuli in the gut.

This chronic granulomatous disease can affect any part of the gastrointestinal tract, but most commonly involves the terminal ileum. Genetically determined predisposition is known to play a part in this condition, but a wide range of aetiological factors have been implicated. These include viral infection, microbial infection, dietary and vascular factors. None of these have been established as causative in the condition and the aetiology is likely to be multifactorial.

Table 11.10 Pancreatic diseases

Condition	Features	Mechanism
Diabetes mellitus	Polyuria and polydipsia	Failure of insulin secretion results in a high blood sugar. This increases the osmotic potential of the filtrate and causes high urine volumes (polyuria). The hypovolaemia and raised serum osmolality stimulate thirst receptors (polydipsia)
	Coma	Deranged glucose and fatty acid metabolism results in a metabolic acidosis. Combined with hypovolaemia this causes a reduced level of consciousness, and death, if not treated promptly
Chronic pancreatitis	Longstanding alcohol abuse	Alcohol is toxic to the pancreatic gland
	Epigastric pain	Inflammation around the autonomic nerves in the coeliac plexus
	Weight loss and diarrhoea	Failure of exocrine function results in incomplete digestion
	Diabetes mellitus	Failure of islet cell function
Cystic fibrosis	Constipation	Failure in the Na/Cl exchange pump results in pancreatic failure and deranged fluid secretion/absorption in the gut. This manifests as mechanical obstruction in the neonate (meconium ileus) and constipation in later life
	Respiratory failure	Abnormal secretions in the alveoli and bronchioli result in airway obstruction and alveolar collapse. Neonates may suffer from impaired lung expansion and adults suffer recurrent respiratory infections

Table 11.11 Small bowel conditions

Condition	Clinical features	Mechanisms
Malabsorption		
Coeliac disease	Chronic diarrhoea, weight loss, anaemia. Most commonly in adults	Autoimmune disease of the small bowel. Malabsorption of fat results in bulky, pale, offensive-smelling stools that often float in the toilet. Failure to absorb protein results in a net loss of protein from the body and loss of muscle bulk. Anaemia may result from failure to absorb folate and iron
Infection		
Salmonella typhus	Sudden profuse watery diarrhoea, which may be blood-stained. Associated with a high fever	The bacillus infection causes acute ulceration of the mucosa throughout the small and large bowel with associated loss of water and protein, resulting in watery diarrhoea. The ulcerated mucosa tends to bleed. The bacillus spreads through the bloodstream via the portal vein, infesting the liver and creating a marked inflammatory response with a high temperature
Cholera	Severe watery diarrhoea with loss of many litres of fluid each day	The *Vibrus cholera* bacterium does not cause ulceration of the mucosa, but causes failure of the salt/water exchange pump allowing profuse amounts of water to pass into the bowel lumen. This results in watery diarrhoea because the colonic mucosa is unable to reabsorb the high volume. Protein loss is not seen
Ischaemia	Abdominal distension, bleeding from the bowel and abdominal pain	Impaired blood supply damages the mucosa first because of its large oxygen requirement and high cell turnover. This results in mucosal ulceration and venous bleeding. The ischaemic bowel loses its normal contractility, resulting in bowel dilatation and abdominal distension

The inflammatory process in Crohn's disease affects the full thickness of the bowel wall. As a consequence, ulceration and secondary fibrosis can result in blockage of the lumen. As the inflammatory process penetrates to the external surface of the bowel (serosa), local abscess formation and perforation into other loops of bowel or other organs, such as the bladder, can occur (fistula). A combination of medical treatment to control the disease, and surgical treatment to deal with its complications, is required. At present there is no curative therapy.

Table 11.12 Crohn's disease

Aetiology	Multifactorial: genetic predisposition has been established through family studies, but only one specific genetic defect has yet been identified (NOD2). Microbiological flora, superimposed infection, and dietary factors have all been implicated. These factors may exert their effect on a genetically predisposed population
Symptoms	*Mechanism*
Abdominal pain/weight loss	Usually from (incomplete) blockage to the passage of food through the small bowel due to narrowing of the lumen. Malnutrition results from reduced nutritional intake, in addition to impaired absorption and protein loss from the diseased mucosa
Diarrhoea	Fluid and protein loss from the ulcerated mucosa is the primary cause. Secondary bacterial overgrowth proximal to the obstruction compounds the symptoms
Fatigue	Anaemia is a common feature of this condition. Poor nutrition combined with chronic bleeding from the ulcerated mucosa results in an iron deficiency. The terminal ileum is commonly involved in this disease and impaired resorption of intrinsic factor may result in B_{12} deficiency
Localized abdominal swelling	Intra-abdominal abscesses are a common feature of this condition. Because the whole thickness of the bowel wall is involved in the inflammatory process deep ulcers or fissures can perforate through to the serosal surface
Painful mouth ulcers and anal canal ulcers	The condition can affect any part of the digestive tract. As the mouth and anal canal are the only regions with a somatic innervation, these lesions are locally painful

Coeliac disease

Coeliac disease is a rare condition that affects the mucosa of the small bowel and, like Crohn's disease, also results in malabsorption. It does not, however, cause ulceration or stricture formation. It is caused by a sensitivity to gluten in the diet. Symptoms are usually completely relieved by adoption of a gluten-free diet.

Like Crohn's disease, there is known to be an inherited predisposition to coeliac disease, with up to 20% of siblings being affected. The genetic determinants of this condition are as yet undefined. The classical histological features are of villous atrophy, which is most marked in the proximal small bowel, associated with a chronic inflammatory infiltrate. Although the disease may present at any age, it is most commonly seen in the third and fourth decades, suggesting that the sensitivity to gluten is in part acquired. In addition to chronic diarrhoea, the most prominent symptoms are weight loss and fatigue, due to malabsorption.

Acute ischaemia

Acute ischaemia of the gastrointestinal tract is a medical emergency. Some 10% of the cardiac output flows to the gastrointestinal tract. Interruption of this blood flow first affects the mucosal layer of the bowel. Fluid collects in the submucosa resulting in oedema and the mucosal cells quickly start to slough into the lumen. This results in blood-stained diarrhoea. These changes are reversible because the mucosa has regenerative properties. It can be associated with a fever, due to an associated bacteraemia, because of

disruption of the mucosal barrier. Persistence of the ischaemic episode will result in secondary damage to the bowel wall by digestive enzymes. Resolution of the ischaemia at this stage can result in secondary fibrosis and stricturing. Ischaemia that persists beyond a few hours results in loss of integrity of the bowel wall (perforation) and ultimately leakage of intestinal contents into the peritoneal cavity (peritonitis), which can be fatal. Acute ischaemia of the gastrointestinal tract is a relatively rare event because of the extensive collateral circulation between the mesenteric arteries. Complete occlusion of the superior mesenteric artery, either by thrombosis or an embolic event, may still not lead to infarction because of the collateral blood supply of the coeliac axis and the inferior mesenteric artery.

Ischaemia of the small bowel is more frequently a result of localized venous occlusion. This is most commonly seen when the bowel is twisted or trapped in a hernia sac. This is made possible because of the mobile nature of the small bowel, the blood supply of which is provided through the mesentry. Here, the arterial pressure is usually sufficient to continue to perfuse the loop of bowel, but the venous drainage which is at a lower pressure is occluded. In this situation, back pressure into the capillary beds results in ischaemia by secondary obstruction to arterial flow.

Infective diarrhoea

Intestinal infections (Table 11.11) have historically been a major cause of morbidity and mortality, and continue to be so in underdeveloped countries. The main causes of death are dehydration and electrolyte loss, making infants and the elderly particularly susceptible.

Cholera is due to infection of the gastrointestinal tract by *Vibrio cholera* and continues to be an important infection in developing countries because of contaminated drinking water. The symptoms of profuse watery diarrhoea are as a consequence of the blockade of the sodium exchange pump by the enterotoxin. Fluid loss can be as high as 1 L/h and rapidly results in hypovolaemic shock, acute renal failure and metabolic acidosis.

In contrast, *Salmonella typhi* and *Shigella* infections directly damage the mucosa of the gastrointestinal tract. *Shigella* infections result in moderate amounts of diarrhoea associated with a high fever. Damage to the bowel mucosa also results in protein and microscopic blood loss. *Shigella dysenteriae* has more effect on the large bowel mucosa, and is associated with frank blood loss in the stool, because the blood is not degraded by proteinases as when it occurs in the small bowel. *Salmonella typhi* infections can be transmitted from contaminated water or food and, like *Shigella*, directly invade the small intestinal mucosa. This initial infection is not, however, directly toxic to the mucosal cells and the organisms spread to the liver via the mesenteric blood supply. Here, a secondary incubation period is followed by a clinical bacteraemia. The accompanying inflammatory reaction to this infection results in ulceration of the bowel mucosa, producing diarrhoea, bleeding and fever. As a consequence of the direct damage to the mucosa, the diarrhoea results in protein loss in addition to salt and water loss. Because these infecting organisms have a different mechanism of action, the incubation period for each infection varies. A cholera infection will manifest symptoms within 12 h, but a *Shigella* infection will usually take several days. Because of the secondary incubation period, a *Salmonella* infection has an incubation period of about 10 days.

Amoebic dysentery remains an important cause of infective diarrhoea in the tropics. It is caused by the ingestion of food and water contaminated by the cysts of *Entamoeba histolytica*. The cysts develop into trophozoites, which invade the mucosa of the colon and can penetrate all the layers of the intestinal wall. This results in ulcer formation and secondary blood-stained diarrhoea. As is the case with many intestinal infestations, some individuals fail to develop invasive disease and remain asymptomatic carriers. The condition can mimic ulcerative colitis because of the mucosa ulceration, but the diagnosis is readily established from biopsy of the ulcer or from examination of fresh stools for the presence of cysts. The condition is readily treated by antibiotics. Because the ulcers penetrate the full thickness of the bowel wall, secondary stricture formation in the large bowel can be seen following treatment.

Large intestine

The most important disease of the large bowel is that of colorectal cancer. Nonetheless, benign disorders of the large bowel also form an important group of clinical disorders (Table 11.13). All large bowel disease results in alteration of bowel habit. The key symptoms are those of a change

Table 11.13 Large bowel disease

Condition	Features	Mechanism
Diverticular disease	Central, lower, abdominal pain	Referred pain from the embryonic hind gut. Muscle hypertrophy in the wall of the bowel results in spasms of pain (colic)
	Fever	The diverticulum can become obstructed and infected. This results in a small abscess in the wall of the colon
	Generalized abdominal pain and tenderness	Rupture of the diverticulum into the peritoneal cavity can cause generalized intraperitoneal infection (peritonitis)
Ulcerative colitis	Diarrhoea and bleeding	Ulceration of the large bowel mucosa results in failure to absorb water from the lumen, and bleeding from the submucosal vessels
	Abdominal distension	Mucosal failure results in loss of peristalsis and a functional obstruction. The proximal bowel can dilate and even perforate causing peritonitis (toxic megacolon)
Dysentery	May follow foreign travel	Infection from ingestion of contaminated food or water
Entamoeba histolytica	Blood-stained diarrhoea	Ulceration of the mucosa results in water/protein loss and bleeding from the submucosal vessels

in bowel habit, which may be either diarrhoea or constipation, together with rectal bleeding and lower abdominal pain. Inflammation of the mucosa of the large bowel usually results in diarrhoea. The important causes are diverticulitis, ulcerative colitis and infection.

Diverticular disease has a high prevalence in the Western world. This is believed to be due to a low-fibre diet, which results in raised intraluminal pressure in the large bowel. This in time leads to muscle hypertrophy in the wall of the colon and pulsion diverticula in the wall of the bowel (Fig. 11.7). The diverticula are outpouchings of the mucosa through the muscle coat of the colon. Without a muscle coat these little mucosal sacs are unable to empty, and faecal residues become lodged in the sac, predisposing the individual to secondary infection. Colonic diverticulae are present in 30% of the population aged 55 years and over, but the majority are asymptomatic. Complications occur because ulceration of the mucosa in the wall of the diverticulum results in bleeding, or obstruction to the neck of the diverticulum results in abscess formation with or without perforation into the peritoneal cavity. These complications are only

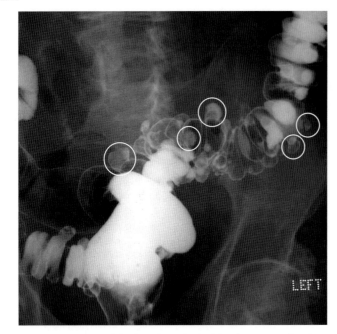

Fig. 11.7 An X-ray of the large bowel, which has been coated with barium. Moderate diverticular disease is apparent in the sigmoid colon. This shows up as small out-pouches filled with barium (circled).

seen in about 1 in 50 patients with diverticular disease, but when they do occur they can be life-threatening.

Obstruction to the flow of faecal contents in the large bowel is life-threatening, because the ileocaecal valve, lying at the proximal end of the colon, creates a closed loop that can only decompress by perforation of the colon. Perforation usually occurs at the caecum where the wall is thin and distends easily. Colorectal cancer is the commonest cause of large bowel obstruction, but obstruction of a diverticular abscess or scarring in the wall of the colon following acute diverticulitis can also cause this problem. The treatment is surgical, and requires resection of the obstructing segment, and where possible, reconstitution of the bowel continuity by anastomosis to the rectum.

Ulcerative colitis

This is an inflammatory condition that is limited to the mucosa of the large bowel. Its incidence has been estimated at approximately 2% per annum in the West, but the vast majority of these patients have disease that is mild and limited only to the rectal mucosa. In a small proportion of cases, the inflammation extends throughout the large bowel mucosa and can result in a more florid illness. The aetiology of this condition is not known, but like Crohn's disease, it is believed to be due to a sensitivity to environmental factors that have yet to be identified. There is an underlying genetic predisposition in at least a proportion of cases. It is interesting to note that ulcerative colitis and Crohn's disease may be seen in the same family, suggesting common aetiological factors.

Extensive mucosal damage results in watery, blood-stained diarrhoea. Infective causes of diarrhoea should always be excluded. Diagnosis is by histological examination of mucosal biopsies. As is the case elsewhere in the digestive tract, extensive ulceration of the mucosa can result in bacteria migrating from the lumen into the portal system. Although the condition is limited to the mucosal lining of the bowel, acute florid attacks will result in transmural inflammation and can lead to secondary perforation and peritonitis. Treatment requires fluid and salt replacement and antibiotics to control any secondary infection.

Immune suppressive therapy is used to dampen down the inflammatory destruction. In a small percentage of patients, medical treatment is unsuccessful and emergency surgery with removal of the large bowel (colectomy) is required. Longstanding disease also increases the risk of secondary colorectal cancer in these patients and occasionally a prophylactic colectomy is necessary to prevent malignant disease developing. Advances in surgical techniques have enabled the development of ileo-anal anastomosis, which reconstitutes bowel continuity and avoids the formation of a permanent stoma in many of these patients.

abetalipoproteinaemia – a rare autosomal recessive disorder characterized by a low plasma level of betalipoprotein.

aborally – in a direction away from the mouth.

achalasia – a motor disorder in which a muscle is unable to relax, particularly the lower oesophagus and the lower oesophageal sphincter (cardiospasm).

achlorhydria – lack of hydrochloric acid secretion in gastric juice.

acholic – absence of bile secretion.

adenocarcinoma – a malignant tumour of the glandular epithelium (e.g. colonic mucosa).

aetiology – the study of the causes of a disease.

aganglionic – displaying an absence of ganglionic cells.

amorphous – without visible structure.

anaemia – a reduction in total blood haemoglobin.

anastomosis – a connection between two vessels or a surgical joining of two bowel segments to allow flux of the contents from one to the other.

aneurysm – a localized dilatation of the wall of a blood vessel.

anorexia nervosa – a condition in which the desire for food is lost.

antidiuretic – a substance which diminishes urine production.

aphagia – a condition in which there is an inability to swallow.

ascites – a fluid collection in the peritoneal cavity.

atony – a lack of contractile function.

atrophy – wasting or shrinking (of an organ or tissue).

autoimmune – pertaining to the development of an immune response (antibody production) to the body's own tissues.

bacteriostatic – tending to restrain the reproduction of bacteria.

benign – non-malignant (pertaining to tumours).

bilirubinuria – the presence of bilirubin in the urine.

calculus – an abnormal stone formed in tissues by an accumulation of mineral salts.

cathartic – a (purgative) medicine which increases evacuation of the bowels.

caveolae – invaginations of the cell membrane extending into its cytoplasm.

chloridorrhoea – excessive loss of chloride ions in the faeces.

cholangitis – a bacterial infection of bile in the bile duct.

cholecystectomy – removal of the gall bladder.

cholecystitis – infection (of bile) in the gall bladder.

cholelithiasis – the presence of gall stones.

cholephilic – attracted to bile; easily dissolved in bile.

cholestasis – interruption of bile flow.

cirrhosis – a progressive inflammatory disease in the liver where there is an increase in non-functioning tissue and disruption of the architecture.

colectomy – removal of part of the large bowel (colon).

colic – cyclical intra-abdominal pain owing to dysfunctional peristalsis of the intestine.

colitis – inflammatory disease of the colon.

colostomy – a surgically created opening of the colon in the wall of the abdomen.

computed tomography (CT) scanning – a radiographic scanning procedure where the detailed structure of a tissue is revealed by densitometry. The body is imaged in cross-sectional slices and the computer quantifies the X-ray absorption by the tissues.

congestive heart failure – a pathological condition that reflects impaired cardiac pumping of the left and right ventricles.

constipation – difficulty in passage of stools or infrequent passage of stools.

cytopemsis – vesicular transport.

deglutition – swallowing.

diarrhoea – an abnormal increase in stool liquidity and in daily stool volume.

diuresis – increased production of urine.

diverticulitis – infection in one or more diverticula, usually of the sigmoid colon.

diverticulosis – the presence of pouch-like herniations (diverticula) in the muscular layer of the colon, especially the sigmoid colon.

dysaesthesia – altered perception of oral sensation.

dysphagia – difficulty in swallowing.

ectasia – dilatation of a duct, vessel or hollow viscus, usually resulting from obstruction to flow or degenerative changes of the wall.

ectopic – present in an abnormal location (e.g. in pregnancy).

embolus – a substance (usually dislodged atheroma or blood clot) lodged in a blood vessel, which blocks the flow of blood.

emetic – a substance which causes vomiting.

emollients – substances which alter the consistency (of the faeces).

encephalopathy – any disease or degenerative condition of the brain.

endocytosis – process whereby a molecule or particle becomes surrounded by the cell membrane and engulfed into the cell in a vesicle.

endogenous – originating within the tissues.

endoscopic retrograde pancreatography (ERCP) – a procedure employing a combination of fibre optic endoscopy and radiography to investigate the presence of biliary and pancreatic disease.

endoscopy – visual examination of a hollow organ (e.g. the gastrointestinal tract) by insertion of an endoscope (an illuminated optical instrument).

enteritis – inflammation of the intestines.

epigastric – in the upper central abdominal region.

excoriation – an injury to the surface of the body, e.g. a scratch.

exocytosis – the process by which vesicles release their contents by fusing with the cell's plasma membrane.

exogenous – originating from outside the tissues.

extrinsic – originating (usually situated) outside the tissue.

exudate – a fluid that has oozed out of a tissue and so has a high protein content.

fenestrae – pores.

fibrosis – proliferation of fibrous connective tissue.

fistula – an abnormal passage from an internal organ to the body surface or between two organs.

gastrectomy – surgical removal of the stomach.

glucagonoma – a glucagon-secreting tumour of the pancreatic islet cells.

glucostatic theory – control of feeding via blood glucose levels.

glycosuria – glucose in the urine.

granuloma – a chronic inflammatory lesion characterized by accumulation of macrophages.

gustation – taste.

haemodynamics – the study of the physical aspects of the blood circulation.

haemolytic – causing the red blood cells to break down and release haemoglobin.

haemorrhoid – a submucosal swelling in the anal canal caused by congestion of the veins of the haemorrhoidal plexus.

hemicolectomy – surgical removal of part of the large bowel with restoration of continuity.

hepatitis – an inflammation of the liver.

hepatoma – a primary tumour of the liver.

homeostasis – constancy of the internal environment of the body.

hydrophilic – attracted to, and easily dissolved in, water.

hydrophobic – not attracted to, and insoluble in, water.

hyperaemia – increased (regional) blood flow.

hyperbilirubinaemia – an abnormally high concentration of bilirubin in the plasma.

hyperglycaemia – increased plasma glucose.

hyperinsulinaemia – increased plasma insulin.

hyperkeratosis – overgrowth of the cornified epithelium layer of the skin, e.g. a wart.

hyperketonaemia – an abnormally high level of ketone bodies in the plasma.

hyperplasia – abnormal growth of a tissue owing to an increased rate of cell division.

hypertension – chronically increased arterial blood pressure.

hypertonic – containing a higher concentration of effectively membrane-impermeable solute particles than normal (isotonic) extracellular fluid.

hypertrophy – enlargement of a tissue or organ because of increased cell size rather than increased cell number.

hypoalbuminaemia – decreased plasma albumin.

hypocalcaemia – decreased plasma calcium.

hypochromia – a low haemoglobin concentration in the erythrocytes.

hypoglycaemia – low plasma glucose.

hypoinsulinaemia – low plasma insulin.

hypokalaemia – decreased plasma K^+ concentration.

hypotension – low blood pressure.

hypotonic – containing a lower concentration of effectively non-penetrating solute particles than normal (isotonic) extracellular fluid.

hypovolaemia – low blood volume.

hypoxia – deficiency of oxygen (in a tissue).

idiopathic – of unknown cause.

ileitis – inflammatory disease of the ileum.

ileus – loss of peristalsis in the small bowel, usually following surgery, that results in a functional obstruction.

inanition – loss of weight.

inspissated – thickened.

insulinoma – a tumour of the insulin-secreting cells of the pancreas.

intrinsic – originating within the tissue.

ischaemia – decreased supply of oxygenated blood to an organ or structure.

isosmotic – having the same total solute concentration as extracellular fluid.

isotonic – containing the same number of effectively non-penetrating solute particles as extracellular fluid.

jaundice – yellowish discolouration of the skin, mucous membranes and sclerae owing to deposition of bilirubin.

ketoacidosis – acidosis accompanied by an accumulation of ketones in the body.

leukocytosis – an increase in the number of white blood cells, usually in response to infection.

lipolysis – breakdown of lipids.

lipostatic theory – control of feeding by lipid metabolites.

lithotripsy – shattering of (gall or kidney) stones by ultrasound waves.

macrocytic – high mean cell volume (usually pertaining to red blood cells).

malignancy – a tumour with the ability to invade and spread to other tissues and organs.

mastication – chewing.

meconium – greenish material which fills the intestines of the fetus and forms the first bowel movement in the newborn.

meconium ileus – obstruction of the small intestine in the newborn by impaction of meconium (usually in cystic fibrosis).

megacolon – a massively enlarged colon.

megaloblast – an abnormally large, nucleated, immature erythrocyte present in large numbers in pernicious anaemia or folate-deficiency anaemia.

metastasis – the process by which tumour cells spread to distant parts of the body.

microcytic – characterized by the presence of cells with low mean cell volume (usually pertaining to red blood cells).

myogenic – pertaining to (cardiac and smooth) muscle that does require nerve impulses to initiate and maintain a contraction.

necrosis – localized tissue death in response to disease or injury.

neoplasm – an abnormal new development of cells (a tumour).

nexus – gap junction; a zone of apposition between two cells where action potentials can be conducted between the cells.

oedema – accumulation of excess fluid in interstitial spaces.

olfaction – smell.

orad – in a direction towards the mouth.

osmolality – total solute concentration per unit weight of solvent (water).

osmolarity – total solute concentration of a solution.

osteopaenia – a reduction in bone mass.

pancreatitis – inflammatory disease of the pancreas.

paracrine – relates to an agent that exerts its effects on cells near its site of secretion (by convention, excludes neurotransmitters).

parenteral – relating to treatment other than through the digestive system (e.g. by intravenous administration).

parietal cells – oxyntic cells; acid-secreting cells of the stomach.

periodontal – pertaining to the area around the teeth.

peritonism – exquisite abdominal tenderness which encourages the patient to lie still. It is indicative of acute inflammation of the parietal peritoneum, usually due to infection and classically associated with appendicitis.

peritonitis – inflammatory disease of the peritoneum, often secondary to perforation of the bowel.

pinocytosis – endocytosis when the vesicle encloses extracellular fluid or specific molecules in the extracellular fluid that have bound to proteins on the extracellular surface of the plasma membrane.

polydipsia – excessive drinking (usually seen in hyperglycaemia).

polyuria – high urine output.

prophylactic – an agent used to prevent the development of a disease.

purgative – a strong medication used to promote evacuation of the bowels.

pyroplasty – division of the pyloric muscle to allow easier emptying of the stomach.

roughage – non-digestible dietary fibre, important to promote gut motility.

ruga – a fold of mucosa in the stomach.

satiety – cessation of the feeling of hunger.

scintigraphy – a clinical procedure consisting of the administration of a radiolabelled agent with a specific affinity for an organ or tissue of interest, followed by determination, with a detector, of the distribution of the radiolabelled compound.

sclerosis – hardening of a tissue, especially by the overgrowth of fibrous tissue.

sclerotherapy – a technique using sclerosing solutions to cause obliteration of pathological blood vessels (as in the treatment of haemorrhoids).

secretagogue – a substance that regulates the release of a secretion.

sigmoidoscope – a rigid tubular instrument used for direct visualization of the rectal and sigmoid colonic mucosa.

somatic – pertaining to one of two major divisions of the peripheral nervous system, consisting of sensory neurones concerned with sensation from the skin and body surface and motor neurones to the skeletal muscles, the other division being the autonomic nervous system.

splenomegaly – enlargement of the spleen.

steatorrhoea – a condition where the faeces have a high fat content.

stenosis – a narrowing or constriction of a tube (e.g. bowel) or aperture (e.g. ampulla of Vater).

stent – a short plastic tube.

submodality – subclass of a stimulus which evokes a sensory response.

submucosal – beneath the mucosa.

tetany – a maintained contraction.

thrombocytopaenia – deficiency of thrombocytes (blood platelets).

thrombocytosis – an abnormal increase in the number of thrombocytes (blood platelets).

thrombus – a clot which attaches to the wall of a vessel.

tonic – undergoing continuous muscular activity.

toxaemia – presence of bacterial toxins in the blood plasma.

transcoelomic – spreading through the peritoneal cavity.

transudate – fluid that has leaked out of a tissue, usually because of increased osmotic/hydrostatic pressure and therefore having a low protein content.

vagotomy – division of the vagus nerves.

varices – dilated veins, usually of the oesophagus, owing to raised portal vein pressure.

vasoconstriction – constriction of blood vessels.

vasodilator – a substance which causes dilatation of arterioles.

viscera – body organs (e.g. liver, pancreas).

xenobiotic – an organic substance which is foreign to the body (e.g. a drug or an organic poison).

xerophthalmia – a disturbance of epithelial tissues.

xerostomia – dry mouth.

Index